NANOTECHNOLOGY FOR NUCLEIC ACID DELIVERY

NANOTECHNOLOGY FOR NUCLEIC ACID DELIVERY

Pankaj Sharma, PhD
Saloni Jain, PhD
Vinay Jain, PhD
Editors

AAP | APPLE ACADEMIC PRESS

First edition published 2026

Apple Academic Press Inc.
1265 Goldenrod Circle, NE,
Palm Bay, FL 32905 USA

760 Laurentian Drive, Unit 19,
Burlington, ON L7N 0A4, Canada

CRC Press
2385 NW Executive Center Drive,
Suite 320, Boca Raton FL 33431

4 Park Square, Milton Park,
Abingdon, Oxon, OX14 4RN, UK

Apple Academic Press exclusively co-publishes with CRC Press, an imprint of Taylor & Francis Group, LLC

Library and Archives Canada Cataloguing in Publication

CIP data on file with Canada Library and Archives

Library of Congress Cataloging-in-Publication Data

CIP data on file with US Library of Congress

ISBN: 978-1-998511-84-6 (hbk)
ISBN: 978-1-998511-85-3 (ebk)
DOI: 10.1201/9781998511853

About the Editors

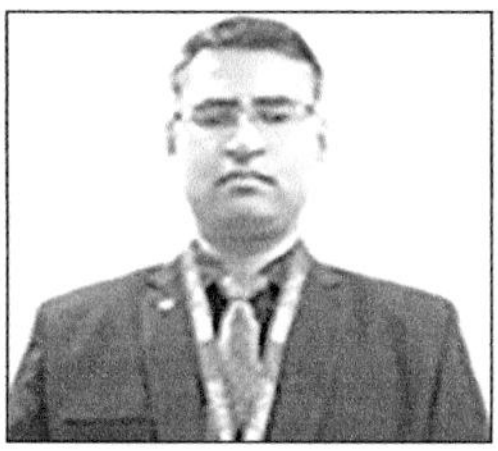

Pankaj Sharma, PhD
Professor and H.O.D, ShriRam College of Pharmacy, Banmore, Morena, Madhya Pradesh, India

Pankaj Sharma, PhD, is currently working as a Professor in the Department of Pharmaceutics at Shri Ram College of Pharmacy, Banmore, Morena, India. He completed his BPharm and MPharm degrees at RGPV University, Bhopal, in 2010 and 2012, respectively. He earned a PhD in the year 2020. He has a total of 11 years of experience in teaching and research. His research interests include the development of transdermal preparations, the role of AI in the healthcare industry, nanocarrier system development, tablets, and other carrier-mediated systems for effective drug delivery. He is actively involved in formulating nanocarriers for the effective delivery of drugs for the treatment of malaria, arthritis, etc. Dr. Sharma has received many awards; a few that stand out are a Young Scientist Award from the Indian Pharmaceutical Education Society, a fellowship from the All India Council for Technical Education (AICTE), New Delhi, as well as several prizes for the best conference papers. Dr. Sharma is a graduate of the Indian Pharmacy Graduate Association and Jiwaji University, Gwalior, India. Dr. Sharma has spoken as a representative or invited speaker at several conferences, seminars, symposiums, and workshops on his research and teaching experiences. He participates actively in a number of university, department, and institute committees. Prof. Sharma has guided 20 MPharm students under his supervision. In national and international publications, he has produced 23 peer-reviewed papers in the field of pharmaceutical sciences, along with 11 book chapters. He also reviews articles for a number of international scientific publications. He belongs to numerous Indian scientific organizations as a member or life member.

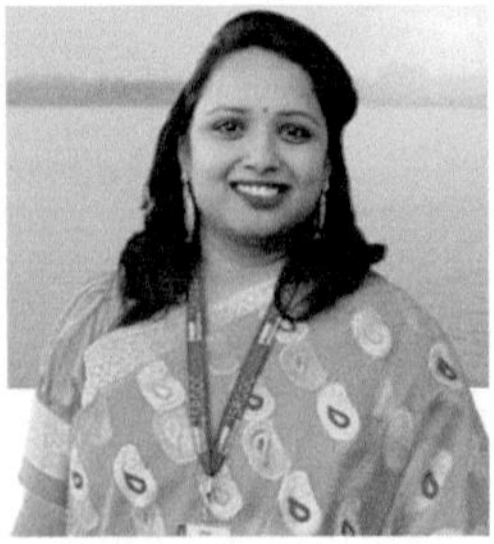

Saloni Jain, PhD
Associate Professor and H.O.D of Pharmacology, ShriRam College of Pharmacy, Banmore, Morena, Madhya Pradesh, India

Saloni Jain, PhD, is currently working as an Associate Professor in the Department of Pharmacology at Shri Ram College of Pharmacy, Banmore, Morena, India. She has seven years of experience in teaching and research. She completed her BPharm and MPharm degrees at RGPV University, Bhopal, India, in 2014 and 2017, respectively. She earned her PhD in February 2023. Her research interests focus on the development of herbal preparations and antidiabetic activities for effective drug delivery, specifically for skin diseases, diabetes, and diuretics. Dr. Jain has presented research papers at international conferences and has been granted a UK patent design. She is an active participant in various university, department, and institute committees. Dr. Jain has guided eight MPharm students and published eight research and review papers in national and international journals. Additionally, she has contributed three book chapters to international publications and attended five faculty development programs. She is a member of numerous Indian scientific organizations, including the Association of Pharmaceutical Teachers of India.

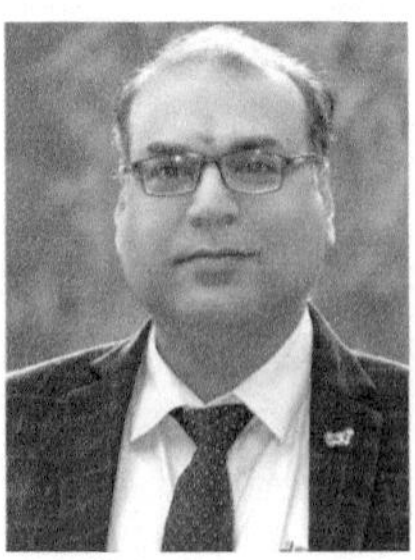

Vinay Jain, PhD
Principal, ShriRam College of Pharmacy, Banmore, Morena, Madhya Pradesh, India

Vinay Jain, PhD, is a highly accomplished academic and administrative professional, currently serving as the Principal of Shri Ram College of Pharmacy, India. He holds an MPharm and PhD degrees in Pharmacognosy and has amassed 20 years of experience in teaching and administration. He has made significant contributions to the field through his research and publications, including peer-reviewed articles, edited and indexed books, and guidance for over 32 research scholars. Dr. Jain completed his MPharm in Pharmacognosy at Barkatullah University in 2007 and began his professional career as an Assistant Professor at Shri Ram College of Pharmacy, Banmore. In 2017, he successfully defended his PhD thesis titled Phytochemical and Pharmacological Investigation of "Arisaema leschenaultia" at Berhampur University, Odisha. In addition to his academic pursuits, Dr. Jain has been an active member of the pharmacy community, serving as Co-convener of the Indo-Caribbean Conference and Organizing Secretary of the national conference on "The Future Prospect in Pharma-Marketing." He is also a lifetime member of the Indian Society of Pharmacognosy and has been recognized for his leadership and mentorship in the field. Dr. Jain has been a strong advocate for the holistic development of society and individuals and has been actively involved in corporate social responsibility initiatives such as health checkup camps, cloth donation drives, and social awareness drives. He has also filed two patents and published over 50 papers in international and national journals. In recognition of his excellence, Dr. Jain has received various awards and honors, including the Dhanvantari Award during SRIJAN 2021. He was granted funding for conducting an international conference by the *All India Council for Technical Education (AICTE)* and a grant by AICTE under the MODROB (Modernisation & Removal of Obsolescence) scheme for laboratory upgradation. He has also been invited as a guest of honor at several conferences and workshops held in Madhya Pradesh. His recent achievements include the Best Principal Award in 2022 by INSC Publishers and the Pharma Rising Star Award in 2022, which he received in New Delhi.

Contents

Contributors

Alam Mohd. Adil
Lovely Institute of Technology (Pharmacy), Lovely Professional University, Phagwara, Punjab, India

Vaibhav Dagaji Aher
Department of Pharmaceutical Medicine, Maharashtra University of Health Sciences, Nashik, Maharashtra, India

P. K. Anjali
Department of Economics, CHRIST (Deemed to Be University), Bangalore, Karnataka, India

Amardeep Ankalgi
Laureate Institute of Pharmacy, Kathog, Himachal Pradesh, India

G. Arpitha
Department of Pharmaceutics, Shridevi Institute of Pharmaceutical Sciences, Tumkur, Karnataka, India

R. Arun
Department of Pharmaceutics, JKKN College of Pharmacy, Kumarapalayam, Tamil Nadu, India

Mahendra Singh Ashawat
Laureate Institute of Pharmacy, Kathog, Himachal Pradesh, India

Astha
Laureate Institute of Pharmacy, Kathog, Himachal Pradesh, India

M. Shamshath Begum
Sharda School of Pharmacy, Sharda University, Agra, Uttar Pradesh, India

Harsh Bhardwaj
Sharda School of Pharmacy, Sharda University, Agra, Uttar Pradesh, India

Himanshu Bhardwaj
Institute of Pharmaceutical Sciences, JS University, Shikohabad, Firozabad, Uttar Pradesh, India

Bhupinder Bhyan
School of Pharmaceutical Sciences, RIMT University, Gobindgarh, Punjab, India

Rajendra Chauhan
School of Studies in Pharmaceutical Sciences, Jiwaji University, Gwalior, Madhya Pradesh, India

Hanish Singh Jayasingh Chellammal
Department of Pharmacology and Pharmaceutical Chemistry, Faculty of Pharmacy, Universiti Teknologi MARA (UiTM), Puncak Alam, Selangor, Malaysia

Rajesh Choudhary
Shri Shankaracharya College of Pharmaceutical Sciences, Junwani, Bhilai, Chhattisgarh, India

Geeta Deswal
Guru Gobind Singh College of Pharmacy, Yamunanagar, Haryana, India

S. Divyadharshini
Department of Pharmaceutics, JKKN College of Pharmacy, Kumarapalayam, Tamil Nadu, India

Shradha Devi Dwivedi
University Institute of Pharmacy, Pandit Ravishankar Shukla University, Raipur, Chhattisgarh, India

Pooja Deshpande
School of Pharmacy, Mody University of Science and Technology, Lakshmangarh, Sikar, Rajasthan, India

Navneet Garud
School of Studies in Pharmaceutical Sciences, Jiwaji University, Gwalior, Madhya Pradesh, India

Hemendra Gautam
School of Pharmaceutical Sciences, Bahra University, Solan, Himachal Pradesh, India

Sailesh Kumar Ghatuary
Department of Pharmacy, Shri R. L. T. Institute of Pharmaceutical Science and Technology, Etawah, Uttar Pradesh, India

Rohit Grover
Guru Gobind Singh College of Pharmacy, Yamunanagar, Haryana, India

Nimisha Jain
Institute of Pharmacy, Rabindranath Tagore University, Bhopal, Madhya Pradesh, India; VNS Group of Institutions, Faculty of Pharmacy, Bhopal, Madhya Pradesh, India

Vincent Jenila Jose Jancy
Department of Pharmacology, S. A. Raja Pharmacy College, Tirunelveli, Tamil Nadu, India

Jayashree
Shri Shankaracharya College of Pharmaceutical Sciences, Junwani, Bhilai, Chhattisgarh, India

Ramakant Joshi
Department of Pharmaceutics, Amity Institute of Pharmacy, Amity University, Gwalior, Madhya Pradesh, India

Shabari Girinath Kala
Central Drugs Standard Control Organization, FDA Bhawan, Kotla Marg, New Delhi, India

Ajay Kumar
Laureate Institute of Pharmacy, Kathog, Himachal Pradesh, India

Pravin Kumar
Laureate Institute of Pharmacy, Kathog, Himachal Pradesh, India

K. Lakshmi
Department of Pharmacy, Chettinad School of Pharmaceutical Sciences, Chettinad Hospital and Research Institute, Chettinad Academy of Research and Education, Kelambakkam, Tamil Nadu, India

Avinash Singh Mandaloi
VNS Group of Institutions, Faculty of Pharmacy, Bhopal, Madhya Pradesh, India

Ankit Mishra
VNS Group of Institutions, Faculty of Pharmacy, Bhopal, Madhya Pradesh, India

Pranali Mishra
Swami Vivekananda College of Pharmacy, Bhopal, Madhya Pradesh, India

Shweta Mishra
Department of Pharmacy, Dr. D. Y. Patil Institute of Pharmaceutical Sciences and Research, Pimpri, Pune, Maharashtra, India

Vishnu Mittal
Guru Gobind Singh College of Pharmacy, Yamunanagar, Haryana, India

Hemant Mourya
School of Studies in Pharmaceutical Sciences, Jiwaji University, Gwalior, Madhya Pradesh, India

Deepesh Parasar
Department of Pharmaceutical Chemistry, Amity Institute of Pharmacy, Amity University, Gwalior, Madhya Pradesh, India

Anasuya Patil
Department of Pharmaceutics, KLE College of Pharmacy, Rajajinagar, Bangalore, Karnataka, India

Rekha Tarasingh Rajput
Sharda School of Pharmacy, Sharda University, Agra, Uttar Pradesh, India

N. G. Raghavendra Rao
Department of Pharmaceutics, KIET School of Pharmacy, KIET Group of Institutions, Delhi-NCR, Muradnagar, Ghaziabad, Uttar Pradesh, India

Kantrol Sahu
Institute of Pharmaceutical Research, GLA University, Mathura, Uttar Pradesh, India

Trapti Sahu
School of Studies in Pharmaceutical Sciences, Jiwaji University, Gwalior, Madhya Pradesh, India

Pranshul Sethi
Department of Pharmacology, College of Pharmacy, Shri Venkateshwara University, Gajraula, Uttar Pradesh, India

Nikhitha Shanmukhan
Department of Pharmaceutics, JKKN College of Pharmacy, Kumarapalayam, Tamil Nadu, India

Anjali Sharma
Guru Gobind Singh College of Pharmacy, Yamunanagar, Haryana, India

Devkant Sharma
Ch. Devi Lal College of Pharmacy, Jagadhari, Haryana, India

Gyanendra Kumar Sharma
Sharda School of Pharmacy, Sharda University, Agra, Uttar Pradesh, India

Pankaj Sharma
VNS Group of Institutions, Faculty of Pharmacy, Bhopal, Madhya Pradesh, India; Shri Ram College of Pharmacy, Banmore, Morena, Madhya Pradesh, India

Anju Singh
Department of Pharmacy, School of Pharmaceutical Sciences, Chhatrapati Shahu Ji Maharaj University, Kanpur, Uttar Pradesh, India

Gurdeep Singh
Lovely Institute of Technology (Pharmacy), Lovely Professional University, Phagwara, Punjab, India

Gurvinder Pal Singh
Sharda School of Pharmacy, Sharda University, Agra, Uttar Pradesh, India

Mahaveer Singh
Department of Pharmaceutics, Dr Karigowda College of Pharmacy, Hassan, Karnataka, India

Manish Pal Singh
Department of Pharmacy, Sharda School of Pharmacy, Sharda University, Agra, Uttar Pradesh, India

Mukesh Kr. Singh
School of Pharmaceutical Sciences, Faculty of Pharmacy, IFTM University, Moradabad, Uttar Pradesh, India

Abhinav Singhal
Guru Gobind Singh College of Pharmacy, Yamunanagar, Haryana, India

Sujith Thomas
Department of Pharmacology, Moulana College of Pharmacy, Malappuram, Kerala, India

Ravindra Singh Tomar
Department of Electronics and Computer Engineering, Anand School of Engineering and Technology, Sharda University, Agra, Uttar Pradesh, India

Komal Tyagi
University Institute of Pharmaceutical Sciences, Panjab University, Chandigarh, India

Goutham Yerrakula
School of Pharmacy, Faculty of Health Sciences, JSS Academy of Higher Education and Research, Mauritius

Preface

In the rapidly evolving landscape of biomedical research and therapeutic development, nanotechnology has emerged as a transformative force, particularly in the field of nucleic acid delivery. The potential to precisely manipulate and deliver genetic material opens new frontiers in treating genetic disorders, cancers, and a myriad of other diseases that have long eluded conventional therapies. This book, *Nanotechnology for Nucleic Acid Delivery*, seeks to explore the intricate interplay between nanotechnology and genetic medicine, offering insights into the latest advancements, methodologies, and applications.

The convergence of nanotechnology and nucleic acid delivery systems represents a paradigm shift in modern medicine. Traditional drug delivery mechanisms often face significant challenges, such as poor bioavailability, limited targeting capabilities, and adverse side effects. Nanotechnology offers innovative solutions to these obstacles, enabling the development of delivery vehicles that can protect nucleic acids from degradation, enhance cellular uptake, and ensure targeted release at the desired site of action. These advancements are not just incremental; they signify a leap toward more efficient, safer, and personalized therapeutic strategies.

This book is designed to serve as a comprehensive resource for researchers, clinicians, and students who are engaged in the field of nanomedicine. It covers a broad spectrum of topics, from the fundamental principles of nanotechnology and nucleic acid chemistry to the design, synthesis, and characterization of various nanocarriers. Special attention is given to the practical aspects of developing nanotechnology-based delivery systems, including scalability, regulatory considerations, and clinical translation.

The chapters within this volume are contributed by leading experts in the field, each bringing a wealth of knowledge and experience. Their insights illuminate the current state of research, highlight key breakthroughs, and offer perspectives on future directions. Whether you are a seasoned researcher or new to the field, this book aims to equip you with a thorough understanding of the critical concepts and technological innovations that are driving progress in nucleic acid delivery.

We are on the cusp of a new era in medical science, where the convergence of nanotechnology and genetic therapy holds the promise of revolutionizing how we diagnose, treat, and ultimately prevent a wide array of diseases. It is my hope that *Nanotechnology for Nucleic Acid Delivery* will not only inform and inspire but also catalyze further advancements in this exciting field. As we navigate through the complexities and challenges of developing these technologies, let us remain guided by the profound potential they hold for improving human health and well-being.

I would like to extend my gratitude to the contributors, reviewers, and all those who have supported this endeavor. Their dedication and expertise have been instrumental in bringing this book to fruition. Finally, I thank you, the reader, for your interest in this field and your commitment to advancing the boundaries of biomedical science.

Welcome to the cutting-edge world of nanotechnology and nucleic acid delivery.

—Pankaj Sharma, PhD
Professor and HOD,
ShriRam College of Pharmacy, Banmore, Morena,
Madhya Pradesh, India

Introduction

In this groundbreaking book, *Nanotechnology for Nucleic Acid Delivery,* the author explores the intersection between nanotechnology and medicine, specifically in the field of nucleic acid delivery. With advancements in artificial intelligence and machine learning technologies, researchers are now able to design more efficient and effective drug delivery systems at an unprecedented scale.

The first part of the book provides an overview of nanomedicine, as well as its applications in various fields such as cancer therapy, gene therapy, etc. The second part delves into how artificial intelligence is changing the game by enabling scientists to develop more targeted therapies that can better penetrate cell membranes while minimizing harmful side effects.

Throughout this book, readers will discover how new technologies like *CRISPR-Cas9* gene editing have revolutionized our understanding of genetic diseases and opened up new avenues for treatment. Additionally, they will learn about cutting-edge research on RNA interference (RNAi), which has shown great promise in treating various diseases including cancer.

Overall, this book offers a comprehensive look at how advances in technology are transforming medicine today—paving the way toward personalized medicine with minimal side effects while maximizing therapeutic benefits—making it essential reading for anyone interested in staying abreast of the latest developments at the intersection between science and technology.

CHAPTER 1

An Overview of Nanomedicine and Its Potentials in Revolutionizing Healthcare

TRAPTI SAHU,[1] HEMANT MOURYA,[1] RAJENDRA CHAUHAN,[1,*] RAMAKANT JOSHI,[2] KANTROL SAHU,[3] DEEPESH PARASAR,[4] NAVNEET GARUD,[1] and KOMAL TYAGI[5]

[1]*School of Studies in Pharmaceutical Sciences, Jiwaji University, Gwalior, Madhya Pradesh, India*

[2]*Department of Pharmaceutics, Amity Institute of Pharmacy, Amity University, Gwalior, Madhya Pradesh, India*

[3]*Institute of Pharmaceutical Research, GLA University, Mathura, Uttar Pradesh, India*

[4]*Department of Pharmaceutical Chemistry, Amity Institute of Pharmacy, Amity University, Gwalior, Madhya Pradesh, India*

[5]*University Institute of Pharmaceutical Sciences, Panjab University, Chandigarh, India*

*Corresponding author

ABSTRACT

The potential of nanomedicine, a science and technology subject, has recently captivated researchers in the domains of physics, biotechnology, chemistry, and medicine. Everything that is done at the nanoscale, or at the level of individual atoms and molecules, is handled by this department. The development of nanotechnology and its introduction have greatly benefited a number of scientific fields. This is particularly significant when it comes to the creation of novel pharmacological compounds

Nanotechnology for Nucleic Acid Delivery: Pankaj Sharma, Saloni Jain, and Vinay Jain (Eds.)

DOI: 10.1201/9781998511853-1

and products. The introduction of nanomedicines to the pharmaceutical industry, the debate surrounding fundamental ideas pertaining to these nanosystems, and the various approaches used to further our understanding are the main topics of this review. The obstacles of implementing nanotechnology, particularly in the pharmaceutical development of novel therapeutic products and related regulatory issues, are critically explored, with a primary focus on the European Union setting, due to the qualities granted by the nanoscale. Issues about the apps that are currently in use, as well as upcoming improvements, are finally discussed.

1.1 INTRODUCTION

Despite being in its early stages, nanomedicine—the use of nanotechnology in medicine—is expected to completely transform the way that healthcare is provided [1]. With significant funding and support from the public sector, nanomedical research is advancing quickly.

As nanomedicines continue to advance, they could offer a host of advantages over traditional medications, such as increased safety, efficacy, bioavailability, dosage response, targeting capability, and personalization [2]. The creation of multifunctional nanoparticle (NP) complexes, which can simultaneously deliver therapeutic and diagnostic chemicals to specified areas, may be the most intriguing idea in nanomedical research [3].

These skills are unheard of and signify enormous advancements in patient diagnosis, care, and follow-up. Nevertheless, despite these possible advantages, there is currently a dearth of important information about the pharmacokinetics, pharmacodynamics, and toxicity of many nanomaterials [4].

1.1.1 NANOTECHNOLOGY

Rapid advancements in the field of nanotechnology are predicted to have a dramatic effect on a variety of industries, including medicine. Many scientific disciplines, including chemistry, biology, physics, mathematics, and engineering, have come together to enable nanotechnology [5]. One billionth of a meter is called a nanometer (nm), and the prefix nano- is derived from the Greek word for dwarf. Scientists can now examine, manipulate, and control atoms, molecules, and submicroscopic objects that are typically between 1 and 100 nm in size with new instruments thanks to nanotechnology. Utilizing naturally occurring quantum phenomena at the nanoscale level that affect biological, physical, chemical, mechanical, and optical aspects is made possible for scientists by nanotechnology [6]. Because of these special characteristics, nanoscale materials frequently have advantageous chemical, physical, and biological qualities that set them apart from their bigger, or bulk, counterparts [7].

1.1.2 NANOMEDICINE

Nanotechnology and medicine have crossed paths to create the multidisciplinary discipline of nanomedicine. The fields of inheritance, proteomics, biochemical and cell biology, materials science, and bioengineering have all contributed to the establishment of this new field, which examines biological functions at the nanoscale. Numerous internal operations of a cell naturally take place on this scale since numerous physiologically important components, such as water, glucose, antibodies, proteins, enzymes, receptors, and hemoglobin, already have sizes that fall into the nanoscale range. Many scientists are now working on medical processes, instruments, and devices that leverage nanotechnology to increase effectiveness, security, sensitivity, and customization [8]. Some of the possible beneficial properties of nanotherapeutics include enhanced solubility, reduced toxicity, higher bioavailability, and greater dose responsiveness as opposed to traditional pharmaceuticals [9].

According to the National Nanotechnology Initiative (NNI), a federal research and development program, nanotechnology is the science of materials and phenomena with diameters between 1 and 100 nm. This term is still in use by a number of federal agencies, such as the FDA and the Patent and Trademark Office (PTO) [10]. Some researchers counter that this artificial and deceptive size restriction is unnecessary because nanomaterials with diameters as small as several hundred nanometers might nevertheless have special features [11].

An alternative definition of nanotechnology, provided by the National Institutes of Health (NIH), does not depend on size; rather, it describes the field as follows:

- Studies that apply concepts and tools from nanotechnology to biology;
- Engineering biological molecules to perform functions different from those found in nature; or

- Manipulation of biological systems using techniques more precise than traditional synthetic, molecular biological, chemical, or biochemical methods [12].

1.1.3 NANOMEDICINE AND ALIGNED TECHNOLOGIES

Understanding the terms listed below is essential to comprehending the principles of Nanomedicine as follows:

1. **Nanotechnology:** It is the scientific field that deals with the modification of atom and molecule sizes to a nanoscale for a variety of purposes.
2. **Nanomaterial:** It's a nanoscale particle, with a size range of 1–100 nanometers. Their smaller size enables them to hinder distinct physical and chemical properties in contrast to their larger counterparts.
3. **Nano Pharmaceutical:** Therapeutic products with nanoparticles are known as nano pharmaceuticals. They could be either a medicine that is a nanoparticle combination with an active ingredient from a pharmaceutical or a drug that is nano sized itself.
4. **Nanomedicine:** A portion of the nanotechnology domain. It is the use of nanotechnology in pharmaceuticals, medical technologies, and healthcare.
5. **Nano Device:** It is the use of nanomaterials and nanotechnologies in medical equipment, including implants, appliances, and instruments [13–18].

1.1.4 APPLICATION OF NANOMEDICINE

Promising and ever-evolving are the medical applications of nanotechnologies, with research being done in fields including molecular imaging, targeted medication delivery, illness diagnostics and detection, and the use of nanomaterials in medical devices. Furthermore, nanoparticles are being applied in a novel way as biomarkers to locate and provide a contrast at the place of interest in the human body to facilitate processes like imaging and component identification in samples taken from the body [2].

Because nanotechnology is a scientific discovery that is founded on the idea of nano-scaling particles, the potential for nanomedicine is enormous. Consequently, any use of nanoparticles in the medical field will inevitably result in a nanomedicine application [20].

While new uses of nanotechnology are being investigated for efficacy and efficiency, the field of healthcare applications of nanotechnology is constantly expanding [21] (Figure 1.1).

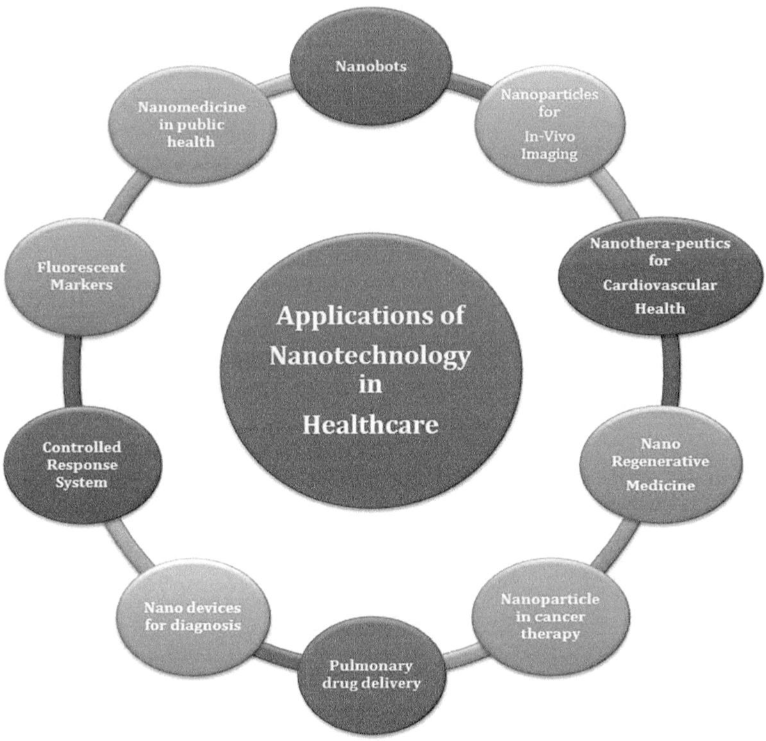

FIGURE 1.1 Application of nanotechnology in healthcare.

A brief discussion of some of the nanotechnology-related healthcare applications are illustrated in the subsections.

1.1.4.1 NANOBOTS

The remarkable engineering achievement of nanobots is among the most significant uses of nanotechnology in medicine. They are being created to have the ability to replicate in order to replace certain molecules, to eradicate sickness in the human body, or to cure a genetic deficit [22].

1.1.4.2 NANOPARTICLE FOR IN VIVO IMAGING

The remarkable engineering achievement of nanobots is among the most significant uses of nanotechnology in medicine. As the name implies, nanobots are tiny surgical helpers that can be utilized to replace intracellular structures in the human body or to repair damaged cells. They are being created to have the ability to replicate in order to replace certain molecules to eradicate sickness in the human body or to cure a genetic deficit [23].

1.1.4.3 NANO THERAPEUTICS FOR CARDIOVASCULAR HEALTH

Targeted medication delivery in the human circulatory system is challenging due to its complexity, making it difficult to image and diagnose the system thoroughly. In order to increase the effectiveness of nanotherapeutics in the treatment of inflammatory and cardiovascular disorders, strategies for leveraging the special qualities of nanoparticles to facilitate targeted drug delivery are being proposed. When using nanoparticles to treat cardiovascular disorders, getting adequate and heterogeneous delivery is still a major problem [24].

1.1.4.4 NANO REGENERATIVE MEDICINE

In the quickly evolving field of life sciences known as stem cell technology, human body stem cells are used as progenitors that can self-renew and differentiate, allowing for *in vitro* manipulation and the replacement of damaged cells in the body to treat illnesses.8 The fusion of nanotechnology and stem cell technologies has given rise to a novel area of medicine called regenerative medicine. For instance, tissue engineering and regenerative medicine can employ nanodiamond polymer composites to repair injured tissue [25]. Likewise, several bioengineered nanoparticles are being investigated for their potential to regenerate bone.

1.1.4.5 NANOPARTICLE IN CANCER THERAPY

While nanoparticles are being developed to treat a wide range of illnesses, the focus on cancer detection and therapy continues to represent a significant advancement in this field. The five CAPIR steps in the drug delivery process for cancer treatment involve circulating the nanoparticle in blood, allowing it to accumulate, and then penetrating the cancer tumor. Internalization within the cell and medication release via nanoparticle application comes next. The fast commencement of effective therapeutic activity is caused by the nonmetals' enhancement of drug solubility and adherence to targeted tumor surfaces [26]. Because they can be actively or passively targeted to cancer tissues to enhance anticancer drug delivery and hence minimize severe side effects, drug-loaded delivery vehicles or nanoparticles are appealing. Another strategy being investigated is the use of nanoparticles to combine multiple medications into a single carrier to solve the issue of inadequate drug delivery brought about by the application of modern medicine and the requirement for improvement. Additionally, this would make it possible to target many tumors for improved cancer diagnosis and treatment [27].

1.1.4.6 PULMONARY DRUG DELIVERY

The microorganisms that cause respiratory infections may live deep within the airways, and the illnesses may be resistant to multiple drugs, making treatment difficult. By using such distinctive nanoparticles and their ease of passage through biological barriers in the human body, drug delivery to such deeper areas of the airway system remains a crucial milestone to be attained in the future for nanomedicine [28].

1.1.4.7 NANO DEVICES FOR DIAGNOSIS

The nanomaterial presents a huge opportunity for advancement as a cutting-edge diagnostic instrument. It may be possible to directly engage with the biological system at the subcellular and molecular level with a nanoscale device or nanomaterial, leading to the development of a molecular probe and biosensor that is more precise and sensitive and facilitates diagnosis. For instance, several businesses are working on creating microchips that can detect the dielectric characteristics of bacteria, viruses, and malignant cells in bodily fluids using electrodes [29].

1.1.4.8 CONTROLLED RESPONSE SYSTEM

Researchers have highlighted concerns about the toxicity and drug release of nanoparticles used in drug delivery in the human body. However, it is possible to build nanoparticles to permit sustained release systems within the body. Because the nanoparticles are designed to release the drug in reaction to certain stimuli, more study is currently being done on this strategy in hopes of applying it to medicine [30].

1.1.4.9 FLUORESCENT MARKERS

In the human body, nanoparticles allow for the use of fluorescent markers for imaging, diagnosis, and screening, even for distant tissues and organs. Through the attachment of quantum dots to specific molecules, nanotechnologies enable the possibility of intracellular imaging, which is encouraging for their use in diagnosis and analysis of extracted human body samples for the detection of potential biological markers as well as changes at the molecular level. Because they aid in the processes of detection and prevention, these nanoparticles are referred to as Nano tools. More potential for enhancing diagnostic accuracy is made possible by this. These nanoparticles can be engineered to perform a variety of tasks on their own, including drug delivery and diagnosis, which aid in the therapeutic process. They can even be left behind at the intended location to track development [31].

1.1.4.10 NANOMEDICINE IN PUBLIC HEALTH

There is a lot of potential to enhance public health in a variety of ways, including increasing overall wellness, addressing and avoiding ailments, and treating serious illnesses, given the advancements being made in the field of nanomedicine. Among the community-based or social health concerns that it may help with include vaccination, prevention of infections, municipal disinfection, ambient infections oversight, early detection, and avoiding infectious illnesses [32].

1.2 CURRENT REGULATORY FRAMEWORK FOR NANOMEDICINE

The same regulations that now extend to medications, medical equipment, and biologics might be applicable to applications involving nanomedicine. The primary legislation governing all forms of nanomedicine is the Drugs and Cosmetics Act (DCA); nevertheless, depending on which of these groups the use fits under, extra-legal issues may need to be considered. Since the area of nanomedicine lacks a defined definition and set of laws, it is designated for control upon its implementation [33].

1.2.1 REGULATION OF NANOMEDICINE AS A DRUG

The DCA is the main law that governs drug use in India. Despite the fact that DCA does not specifically define or regulate nanomedicine, it does govern the production, importation, distribution, and sale of medications. DCA is implemented by the Central Drugs Standard Control Organization (CDSCO), which is led by the Drug Controller General of India (DCGI). In addition, the CDSCO creates standards, manages product approvals, and grants licenses in accordance with the DCA. State Drug Licensing Authorities (SLA) under the CDSCO are another entity that assists in performing these duties within particular states. A license is required for both the medicine and the manufacturing facility in order to produce a Nano pharmaceutical product [34]. Any procedure (or component) used to create, modify, embellish, finish, package, label, split, or otherwise handle any medication with the intention of selling or distributing it is referred to as manufacturing. It does not, however, include packing or dispensing at the retail sale level. Therefore, a second license will need to be obtained in order to retail a Nano pharmaceutical, that is, make it available to an end user [35].

1.2.2 REGULATION OF NANOMEDICINE AS A MEDICAL DEVICE

Medical devices in India are governed by the MDR, notified under the DCA, which places enforcement of the MDR under the purview of the CDSCO and SLAs. The term "medical device," as defined by the government, does not apply to all medical devices; rather, only those that have received notification from the government fall under the purview of MDR.

As a result, non-notified medical devices [36] utilizing nanotechnology will be regulated like medicines in accordance with the guidelines covered in the section before this one. Notified medical devices based on nanotechnology will fall under the MDR's jurisdiction.

1.2.3 REGULATION OF NANOMEDICINE AS A BIOLOGIC

Biologics are synthetic pharmaceuticals derived from biological organisms. These include antitoxins, serums, immunizations, and so forth. A list of them may be found in DCA Schedule C. Identical drugs and genetically modified drugs are governed by the Guidance for Identical Drugs, 2016 (Biosimilar Guidelines) and the Regulations for the Production, Usage, Export, Import, and Preservation of Dangerous Microorganisms/ Genetically Designed Living Things or Cells, 1989 (By Genes Designed Microorganisms Rules), which were issued according to the Environment Protection Act, 1986 (EPA) [37].

1.2.4 PRICE REGULATION OF NANOMEDICINE

All medicine prices in India are governed by the Medicine Price Control Order (DPCO), which was issued in accordance with Section 3 of the Essential Commodities Act, 1955. It outlines the processes for setting medicine pricing, how those prices are to be implemented, and the consequences of breaking the rules [38]. The body that carries out the DPCO's duties is the National Pharmaceutical Pricing Authority (NPPA) [39].

1.2.5 SAFETY STANDARDS

The Environmental Protection Agency (EPA) and its regulations provide a comprehensive regulatory framework for applications of nanotechnology in the lack of a specific statute [40]. The EPA is a broad body of law that aims to forbid and prevent actions that could endanger the environment. Any preparation or material that has the potential to harm people, other living things, plants, microorganisms, property, the environment, or any combination of these due to its handling, chemical, or physio-chemical qualities is considered hazardous [41]. This concept is sufficiently broad to include nanoparticles within the EPA's regulatory purview. The EPA's operations and the regulations it issues are within the purview of the Central and State Pollution Control Boards [42].

1.2.6 NANOTECHNOLOGY PRODUCTS

Nanotechnology has tremendous possibilities for use in a wide range of products, including food, electronics, cosmetics, and pharmaceuticals. As per The Woodrow Wilson Worldwide Center for Research' Program for Developing Nanotechnology [43], there are presently over 800 products on the market that are manufactured using nanotechnology. Nanomaterials have been used in digital cameras, mobile devices, laptops, filters for water, and aesthetics. Nanotechnology study is additionally underway to improve the bioavailability of food ingredients and develop packaging for food that can recognize and prevent rotting. The use of nanoscale has also helped a wide range of medical processes and goods, including drugs, imaging for healthcare, antimicrobial substances, medical equipment, sun protection products, burning and healing dressings, dental-bonding substances, and coatings that protect eyeglasses [44]. Nanotechnology has improved bioavailability and aiming for, drug delivery effectiveness, detecting biomarker sensibility, and imaging for diagnosis. Current nanomedicines involve doxorubicin HCl liposome injection (Doxil, Ortho Biotech) for cancer of the ovary, daunorubicin citrate the liposome the injection (DaunoXome, Diatos) for developed AIDS-related Kaposi's tumor, and amphotericin B lipid particles administration (AmBisome, Gilead) for fungal infections (Table 1.1). Moreover, indoor medical settings like hospitals employ antibacterial paints containing silver NPs [45].

1.2.7 PRODUCT GROWTH OF NANOTECHNOLOGY

The science of nanotechnology is expanding quickly. Because of its widespread use in everyday items, nanomaterials were expected to be a $10.5 billion business in the United States in 2008. By 2015, the nanotechnology sector was expected to have grown to $1 trillion, a growth of roughly 100 times in just seven years. One of nanotechnology's main uses is currently in nanomedicine. The National Science Foundation (NSF) projects that by 2020, medical uses will account for one-third of inventions and new

TABLE 1.1 Nanotechnology Products

Product	Company Name	Therapeutic Agent	Nanotechnology	Therapeutic Role	Route of Administration
Pacliall	Panacea	Paclitaxel	Nanoparticles	Lung cancer	(i.v)
Myocet	Zencus Pharma, Sophenion	Doxorubicin	Liposome	breast cancer	(i.v)
LEP-ETU	Ncopharm	Paclitaxel	Neolipid	Advanced Cancer	(i.v)
Clinical trial	–	SN38	PAMAM dendrimers	Hepatic colorectal cancer	Oral
Allovectin	VICAL	Plasmid DNA	Liposomal DNA/Lipidic complex	Melanoma	(i.v)
DepoCy	Skyc Pharma Enzon	Cytarabine	Liposome	Lymphomatous meningitis	(i.v)
Avinza	King Pharma. Elan	Morphine Sulfate	Nano Crystal	psycho-stimulant	Oral
Tricor	Abbott Lab (USA)	Fenofibrate	Nanocrystal particles	Primary lipidemia	Oral
Clinical trial	AlphaRx	Streptomycin	Nanocapsule	tuberculosis	(i.m)
MiKasome	NeXstar Pharmceutica 1	Amikacin	Liposome	tuberculosis	(i.v)
Clinical trial	-	Rifampicin + isoninzide	SLN Nebulization	tuberculosis	Inhalation
Emend	Merck, Elan	Aprepitan	DepoFoam	antiemetic	Oral

businesses in the nanomaterials industry. The NSF also projects that nanotechnology will be a part of about half of medications produced in the foreseeable future [46].

1.2.8 REGULATION OF NANOMEDICINE AS MEDICAL DEVICES

A combination product combines two or more application categories, such as biologic, device, and medication. As was said above, because of their varied properties, items related to nanomedicine are hard to categorize into a single application area. As a result, licensing and regulating nanomedicine items as combination products will allow regulators to adequately consider the product's distinctive qualities and tailor their regulations accordingly [47].

1.3 NANOPARTICLES (NPS)

A nanoparticle is a nano-object that has all of its exterior dimensions in the nanoscale and whose longest and shortest axes have lengths that are not significantly different from one another. In cases when there is a considerable difference in dimensions (usually greater than three times), it may be more appropriate to use terminology like nanofibers or nanoplates instead of nanoparticles [48]. Nanoparticles come in a variety of sizes, forms, and configurations. They can have unusual shapes such as spherical, cylindrical, conical, tubular, hollow core, spiral, and so forth. NPs can range in size from 1–100 nm. When nanoparticles are smaller than 1 nm, the phrase atom clusters is typically used. Nanoparticles can be amorphous or crystalline, containing single or many crystal solids. NPs may aggregate or remain loose [49].

Nanoparticles might consist of many layers or be uniform. In the latter instance, the layers are typically:

- The surface layer, which is typically made up of metal ions, polymers, surfactants, and a variety of tiny molecules.
- The outermost layer is composed of a material that differs chemically from the innermost layer. The core layer or the middle part of the Nanoparticles [50].

1.3.1 PHYSICAL FEATURES OF NANOPARTICLES

There are numerous variations in the physical properties of NPs that affect their functionality. Following is a discussion of a few of these physical characteristics [51].

1.3.1.1 SIZE

Nanoparticles (NPs) have a minimum dimension of 1–100 nm. However, they can also have a size of micrometers (μm). Many larger molecules or bulk materials lack the unique structural, optical, and electrical features that NPs possess. Additionally, because of their increased solubility, they might be utilized to reexamine bulk medication counterparts that have a history of low solubility. This characteristic would make it possible to turn weakly soluble or insoluble medications into soluble aqueous solutions, doing away with the requirement for hazardous organic solvents. The enhanced bioavailability and circulation time of NPs is another important advantage associated with their tiny size. Research has demonstrated that, regardless of any surface changes, particles smaller than 200 nm circulate more slowly than larger particles [52].

1.3.1.2 SHAPE

NPs are shaped like spheres, discs, hemispheres, cylinders, cones, tubes, and wires, among other shapes. Moreover, NPs may be solid, porous, or hollow. These NP properties can be chosen based on transit capability, loading capacity, and interaction. For instance, a hollow nanoparticle could be a desirable delivery system for medication or contrast chemicals for imaging [53].

1.3.1.3 SURFACE AREA

NPs have distinct physical features, one of which is their enormous surface area to size ratio. The overall surface area increases exponentially with decreasing particle size. A higher percentage of atoms are found on the particle surface compared to the center when the surface area of the particle increases. When NPs are compared to their bulk solid or traditional bigger molecule counterparts, this effect increases their reactivity. Moreover, increased surface area is in charge of NPs' frequently observed improved water solubility and bioavailability [54].

Because of their vast surface area, NPs can be engineered to have a variety of surface properties, such as conjugation with proteins or electrostatic charges. These surface characteristics are chosen based on their potential for strategic targeting and other uses.

1.3.1.4 PERMEABILITY

Because of their small size, NPs have the potential to deliver medications to locations that are inaccessible by conventional methods if they are appropriately constructed to overcome physiological obstacles. For instance, an NP's enhanced permeability might enable it to enter a tumor and deliver cancer-fighting agents by squeezing through neovessel pores with a diameter of less than 1 μm. Through the use of several uptake mechanisms, NPs may be able to traverse the blood–brain barrier due to their increased permeability [55].

1.3.2 SPECIFIC NANOPARTICLES AND MATERIALS

Depending on the application, a wide range of NPs and materials are employed in nanomedicine. Liposomes, polymers, iron oxide (IO) particles, quantum dots (QDs), carbon nanotubes, and nanoshells are a few of the most commonly used materials [56].

1.3.2.1 LIPOSOMES

A liposome is a spherical vesicle that typically contains an aqueous solution and is made up of an empty core and a lipid bilayer membrane. Liposomes are often slightly bigger than ordinary NPs because of their 90–150 nm diameters. Liposomes are frequently made to transport biomolecules that are attached to the surface as ligands, such as monoclonal antibodies and antigens. Because liposomes have so many special qualities, they are frequently used in nano medical research. Because liposomes' constituent parts resemble those of human cell membranes in their natural state, liposomal drug delivery is endowed with a number of inherent advantages [57]. Unlike non-liposomal medications, liposomes circulate in the bloodstream for a longer period of time, resulting in a longer duration of therapeutic impact.

Additionally, liposomes gather in the location of an infection or tumor, where they naturally locate and transport larger medication concentrations to these targets. Hydrophilic or hydrophobic medicines can be delivered by liposomes and preserved in their empty cores. Scientists can create temperature- or pH-sensitive liposomes that allow for the regulated release of their contents only when exposed to particular environmental conditions by utilizing lipids with varying fatty acid chain lengths [58].

1.3.2.2 POLYMERS

Compared to other materials, polymer NPs are commonly used in nanomedical research since data regarding their safety and effectiveness are already available for many of them. Polymer NPs can be produced in an extensive array of shapes and dimensions, spanning from 10 nm–1 μm. Some polymer NPs do not build up in the body and can help release drugs for weeks at a time [59]. Therefore, polymeric NPs are thought to be promising carriers for a variety of drugs, such as those used in the treatment of diabetes, cancer, and cardiovascular disease, as well as bone-healing therapies and vaccines. Polymeric NPs can also be conjugated to the surface of contrast agents, making them suitable for use in diagnostic imaging [60].

1.3.2.3 QUANTUM DOTS

Quantum dots, also known as semiconductor nanocrystals, are typically composed of 10–50 atoms and range in size from 2–10 nm. Quantum dots (QDs) have been utilized for 20 years in electronics and optics, but their application in nanomedical research is relatively new [61]. For biological applications, cadmium telluride (CdTe) or cadmium selenide (CdSe) are the most often employed QDs. Additionally, widely utilized QDs include those containing indium arsenide (InAs) and indium phosphide (InP).

Because of their special optical and electrical characteristics, QDs are useful as luminous probes and offer enormous potential in a variety of biomedical applications. Due to their inherent fluorescence, QDs may generate light in a wide spectrum, spanning from the mid-infrared to the near-ultraviolet (UV). Their exceptional photostability, size-dependent optical characteristics, and adjustable surface qualities make them perfect for optical imaging [61].

1.3.2.4 CARBON NANOTUBES (CNT)

The unique molecular structure of carbon atoms that makes up carbon nanotubes endows them with exceptional mechanical, electrical, and thermal characteristics. They are, for instance, 100 times stronger than steel that is six times their weight. 5. Polyethylene glycol (PEG)-modified carbon nanotubes exhibit remarkable stability *in vivo*, exhibiting extended circulation durations and minimal absorption by the reticuloendothelial system (RES). Carbon nanotubes have been employed in the administration of medicinal and diagnostic substances, as well as in the intracellular delivery of DNA molecules. Because of their huge surface area and electro catalytic capabilities, the single-walled and multiwalled carbon's nanoscale dimensions have forced researchers to use nanotubes as tiny electrodes [62].

1.3.2.5 CARBON NANO SHELLS

The silica core of carbon nanoshells is encased in a thin metallic shell, often made of gold. Light scattering is a property of carbon nanoshells that makes them valuable for imaging cancer. They are still mostly used in thermal ablation therapy, though. On the other hand, targeted lasers have shown effective in cancer thermotherapy; nevertheless, they are unable to distinguish between sick and healthy tissue. In contrast, heat energy flows through healthy tissue without harming it when carbon nanoshells are utilized for targeting in thermal ablation therapy, destroying only the targeted tumor cells. Colon cancer cell tumors were totally eradicated *in vivo* in mice using carbon nanoshells and near-infrared spectroscopy (NIRS) thermal ablation therapy [63].

1.4 POTENTIAL ADVANTAGES OF NANOMEDICINE

Someday, nanomedicines may be able to address persistent issues in medical research, such as low drug solubility and a lack of target specificity for therapeutic mixtures [63]. Because NPs have special optical, magnetic, and structural qualities that conventional tools do not, nanomedicine also holds great potential as a noninvasive tool for drug administration, tumor detection, and diagnostic imaging. Nanomedicine offers fresh chances to raise the efficacy and safety of traditional treatments. It is now possible to target drugs with low bioavailability directly to the needed spot. A drug's dose may be able to be reduced thanks to the wide surface area and increased reactivity of NPs, which can enhance toxicity profiles and patient compliance [64].

In addition to increasing the rate of drug dissolution, saturation solubility, and intracellular absorption, NPs' vast surface area can also enhance *in vivo* performance. The efficacy of NP formulations could be increased several times over when encapsulation, release modalities, and surface changes are combined to enhance therapeutic targeting or bioavailability. This would be in comparison to bulk counterparts. Targeted nanoparticles have the ability to deliver substantial dosages of medicinal substances to cancerous cells while preserving healthy, normal cells [64].

Using multifunctional NP complexes for simultaneous non-invasive targeting, imaging, and treatment is one of the most promising uses of nanomedicine. Multifunctional NPs for cancer treatment may comprise therapeutic compounds and imaging agents that enable noninvasive treatment and monitoring, along with a range of tumor-targeting ligands. Multifunctional NPs with fluorescence dyes can potentially serve as possible diagnostic markers for the early identification and localization of malignancies, as well as *in vivo* imaging of biologic events during medication delivery.

The development of magnetic NPs for the targeted administration of different medicinal or diagnostic substances is another area of recent scientific attention. The prospect of using magnetic resonance imaging (MRI) to identify the particles and subsequently comparing the results with histology findings following therapy has sparked interest in magnetic nanoparticle targeted applications. The most popular NPs employed in theranostics (diagnostics) are Polymer/SPIO composites. A polymer/IO conjugate backbone can also include many cancer drugs. The medications can be released at the location of the tumor, enabling them to work in concert and possibly achieving greater efficacy. Since SPIO NPs produce heat when they come into contact with an alternating current, external electromagnetic fields can also be used to remotely activate SPIO NPs for the purpose of thermal ablation therapy [65]. Devices that look for molecular biomarkers have already revolutionized biological and genetic studies thanks to nanotechnologies. These tests can be carried out more quickly, accurately, and affordably than with traditional modalities thanks to *in vitro* and *in vivo* diagnostic technologies, which could make use of QDs or Nano chips, among other things. Additionally, nanotechnologies can be used to create more sensitive diagnostic tools that can identify metabolic imbalances early on and help avoid disorders like diabetes and obesity. Personalized medicine will become more commonplace if nanotechnologies are used to provide more efficient and affordable methods of identifying molecular biomarkers.

Since the antigen nanoparticle delivery system is intended to be supplied directly to the colon, Sahu and Pandey created a novel, straightforward, and effective method that does not require the use of any unique polymers. Strong humoral and cellular immunological responses were elicited by it, with mucosal IgA levels being much higher than those of normal subjects. The immunological response was noticeably enhanced, which justifies the use of a more affordable vaccine in place of the traditional ones.

1.5 CHALLENGES FOR NANOMEDICINE

Even with all of nanomedicine's advantages, a great deal of research is still needed to determine the safety and toxicity of many NPs. Much of the study on nanomedicines has focused mostly on medication delivery, with comparatively little research on NPs' toxicity or pharmacokinetics. It's critical to look into the pharmacokinetics, pharmacodynamics, and possible long-term toxicity of NPs *in vivo* while tracking their effects on patient populations [66]. Researchers and the FDA face a great deal of difficulty in validating each nanotherapeutic agent for safety and efficacy, whether it be a medication, device, biologic, or combination product. The FDA is currently having difficulty developing testing criteria and gathering safety data. Additionally, research is required to evaluate the immunogenicity of NPs.

Since nanotherapeutics and diagnostics are more reactive than their bulk counterparts, they may have unanticipated harmful effects. Hypersensitivity reaction following injection of a nanotherapeutic drug appears to be the most commonly reported adverse effect, possibly due to immunological complement system activation. It is believed that the primary chemical mechanism underlying *in vivo* nanoparticle toxicity is the generation of free radicals, which induces oxidative stress. When free radicals are present in excess, they can oxidize proteins, lipids, DNA, and other biological components. According to a number of writers, NPs' inherent properties, like aspect ratio and surface area, may have pro-inflammatory and pro-oxidant effects.

Free radical production in response to NPs, however, can also result from other variables, including the phagocytic cells' response to foreign material, an inadequate amount of antioxidants, the presence of transition metals, ambient conditions, and other inherent chemical or physical characteristics.

Finding the threshold dimensions at which NPs are likely to aggregate considerably in the body may also be aided by research evaluating the size and surface characteristics of NPs. Because of their small size, NPs have the potential to concentrate in tissues and cells due to their enhanced capacity to overcome biological barriers.

The propensity for these potentially free radical-producing particles to accumulate, store, and clear slowly from tissue, as well as the high phagocyte predominance, may make the liver and spleen the primary targets of oxidative stress in the RES. Since there is a dearth of information on possible toxicity concerns, nanomedical research is forced to concentrate mostly on polymer NPs, for which safety and efficacy data are already available. In reality, the FDA has previously approved a number of nanomedicines that contain polymer NPs. Lipid NPs are likewise thought to be biocompatible and bearable, in contrast to other substances that could turn hazardous when in the form of nanoparticles.

Therefore, it is far preferable to employ biodegradable, soluble, nontoxic NPs in nanomedicines rather than biopersistent ones, such as polymers, liposomes, and IO particles [67]. The application of non-biodegradable NPs such as QDs, carbon nanotubes, and certain metallic Nano carriers may provide more challenges. This property shouldn't prevent scientists from using these NPs in nanomedical research; rather, it should motivate researchers to find more biodegradable forms, substances, and surface treatments.

1.6 CLASSIFICATION OF NANOPARTICLES

Most of the current nanomaterial's can be grouped into following categories, and they are discussed in the subsections.

1.6.1 ORGANIC NANOPARTICLES

Micelles, ferritin, liposomes, dendrimers, and so forth are examples of organic nanoparticles or polymers in general. Naturally breaking down, these nanoparticles pose no threat. Micelles and liposomes are sometimes known as nanocapsules because of their hollow cores. Moreover, these particles are susceptible to the effects of light, heat, and other types of thermal and electromagnetic radiation [68]. Their distinct qualities provide them with the perfect option for dispensing drugs. Apart from the usual characteristics such as size, content, surface form, and so forth, the drug's efficacy and range of applications are determined by its stability, carrying capacity, and delivery mechanisms (adsorbed or entrapped). The biomedical sector, particularly in drug delivery systems, is where organic nanoparticles are most frequently used due to their effectiveness and ability to be injected into specific bodily regions. Targeted medication delivery is the term for this methodology.

1.6.2 INORGANIC NANOPARTICLES

Non-carbon-based particles are known as inorganic nanoparticles. A common definition of inorganic nanoparticles is those that are composed of metals and metal oxides.

1.6.2.1 METAL BASED

Metal-based nanoparticles are those that are made from metals, either constructively or destructively. It is possible to synthesize nearly every metal into a nanoparticle [68]. When making nanoparticles, the following metals are commonly used: aluminum (Al), cadmium (Cd), cobalt (Co), copper (Cu), gold (Au), iron (Fe), lead (Pb), silver (Ag), and zinc (Zn). Sizes between 10 and 100 nm, high surface area to volume ratios, pore sizes, surface charges, and surface charge densities are some characteristics that distinguish the nanoparticles. Other characteristics include crystalline and amorphous structures, spherical and cylindrical shapes, color, and reactivity and sensitivity to different environmental stimuli, including heat, moisture, air, and sunlight.

1.6.2.2 METAL OXIDES BASED

To alter the relevant metal-based nanoparticles' properties, metal oxide-based nanoparticles are synthesized. As an example, iron (Fe) nanoparticles at ambient temperature oxidize fast to form iron oxide (Fe_2O_3), which makes them more reactive than other forms of iron nanoparticles. Since they are highly reactive and efficient, metal oxide nanoparticles are mostly manufactured [69]. The most often generated oxides are aluminum oxide (Al_2O_3), cerium oxide (CeO_2), iron oxide (Fe_2O_3), magnetite (Fe_3O_4), silicon dioxide (SiO_2), titanium oxide (TiO_2), and zinc oxide (ZnO). These nanoparticles exhibit notable properties in contrast to their metal counterparts.

1.6.2.3 CARBON BASED

Nanoparticles that are totally made of carbon are called carbon-based nanoparticles [69]. They come into the following categories: fullerenes, graphene, CNT, carbon nanofibers, carbon black, and seldom activated carbon. They are displayed at nanoscale as follows:

1. **Fullerenes:** Carbon atoms joined together by sp2 hybridization form fullerenes (C60), spherical carbon molecules. Fullerenes are spherical materials with diameters ranging from 8.2 nm for single layers and 4–36 nm for multi-layered fullerenes. They are composed of 28–1500 carbon atoms [70].
2. **Graphene:** One kind of carbon allotrope is graphene. Graphene is made of carbon atoms arranged in a hexagonal honeycomb lattice on a two-dimensional planar surface. A graphene sheet is typically one nanometer thick.
3. **Carbon Nano Tubes (CNT):** Often known as CNTs, they are hollow cylinders composed of a honeycomb lattice of twisted carbon atoms constructed of graphene Nano foil. The diameter

of a single-layered carbon nanotube can be as small as 0.7 nm, whereas the diameter of a multi-layered carbon nanotube can reach up to 100 nm. Their length varies from a few micrometers to many millimeters. A half-fullerene molecule has the potential to have both hollow and closed ends.

4. **Carbon Nanofibers:** Carbon nanofibers are made using graphene Nano foils, but instead of being twisted into a typical cylindrical tube, they take the form of a cup or cone.

5. **Carbon Black:** It is a spherical, amorphous substance composed of carbon that has sizes between 20 and 70 nm. Agglomerates, which are around 500 nm in size, are formed when particles have such strong contacts with one another [19].

1.7 CONCLUSION

Through increased daily object usefulness and efficiency, nanotechnology is improving our lives. Together with better air and water quality, it offers clean, renewable energy for a sustainable future and a clean environment. Because of the increasing interest in nanotechnology, major institutions, businesses, and organizations are investing more in this field's research and development. Much research is done in the cutting-edge field of nanotechnology in order to use the technology. In an attempt to increase the objects' or process's performance and efficiency while bringing down its cost to make it accessible to everyone, it is being tested for a number of innovative purposes. Nanotechnology has a promising future since it is both ecologically friendly and effective.

ACKNOWLEDGMENT

None

CONFLICT OF INTEREST

The authors declare no conflict of interest

FUNDING

None

KEYWORDS

- **nanobots**
- **nanomaterial**
- **nanomedicine**
- **nanoparticles**
- **nanoscale**
- **nanotechnology**
- **pharmaceutical development**

REFERENCES

1. Poirot-Mazères, I. (2011). Chapter 6. Legal aspects of the risks raised by nanotechnologies in the field of medicine. *Journal International de Biotechnique, 22*(1), 99. https://doi.org/10.3917/jib.221.0099 (accessed on 23rd June 2025).
2. Bawa, R. (2011). Regulating nanomedicine–Can the FDA handle it? *Current Drug Delivery, 8*(3), 227–234. https://doi.org/10.2174/156720111795256156 (accessed on 23rd June 2025).
3. Galvin, P., Thompson, D., Ryan, K. B., McCarthy, A., Moore, A. C., Burke, C. S., Dyson, M., MacCraith, B. D., Gunko, Y. K., Byrne, M. T., Volkov, Y., Keely, C., Keehan, E., Howe, M., Duffy, C., & MacLoughlin, R. (2011). Nanoparticle-based drug delivery: Case studies for cancer and cardiovascular applications. *Cellular and Molecular Life Sciences, 69*(3), 389–404. https://doi.org/10.1007/s00018-011-0856-6 (accessed on 23rd June 2025).
4. Bharali, D. J., & Mousa, S. A. (2010). Emerging nanomedicines for early cancer detection and improved treatment: Current perspective and future promise. *Pharmacology & Therapeutics, 128*(2), 324–335. https://doi.org/10.1016/j.pharmthera.2010.07.007 (accessed on 23rd June 2025).
5. Sajja, H., East, M., Mao, H., Wang, Y., Nie, S., & Yang, L. (2009). Development of multifunctional nanoparticles for targeted drug delivery and noninvasive imaging of therapeutic effect. *Current Drug Discovery Technologies, 6*(1), 43–51.
6. Seigneuric, R., Markey, L., Nuyten, D. S. A., Dubernet, C., Evelo, C. T. A., Finot, E., & Garrido, C. (2010). From nanotechnology to nanomedicine: Applications to cancer research. *Current Molecular Medicine, 10*(7), 640–652.
7. Bhaskar, S., Tian, F., Stoeger, T., Kreyling, W., de la Fuente, J. M., Grazú, V., Borm, P., Estrada, G., Ntziachristos, V., & Razansky, D. (2010). Multifunctional nanocarriers for diagnostics, drug delivery and targeted treatment across blood-brain barrier: Perspectives on tracking and neuroimaging. *Particle and Fiber Toxicology, 7*(1), 1–25. https://doi.org/10.1186/1743-8977-7-3 (accessed on 23rd June 2025).

8. McGrady, E., Conger, S., Blanke, S., & Landry, B. J. L. (2010). Emerging technologies in healthcare: Navigating risks, evaluating rewards. *Journal of Healthcare Management, 55*(5), 353–365.
9. Godin, B., Sakamoto, J. H., Serda, R. E., Grattoni, A., Bouamrani, A., & Ferrari, M. (2010). Emerging applications of nanomedicine for the diagnosis and treatment of cardiovascular diseases. *Trends in Pharmacological Sciences, 31*(5), 199–205. https://doi.org/10.1016/j.tips.2010.01.003 (accessed on 23rd June 2025).
10. Webster, T. J., & Taylor. (2011). Reducing infections through nanotechnology and nanoparticles. *International Journal of Nanomedicine*, 1463. https://doi.org/10.2147/IJN.S22021 (accessed on 23rd June 2025).
11. Ferrari, M. (2005). Cancer nanotechnology: Opportunities and challenges. *Nature Reviews Cancer, 5*(3), 161–171. https://doi.org/10.1038/nrc1566 (accessed on 23rd June 2025).
12. Vaddiraju, S., Tomazos, I., Burgess, D. J., Jain, F. C., & Papadimitrakopoulos, F. (2010). Emerging synergy between nanotechnology and implantable biosensors: A review. *Biosensors and Bioelectronics, 25*(7), 1553–1565. https://doi.org/10.1016/j.bios.2009.12.001 (accessed on 23rd June 2025).
13. Prasenjit, S., Tanvi, G., & Sandeep, R. (2022). *Colocasia plants used treat waste water from homes*. *Applied Science and Engineering Journal for Advanced Research, 1*(1), 14–21.
14. Salavati-Niasari, M., Davar, F., & Mir, N. (2008). Synthesis and characterization of metallic copper nanoparticles via thermal decomposition. *Polyhedron, 27*(17), 3514–3518. https://doi.org/10.1016/j.poly.2008.08.020 (accessed on 23rd June 2025).
15. Tai, C. Y., Tai, C. T., Chang, M. H., & Liu, H. S. (2007). Synthesis of magnesium hydroxide and oxide nanoparticles using a spinning disk reactor. *Industrial & Engineering Chemistry Research, 46*(17), 5536–5541. https://doi.org/10.1021/ie060869b (accessed on 23rd June 2025).
16. Bhaviripudi, S., Mile, E., Steiner, S. A., Zare, A. T., Dresselhaus, M. S., Belcher, A. M., & Kong, J. (2007). CVD synthesis of single-walled carbon nanotubes from gold nanoparticle catalysts. *Journal of the American Chemical Society, 129*(6), 1516–1517. https://doi.org/10.1021/ja0673332 (accessed on 23rd June 2025).
17. Sahu, K. K., & Pandey, R. S. (2016). Immunological evaluation of colonic delivered Hepatitis B surface antigen loaded TLR-4 agonist modified solid fat nanoparticles. *International Immunopharmacology, 39*, 343–352. https://doi.org/10.1016/j.intimp.2016.08.007 (accessed on 23rd June 2025).
18. Hua, S., & Wu, S. Y. (2018). Editorial: Advances and challenges in nanomedicine. *Frontiers in Pharmacology, 9*. https://doi.org/10.3389/fphar.2018.01397 (accessed on 23rd June 2025).
19. Reed, M. A. (2005). Book review: *Springer Handbook of Nanotechnology* by Bharat Bhushan (Ed.). *Advanced Materials, 17*(14), 1804–1804. https://doi.org/10.1007/978-3-662-54357-3_1 (accessed on 23rd June 2025).
20. Jeevanandam, J., Barhoum, A., Chan, Y. S., Dufresne, A., & Danquah, M. K. (2018). Review on nanoparticles and nanostructured materials: History, sources, toxicity and regulations. *Beilstein Journal of Nanotechnology, 9*, 1050–1074. https://doi.org/10.3762/bjnano.9.98 (accessed on 23rd June 2025).

21. Bayda, S., Adeel, M., Tuccinardi, T., Cordani, M., & Rizzolio, F. (2019). The history of nanoscience and nanotechnology: From chemical–physical applications to nanomedicine. *Molecules, 25*(1), 112. https://doi.org/10.3390/molecules25010112 (accessed on 23rd June 2025).
22. Rani, K., Devi, N., Banakar, P., Kharb, P., & Kaushik, P. (2022). Nematocidal potential of green silver nanoparticles synthesized using aqueous root extract of *Glycyrrhiza glabra*. *Nanomaterials, 14*(7), 585. https://doi.org/10.1016/bs.coac.2020.12.011 (accessed on 23rd June 2025).
23. Griffin, S., Masood, M., Nasim, M., Sarfraz, M., Ebokaiwe, A., Schäfer, K. H., Keck, C., & Jacob, C. (2017). Natural nanoparticles: A particular matter inspired by nature. *Antioxidants, 7*(1), 3. https://doi.org/10.3390/antiox7010003 (accessed on 23rd June 2025).
24. Boverhof, D. R., Bramante, C. M., Butala, J. H., Clancy, S. F., Lafranconi, M., West, J., & Gordon, S. C. (2015). Comparative assessment of nanomaterial definitions and safety evaluation considerations. *Regulatory Toxicology and Pharmacology, 73*(1), 137–150. https://doi.org/10.1016/j.yrtph.2015.06.001 (accessed on 23rd June 2025).
25. Kumar, P., Saini, M., Dehiya, B. S., Sindhu, A., Kumar, V., Kumar, R., Lamberti, L., Pruncu, C. I., & Thakur, R. (2020). Comprehensive survey on nano biomaterials for bone tissue engineering applications. *Nanomaterials, 10*(10), 2019. https://doi.org/10.3390/nano10102019 (accessed on 23rd June 2025).
26. Mabrouk, M., Das, D. B., Salem, Z. A., & Beherei, H. H. (2021). Nanomaterials for biomedical applications: Production, characterizations, recent trends and difficulties. *Molecules, 26*(4), 1077. https://doi.org/10.3390/molecules26041077 (accessed on 23rd June 2025).
27. Salah, N., Habib, A., Khan, Z., Memic, A., Azam, A., Al-Hamedi, S., Zahed, M., & Habib, S. S. (2011). High-energy ball milling technique for ZnO nanoparticles as antibacterial material. *International Journal of Nanomedicine*, 863–869. https://doi.org/10.2147/IJN.S18267 (accessed on 23rd June 2025).
28. Thiruvengadam, M., Rajakumar, G., & Chung, I. M. (2018). Nanotechnology: Current uses and future applications in the food industry. *Biotech, 8*(1), 1–13. https://doi.org/10.1007/s13205-018-1104-7 (accessed on 23rd June 2025).
29. Sechi, M., Sanna, V., & Pala, N. (2014). Targeted therapy using nanotechnology: Focus on cancer. *International Journal of Nanomedicine*, 467–483. https://doi.org/10.2147/IJN.S36654 (accessed on 23rd June 2025).
30. Zielińska, A., Carreiró, F., Oliveira, A. M., Neves, A., Pires, B., Venkatesh, D. N., Durazzo, A., Lucarini, M., Eder, P., Silva, A. M., Santini, A., & Souto, E. B. (2020). Polymeric nanoparticles: Production, characterization, toxicology and ecotoxicology. *Molecules, 25*(16), 3731. https://doi.org/10.3390/molecules25163731 (accessed on 23rd June 2025).
31. Tomao, S. (2009). Albumin-bound formulation of paclitaxel (Abraxane® ABI-007) in the treatment of breast cancer. *International Journal of Nanomedicine, 99*, 99–105. https://doi.org/10.2147/ijn.s3061 (accessed on 23rd June 2025).
32. Bao, Y., Wen, T., Samia, A. C. S., Khandhar, A., & Krishnan, K. M. (2015). Magnetic nanoparticles: Material engineering and emerging applications in lithography and biomedicine. *Journal of Materials Science, 51*(1), 513–553. https://doi.org/10.1007/s10853-015-9324-2 (accessed on 23rd June 2025).

33. Sowa, P., Rutkowska-Talipska, J., Rutkowski, K., Kosztyła-Hojna, B., & Rutkowski, R. (2013). Optical radiation in modern medicine. *Advances in Dermatology and Allergology, 4*, 246–251. https://doi.org/10.5114/pdia.2013.37035 (accessed on 23rd June 2025).
34. Hirsch, L. R., Stafford, R. J., Bankson, J. A., Sershen, S. R., Rivera, B., Price, R. E., Hazle, J. D., Halas, N. J., & West, J. L. (2003). Nano shell-mediated near-infrared thermal therapy of tumors under magnetic resonance guidance. *Proceedings of the National Academy of Sciences, 100*(23), 13549–13554. https://doi.org/10.1073/pnas.2232479100 (accessed on 23rd June 2025).
35. Bozzuto, G., & Molinari, A. (2015). Liposomes as nanomedical devices. *International Journal of Nanomedicine*, 975–999. https://doi.org/10.2147/IJN.S68861 (accessed on 23rd June 2025).
36. Akbarzadeh, A., Rezaei-Sadabady, R., Davaran, S., Joo, S. W., Zarghami, N., Hanifehpour, Y., Samiei, M., Kouhi, M., & Nejati-Koshki, K. (2013). Liposome: Classification, preparation, and applications. *Nanoscale Research Letters, 8*(1), 1–9. https://doi.org/10.1186/1556-276X-8-102 (accessed on 23rd June 2025).
37. Bulbake, U., Doppalapudi, S., Kommineni, N., & Khan, W. (2017). Liposomal formulations in clinical use: An updated review. *Pharmaceutics, 9*(4), 12. https://doi.org/10.3390/pharmaceutics9020012 (accessed on 23rd June 2025).
38. Petre, C. E., Sin, S. H., & Dittmer, D. P. (2007). Functional p53 signaling in Kaposi's sarcoma-associated herpesvirus lymphomas: Implications for therapy. *Journal of Virology, 81*(4), 1912–1922. https://doi.org/10.2147/IJN.S2.3.277 (accessed on 23rd June 2025).
39. Luk, B. T., Fang, R. H., & Zhang, L. (2012). Lipid- and polymer-based nanostructures for cancer. *Theragnostic, 2*(12), 1117–1126. https://doi.org/10.7150/thno.4381 (accessed on 23rd June 2025).
40. Mohammed, A. M., Rahim, R. A., Ibraheem, I. J., Loong, F. K., Hisham, H., Hashim, U., & Al-Douri, Y. (2014). Application of gold nanoparticles for electrochemical DNA biosensor. *Journal of Nanomaterials*, 1–7. https://doi.org/10.1155/2014/683460 (accessed on 23rd June 2025).
41. Douloudi, M., Nikoli, E., Katsika, T., Vardavoulias, M., & Arkas, M. (2020). Dendritic polymers as promising additives for the manufacturing of hybrid organ ceramic nanocomposites with ameliorated properties suitable for an extensive diversity of applications. *Nanomaterials, 11*(1), 19. https://doi.org/10.3390/nano11010019 (accessed on 23rd June 2025).
42. Kraatz, H. (2005). [Review of the book *Bioconjugation Protocols: Strategies and Methods*, by C. M. Niemeyer (Ed.)]. *Angewandte Chemise, 117*(6), 869–869. https://doi.org/10.1007/978-1-61779-151-2_32 (accessed on 23rd June 2025).
43. Zhao, C. Y., Cheng, R., Yang, Z., & Tian, Z. M. (2018). Nanotechnology for cancer therapy based on chemotherapy. *Molecules, 23*(4), 826. https://doi.org/10.3390/molecules23040826 (accessed on 23rd June 2025).
44. Barroso, M. M. (2011). Quantum dots in cell biology. *Journal of Histochemistry & Cytochemistry, 59*(3), 237–251. https://doi.org/10.1369/0022155411398487 (accessed on 23rd June 2025).

45. Sapsford, K., Pons, T., Medintz, I., & Mattoussi, H. (2006). Biosensing with luminescent semiconductor quantum dots. *Sensors, 6*(8), 925–953. https://doi.org/10.3390/s6080925 (accessed on 23rd June 2025).
46. Jamieson, T., Bakhshi, R., Petrova, D., Pocock, R., Imani, M., & Seifalian, A. M. (2007). Biological applications of quantum dots. *Biomaterials, 28*(31), 4717–4732. https://doi.org/10.1016/j.biomaterials.2007.07.014 (accessed on 23rd June 2025).
47. Yezhelyev, M. V., Qi, L., O'Regan, R. M., Nie, S., & Gao, X. (2008). Proton-sponge coated quantum dots for siRNA delivery and intracellular imaging. *Journal of the American Chemical Society, 130*(28), 9006–9012. https://doi.org/10.1021/ja800086u (accessed on 23rd June 2025).
48. Patra, J. K., Das, G., Fraceto, L. F., Campos, E. V. R., Rodriguez-Torres, M. del P., Acosta-Torres, L. S., Diaz-Torres, L. A., Grillo, R., Swamy, M. K., Sharma, S., Habtemariam, S., & Shin, H. S. (2018). Nano based drug delivery systems: Recent developments and future prospects. *Journal of Nanobiotechnology, 16*(1), 1–33. https://doi.org/10.1186/s12951-018-0392-8 (accessed on 23rd June 2025).
49. Wang, L. W., Peng, C. W., Chen, C., & Li, Y. (2015). Quantum dots-based tissue and *in vivo* imaging in breast cancer researches: Current status and future perspectives. *Breast Cancer Research and Treatment, 151*(1), 7–17. https://doi.org/10.7497/j.issn.2095-3941.2012.03.001 (accessed on 23rd June 2025).
50. Murar, M., Albertazzi, L., & Pujals, S. (2022). Advanced optical imaging-guided nanotheranostics towards personalized cancer drug delivery. *Nanomaterials, 12*(3), 399. https://doi.org/10.3390/nano12030399 (accessed on 23rd June 2025).
51. Kelkar, S. S., & Reineke, T. M. (2011). Theragnostic: Combining imaging and therapy. *Bioconjugate Chemistry, 22*(10), 1879–1903. https://doi.org/10.1021/bc200151q (accessed on 23rd June 2025).
52. Theek, B., Rizzo, L. Y., Ehling, J., Kiessling, F., & Lammers, T. (2014). The theragnostic path to personalized nanomedicine. *Clinical and Translational Imaging, 2*(1), 67–76. https://doi.org/10.1007/s40336-014-0051-5 (accessed on 23rd June 2025).
53. Modi, S., Prajapati, R., Inwati, G. K., Deepa, N., Tirth, V., Yadav, V. K., Yadav, K. K., Islam, S., Gupta, P., Kim, D. H., & Jeon, B. H. (2021). Recent trends in fascinating applications of nanotechnology in allied health sciences. *Crystals, 12*(1), 39. https://doi.org/10.3390/cryst12010039 (accessed on 23rd June 2025).
54. Avula, L. R., & Grodzinski, P. (2022). Nanotechnology-aided advancement in the combating of cancer metastasis. *Cancer and Metastasis Reviews, 41*(2), 383–404. https://doi.org/10.1007/s10555-022-10025-7 (accessed on 23rd June 2025).
55. Nasra, S., Bhatia, D., & Kumar, A. (2022). Recent advances in nanoparticle-based drug delivery systems for rheumatoid arthritis treatment. *Nanoscale Advances, 4*(17), 3479–3494. https://doi.org/10.1039/d2na00229a (accessed on 23rd June 2025).
56. Erkoc, P., & Ulucan-Karnak, F. (2021). Nanotechnology-based antimicrobial and antiviral surface coating strategies. *Prosthesis, 3*(1), 25–52. https://doi.org/10.3390/prosthesis3010005 (accessed on 23rd June 2025).
57. Hulla, J., Sahu, S., & Hayes, A. (2015). Nanotechnology. *Human & Experimental Toxicology, 34*(12), 1318–1321. https://doi.org/10.1177/0960327115603588 (accessed on 23rd June 2025).

58. Wong, I. Y., Bhatia, S. N., & Toner, M. (2013). Nanotechnology: Emerging tools for biology and medicine. *Genes & Development, 27*(22), 2397–2408. http://www.genesdev.org/cgi//10.1101/gad.226837.113 (accessed on 23rd June 2025).
59. Misra, R., Acharya, S., & Sahoo, S. K. (2010). Cancer nanotechnology: Application of nanotechnology in cancer therapy. *Drug Discovery Today, 15*(19, 20), 842–850. https://doi.org/10.1016/j.drudis.2010.08.006 (accessed on 23rd June 2025).
60. Mourya, H., Garud, N., Joshi, R., Akram, W., & Singh, N. (2023). Formulation and optimization of propranolol bilayer tablets: A potential approach for effective management of hypertension. *Indian Journal of Pharmaceutical Sciences, 85*(1). https://doi.org/10.36468/pharmaceutical-sciences.1081 (accessed on 23rd June 2025).
61. Balaji, V. (2010). Applications of nanotechnology in veterinary medicine. *Veterinary World*, 477–480. https://doi.org/10.5455/vetworld.2010.477-480 (accessed on 23rd June 2025).
62. Pramanik, P. K. D., Solanki, A., Debnath, A., Nayyar, A., El-Sappagh, S., & Kwak, K. S. (2020). Advancing modern healthcare with nanotechnology, nano biosensors, and Internet of Nano Things: Taxonomies, applications, architecture, and challenges. *IEEE Access, 8*, 65230–65266. https://doi.org/10.1109/ACCESS.2020.2984269 (accessed on 23rd June 2025).
63. Gana, A. I., Vlad, I. C., & Achimaş-Cadariu, P. A. (2022). Quality of life in patients with colorectal cancer: A review. *Health, Sports & Rehabilitation Medicine, 23*(2), 94–100. https://jclmm.com/index.php/journal/article/view/295 (accessed on 23rd June 2025).
64. Vaishampayan, V., Kapoor, A., & Gumfekar, S. P. (2023). Enhancement in the limit of detection of lab-on-chip microfluidic devices using functional nanomaterials. *The Canadian Journal of Chemical Engineering, 101*(9), 5208–5221. https://doi.org/10.1002/cjce.24915 (accessed on 23rd June 2025).
65. Dessale, M., Mengistu, G., & Mengist, H. M. (2022). Nanotechnology: A promising approach for cancer diagnosis, therapeutics and theragnosis. *International Journal of Nanomedicine, 17*, 3735–3749. https://doi.org/10.2147/IJN.S378074 (accessed on 23rd June 2025).
66. Mbunge, E., Muchemwa, B., Jiyane, S., & Batani, J. (2021). Sensors and healthcare 5.0: Transformative shift in virtual care through emerging digital health technologies. *Global Health Journal, 5*(4), 169–177. https://doi.org/10.1016/j.glohj.2021.11.008 (accessed on 23rd June 2025).
67. Yang, Y. (2013). Translational medicine: From translational research to targeted therapy and personalized medicine. *Academic Journal of Second Military Medical University, 32*(12), 1277–1283. https://doi.org/10.1016/B978-0-12-813477-1.00008-6 (accessed on 23rd June 2025).
68. Singh, A., & Amiji, M. M. (2022). Application of nanotechnology in medical diagnosis and imaging. *Current Opinion in Biotechnology, 74*, 241–246. https://doi.org/10.1016/j.copbio.2021.12.011 (accessed on 23rd June 2025).
69. Amiri, M. R., Alavi, M., Taran, M., & Kahrizi, D. (2022). Antibacterial, antifungal, antiviral, and photocatalytic activities of TiO_2 nanoparticles, nanocomposites, and bio-nanocomposites: Recent advances and challenges. *Journal of Public Health*

Research, 11(2). https://doi.org/10.1177/22799036221104151 (accessed on 23rd June 2025).

70. Mourya, H., Chauhan, R., Joshi, R., Akram, W., & Garud, N. (2023). Bilayer tablets: A promising novel drug delivery system. *Research Journal of Pharmacy and Technology*, 2517–2521. https://doi.org/10.52711/0974-360X.2023.00414 (accessed on 23rd June 2025).

CHAPTER 2

Current Advancements and Upcoming Possibilities of Nanotechnology in Nucleic Acid Delivery

ABHINAV SINGHAL,[1] ANJALI SHARMA,[1,*] VISHNU MITTAL,[1] GEETA DESWAL,[1] DEVKANT SHARMA,[2] and ROHIT GROVER[1]

[1]*Guru Gobind Singh College of Pharmacy, Yamunanagar, Haryana, India*

[2]*Ch. Devi Lal College of Pharmacy, Jagadhari, Haryana, India*

*Corresponding author

ABSTRACT

Nanotechnology has emerged as a transformative tool in the field of drug delivery, offering unprecedented control over the delivery of therapeutic agents for various clinical applications. The study focuses on various challenges associated with nucleic acid delivery, including enzymatic degradation and off-target effects, and discusses how nanotechnology-based approaches address these challenges through precise control over delivery systems. The recent advancements in nanocarrier design, with a focus on metal-based nanoparticles (MNPs) and their unique properties for nucleic acid delivery, are also discussed. Moreover, the chapter examines innovative strategies, such as DNA origami and RNA aptamers, which hold promise in enhancing the specificity and efficiency of nucleic acid delivery. Furthermore, the potential of nanotechnology in enabling targeted delivery to specific tissues or cells is explored, highlighting the role of surface modification and functionalization techniques in achieving site-specific delivery. The chapter also discusses the translational potential

Nanotechnology for Nucleic Acid Delivery: Pankaj Sharma, Saloni Jain, and Vinay Jain (Eds.)

DOI: 10.1201/9781998511853-2

of these advancements, emphasizing the importance of bridging the gap between preclinical research and clinical application.

2.1 INTRODUCTION

Nanotechnology has garnered significant attention in recent years, particularly regarding its potential medical applications. By utilizing nanoscale manipulation, it is possible to release drugs or imaging agents under controlled conditions, thereby enabling a targeted and precise distribution. The development of nanocarrier-assisted medication delivery systems has immense translational value and has attracted considerable interest from researchers in various fields. Furthermore, nanocarriers can improve the bioavailability of poorly soluble drugs and protect against the degradation of readily degradable medications [1]. The tunable surfaces of nanocarriers also increase their utility in various biological contexts, particularly in targeted therapy. Moreover, altering the surface properties of nanocarriers allows them to react to various stimuli, thereby augmenting the efficacy of treatment [2]. In this section, we explore recent progress in the design and application of a range of nanocarriers, emphasizing their distinct compositions and methods of functionalization. Following an introduction to the different classes of nanocarriers, we aim to present a comprehensive examination, recognizing the expansive and evolving landscape of nanocarrier-mediated drug delivery systems [3, 4].

2.2 TYPES OF NUCLEIC ACIDS

Nucleic acids, which are the primary molecules responsible for transmitting information and regulating protein synthesis, comprise sugars, phosphoric acids, and a mixture of organic bases, including purines and pyrimidines [5]. DNA, acting as the genetic material and fundamental blueprint for life, is found in all organisms that are free-living, as well as in the majority of viruses. On the other hand, RNA is essential for several cellular processes, such as protein synthesis, and is found in all living cells, although it is the genetic material of some viruses [6].

2.2.1 DEOXYRIBONUCLEIC ACID (DNA)

DNA is a vital molecule in living cells that serves as a blueprint for life. The genome comprises the entire DNA content within an organism, which includes 23 pairs of chromosomes in the nucleus and a smaller mitochondrial genome in humans. Humans possess a diploid genome that is inherited from both parents and is necessary for proper growth and maintenance of life [7].

In 1869, Miescher, a Swiss biologist, made a groundbreaking discovery when he identified DNA. By employing pus from surgically treated bandages as a source of leukocytes, he aimed to investigate the chemical makeup of blood cells. Initially, Miescher was fascinated with every aspect of the cell, but ultimately narrowed his focus to the nucleus after observing that, in the presence of acid, a precipitate referred to as "nuclein" was produced [8]. A considerable number of molecular biology graduates have likely conducted experiments similar to this one, in which DNA is extracted from cells during laboratory classes [9]. Albrecht Kossel, Richard Altmann, and Miescher further characterized "nuclein," with Altmann subsequently changing the term to nucleic acid. Kossel demonstrated the presence of sugar, phosphate, purine, and pyrimidine bases in the nucleic acids. During the 1930s, numerous scientists attempted to elucidate the nature of nucleic acids [10].

DNA is a polymer composed of sugars, deoxyribose, nitrogenous bases, and phosphate groups, which are linked together to form nucleotides. During DNA synthesis, each nucleotide contains one phosphate group [11]. Griffith's research in 1928 demonstrated that extracts from heat-killed cells could transform living cells, and that this transformation could permanently alter the recipient cell's genetic makeup. Griffith's experiment used Streptococcus pneumoniae strains two and three, with the noncapsulated R strain being nonvirulent, whereas the encapsulated S strain is virulent. MacLeod and McCarty's research in 1944 further demonstrated that dead bacteria could be altered by DNA. Bacteriophages have a protein capsid that surrounds DNA molecules. Hershey and Chase demonstrated when bacteriophage T2 infects *Escherichia coli*, bacterial cells take in phage DNA instead of proteins [12,13].

2.2.2 RIBONUCLEIC ACID (RNA)

The backbone of RNA, a single-stranded nucleic acid polymer, comprises alternating phosphate and ribose sugar residues that connect four nucleotides: A, C, G, and U. This fundamental step in the translation of genetic information into proteins is critical for cellular activity [14]. In addition, some RNAs directly contribute to cellular metabolism. The types of RNA are shown in Figure 2.1. Nucleotides, which are composed of nitrogenous bases, phosphate, and the 5-carbon sugar ribose, are building blocks. François Jacob and Jacques Monod created the concept of mRNA, a genetic messenger during protein synthesis, based on characteristics of RNA that made it perfect for this purpose [15].

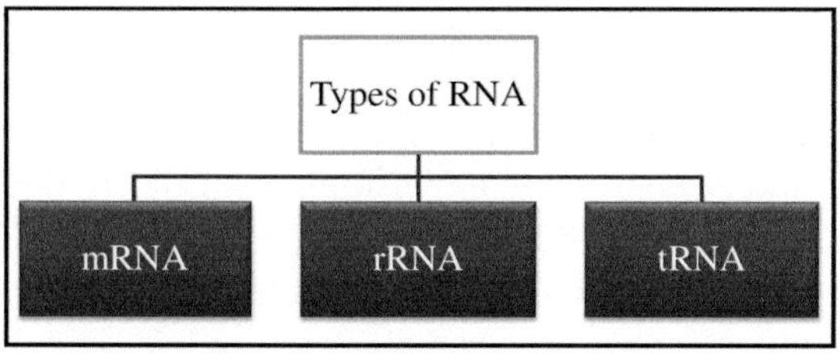

FIGURE 2.1 Types of ribonucleic acid (RNA).

2.2.2.1 MESSENGER RNA (mRNA)

mRNA serves as an intermediate between DNA and ribosomes, translating genetic information into proteins. In prokaryotes, mRNA is a direct replica of original DNA sequence, featuring a terminal 5′-triphosphate group and a 3′-hydroxyl residue [16]. In eukaryotes, mRNA molecules are notably more intricate, characterized by presence of a 5′-triphosphate residue that is esterified to create a cap structure, along with extended sequences of adenosine residues (polyA) that are enzymatically added subsequent to transcription. These modifications enhance the stability of eukaryotic mRNAs, while prokaryotic mRNAs are rapidly degraded [17].

2.2.2.2 RIBOSOMAL RNA (rRNA)

Ribosomal RNA (rRNA) molecules are integral constituents of ribosomes, playing a crucial role in the process of protein synthesis. rRNA molecules have extensive secondary structures that help them recognize mRNA and tRNA sequences. This recognition process is crucial for catalyzing protein synthesis [18]. In prokaryotes such as E. coli, approximately 15,000 ribosomes are produced per cell from seven rRNA gene copies. In eukaryotes, the number of ribosomes varies greatly, with some cells containing up to

10 million ribosomes. In eukaryotes, rRNA genes are located outside main chromosomal fibers and form a nucleolus when coalesced with proteins [19, 20].

2.2.2.3 TRANSFER RNA (tRNA)

tRNA plays a crucial role in the assembly of amino acids into proteins within the ribosome. tRNA molecules are approximately 70–80 nucleotides in length and have a characteristic cloverleaf structure. For each of the 20 amino acids necessary for protein synthesis, there exists a specialized tRNA molecule, often with multiple tRNAs carrying the same amino acid [21]. However, certain species require fewer synthetases than the total number of amino acids (20) due to the ability of glutamine and asparagine to be synthesized directly on their respective tRNAs. Because tRNAs attach to the same ribosome sites, their shapes are similar [22].

2.3 TYPES OF CARRIERS

In the realm of biomedicine, the use of drug delivery methods aided by nanocarriers has recently attracted considerable attention. Different nanocarrier designs are being created to fulfill unique needs, given the diversity of therapeutic needs. Based on their composition and structure, many types of nanocarriers used for drug administration can be divided into groups [23, 24].

2.3.1 LIPOSOMAL NANOCARRIERS

Phospholipid vesicles, called liposomes, are composed of lipid bilayers that are separated by distinct aqueous gaps. Liposomes possess several characteristics that make them attractive options for drug delivery. Self-assembled nanocarriers may have substantial therapeutic payloads and are readily customizable and biocompatible. Hydrophilic drugs and imaging agents can be enclosed within the aqueous cores and lipid membranes of liposomes, respectively [25]. In addition, they are typically considered to exhibit good safety characteristics. Typical liposomal nanocarriers consist of basic lipid bilayers that assemble and contain drugs within their aqueous centers. PEGylation, or the addition of PEG to the surface, is a modification that can further stabilize lipid bilayers [26]. Moreover, liposomes can be functionalized by applying ligands to their surfaces. Additionally, they can have both therapeutic and diagnostic (theranostic) qualities and can be surface-equipped with imaging agents in addition to targeting ligands to maximize targeting efficiency [27]. Liposomal carriers present a notable biological challenge. It is not possible to completely prevent the clearance of liposomes, even if PEGylation of their surface can greatly reduce the amount of RES uptake [28]. Liposomal targeting efficiency and therapeutic efficacy have been continuously improved, while liposome toxicity has been reduced. This strategy was made possible by the discovery that some cancer cells express higher levels of CD47 on their surfaces to evade phagocytosis [29, 30].

Liposomal carriers are extensively employed in drug delivery owing to their capacity to improve therapeutic efficacy. A significant advancement in the clinical application of nanocarriers occurred with the approval by the FDA of Doxil, a liposomal formulation containing the anticancer agent doxorubicin hydrochloride [31]. Liposomes have been the most frequently employed nanocarriers for FDA-approved drugs, demonstrating their effectiveness and safety. Most liposomal nanocarriers in the market today are intended to be administered intravenously. Liposomal nanocarriers are the most widely utilized nanocarriers in cancer therapy, but their limited capacity to achieve the requisite transport efficiency and their inevitable off-target accumulation still prevent their widespread use [32].

Liposomal nanocarriers have been investigated for their potential in nucleic acid and medication delivery. The fact that systemic treatment with liposomal nanocarriers containing nucleic acids mostly results in hepatic absorption presents a significant obstacle for targeted therapy employing these nanocarriers. This innovative method directed nanocarriers to the targeted tissues and significantly decreased hepatic uptake, using a similar method [33].

2.3.2 CARBON NANOTUBES

A carbon allotrope in a hollow, cylindrical form is called a carbon nanotube (CNT). SWNTs with a diameter of one nanometer and multi-walled nanotubes (MWNTs) with an outer diameter ranging from 5–20 nm and an inner diameter of 2–6 nm are the two categories into which they are divided [34]. Raw CNTs are unsuitable for biological applications due to their hydrophobic nature. Functionalization is necessary to render them biocompatible and soluble in water [35]. PEGylation is a functionalization technique that can significantly increase CNTs' ability to load drugs. Subsequent supramolecular π–π stacking allows aromatic molecular medications such as doxorubicin to attach to the surface of the CNTs. Depending on their functionalization type and reactivity to different stimuli, functionalized CNTs have the capability to serve as carriers for various therapies such as peptides, nucleic acids, and small molecules, delivering them to diverse organs [36]. In addition to their extensive use in cancer treatments, CNTs may also be used to treat other illnesses, according to ongoing research. Owing to their easy cell penetration, CNTs have the potential to cure neurological illnesses by bridging the BBB. The best transportation rate of functionalized anionic MWNTs across the human blood-brain barrier was discovered by Porter's group [37]. Regarding the safety profile of CNTs, research indicates that their endocytosis causes oxidative stress in cells, indicating a strong correlation between CNTs and cancer, fibrosis, and inflammation. This suggests that the translational usefulness of CNTs is hindered [38].

2.3.3 CARBON DOTS

Xu et al. reported the coincidental discovery of carbon dots (CDs) while purifying single-walled CNTs. Sun and colleagues subsequently synthesized carbon nanoparticles that exhibited light emission throughout visible and near-infrared spectra. At that point, fluorescent carbon nanoparticles were first identified using the phrase "carbon dots," which were created. Therefore, CDs are the newest members of the carbon family [39]. Drugs can be conjugated to CDs by electrostatic interactions via functional groups or noncovalent bonding using the carboxyl group on the CDs. Conjugated drugs are released passively into the cells by CDs after they are inside by endocytosis and passive diffusion [40]. For the treatment of neurological disorders, carbon dots, which have diameters less than 10 nm, present a promising way to overcome the problem of getting medication past the BBB. To heal glioblastoma brain tumors, LeBlanc's group of researchers created carbon dots conjugated with therapeutic agents and targeted ligands [41]. Additionally, they created carbon nitride dots that could be used in juvenile glioblastoma therapy. The BBB-piercing capability of carbon nitride dots was demonstrated using zebrafish models. Nevertheless, additional verification is required to evaluate safety profiles [42].

2.3.4 NANOGELS

Nanogels are minute particles composed of cross-linked polymers that absorb water, commonly utilized in drug delivery systems. They possess characteristics of being non-toxic, biocompatible, and capable of encapsulating multiple drugs. They can release drugs either by swelling or upon contact with other substances. However, there are still some problems with the use of nanogels in clinical settings [43]. For example, when they are damaged, they may not work. Scientists are working to improve their performance by controlling how they are made and how they break down. Recently, researchers led by Myerson developed a new type of nanogel that is cross-shaped and has antibodies that can target specific cells in the body. This could help improve drug delivery to the right side of the body [44].

2.3.5 HYBRID NANOCARRIERS

In addition, hybrid nanocarriers are being developed as technology progresses. For example, carbon-based hybrid nanogels provide real-time imaging through fluorescent carbon dots and serve as platforms for drug administration. Furthermore, liposome- and polymer-based hybrid nanogels have been developed to improve biocompatibility [45]. Scientists are experimenting with different arrangements of nanomaterials to attain the best possible drug delivery effectiveness. Among these pairings, polymers and liposomes are frequently used. Recently, Cao et al. [59] created a hybrid nanocarrier that inserts PLGA polymeric cores containing hydrophobic HIV medications into lipid bilayers. To target CD4+ T cells, the hybrid nanocarrier was coupled with several antibodies. This strategy decreased the toxicity of several HIV medications and increased their latencies [46].

2.3.6 DENDRIMERS

On the nanoscale, dendrimers are three-dimensional branched polymeric structures. Medications can be covalently attached to dendrimers or physically trapped through non-covalent interactions. By altering the dendrimer surface, drug entrapment and release can be managed [47]. Enhancing the targeting efficacy of dendrimers can also be accomplished. Due to their substantial surface-to-volume ratio and capacity to encapsulate molecules of high molecular weight, both hydrophilic and hydrophobic, dendrimers hold considerable promise for various biological applications [48]. They can also be used as carriers for gene therapy. Additionally, they improve the oral bioavailability, stability, and solubility of several drugs. Future cancer treatments are hopeful, owing to such technological advancements [49].

2.3.7 IRON OXIDE NANOPARTICLES

Iron oxide nanoparticles, which are biocompatible and exhibit supramagnetism, are widely used in medicine as contrast agents and drug carriers. Nevertheless, bare nanoparticles tend to group together, causing the reticuloendothelial system to absorb them [50]. Addressing this issue can be achieved through surface functionalization and coating nanoparticles with stabilizing agents like PEG, gelatin, or chitosan. Hepatic metastasis can be avoided using iron oxide nanoparticles as a preventative measure *in vivo* [51].

2.4 STRATEGIES TO ENHANCE DRUG DELIVERY EFFICIENCY

Most nanocarriers rely on their small size to passively accumulate and remain at disease sites without specialized targeting functionalization. Even if this drug delivery method is already better than others, there is still considerable work to be done to obtain the best possible therapeutic results, which include focused drug release at controlled rates. Passive diffusion out of nanocarriers collected in the diseased tissue is a frequent way for carried-on medications to reach the affected area in nanomedicine [52]. Incorporating ligands onto the surface of nanocarriers specific to receptors overexpressed in cancer cells is a common approach to enhance their targeting capability, particularly in cancer therapy [53]. Advancements of nanotechnology in nucleic acid delivery are shown in Table 2.1.

TABLE 2.1 Advancements of Nanotechnology in Nucleic Acid Delivery

Advancements	Description
Lipid Nanoparticles	Utilized for delivering nucleic acids, like mRNA and siRNA, into cells. They offer high encapsulation efficiency, stability, and low toxicity.
Polymeric Nanoparticles	Polymeric nanoparticles protect nucleic acids from degradation and enhance cellular uptake. They can be engineered for controlled release and response to specific stimuli [54].
Inorganic Nanoparticles	Inorganic nanoparticles, such as gold and silica nanoparticles, efficiently deliver nucleic acids. Surface modifications improve biocompatibility and target specificity.
Exosome-based Delivery	Natural nanovesicles, exosomes, are explored as carriers for nucleic acids. They offer targeted delivery, can evade the immune system, and possess inherent biocompatibility [55].
RNA Interference (RNAi)	Utilizes small RNA molecules to silence target genes. Nanoparticle delivery systems enhance stability and efficacy, promising for therapeutic applications in gene regulation.
CRISPR/Cas Delivery	Nanoparticles deliver CRISPR/Cas gene editing tools into target cells, enabling precise genetic modifications. Advancements aim at improving delivery efficiency and accuracy [56].
Targeted Delivery	Nanotechnology enables targeted delivery of nucleic acids to specific tissues or cells, reducing off-target effects and enhancing therapeutic outcomes for various diseases.
Stimuli-responsive Nanoparticles	Engineered to release nucleic acids in response to external stimuli like pH, temperature, or enzymes, improving efficacy and minimizing side effects in targeted delivery strategies [57].

2.4.1 THERMO-RESPONSIVE

The way these nanocarriers work is to hold onto their payload at a normal body temperature of 37 °C, but they quickly release it at the tumor location, which is usually between 40 and 42 °C. Polymeric nanocarriers with a lower and upper critical solution temperature provide better control over medication release as nanotechnology develops [58]. This method is very helpful in treating solid tumors because medications may be loaded at 37°C and subsequently released by either heating or cooling the tumor after injection, depending on LCST or UCST. *Thermoresponsive* polymers have been incorporated into liquid crystals to create a pulsatile drug release system that is synchronized with the body's circadian rhythm. This innovation builds upon the existing thermo-responsive technology and holds great promise for improving cancer therapy [59].

2.4.2 PH RESPONSIVE

As various biological compartments have varying pH values, pH-responsive nanocarriers are a viable method for regulating site-specific medication release. Because of the acidic nature of tumor areas and the pH changes between the intracellular and extracellular matrices, this approach is very helpful in targeted cancer therapy [60]. It is possible to prepare a broad variety of pH-responsive nanocarriers, including polymeric micelles under investigation for chemotherapeutic applications and pH-responsive liposomes being developed for hepatitis B virus vaccinations. Additionally, non-polymeric pH-sensitive carbon dots have been engineered to address certain drawbacks associated with pH-sensitive polymers, such as unregulated drug-loading or drug-release rates and potential toxicity concerns [61].

2.5 DELIVERY OF NUCLEIC ACIDS USING NANOMATERIALS

A unique treatment approach for both congenital and acquired disorders, nucleic acid therapy involves the introduction of exogenous nucleic acids into lesions to alter protein expression. Nucleic acid medications have several benefits over traditional small-molecule and antibody treatments, including a brief development cycle, wide range of target selection, and exceptional curative efficiency [62]. Moreover, nucleic acid medications can overcome a way around the restrictions imposed by undruggable targets. These developments offer possible alternatives to the treatment of diseases that were previously thought to be incurable. When delivered *in vivo*, naked nucleic acids encounter several difficulties. The selection of delivery vectors is crucial to ensure that nucleic acid medications perform to their full potential. These vectors should ideally show minimum toxicity, promote cellular uptake and endosomal escape, and shield nucleic acids from enzymatic destruction. To facilitate effective cellular absorption, viral vectors, including lentivirus, adenovirus, and adeno-associated viruses, have been created [63]. Viral vector-based nucleic acid therapies typically outperform conventional treatments in terms of their long-term effectiveness. These drugs require only one injection to achieve therapeutic efficacy for extended periods. However, viral vectors may elicit antiviral immune responses, which present a problem for repeated delivery [64]. Additionally, in a few cases of therapeutic use of viral vector nucleic acid medications, adverse reactions included irregular blood clots. Non-viral vectors are easier to produce on a large scale and have lower immunogenicity than viral vectors, without risk of insertional mutagenesis. Traditional non-viral vectors have poor tissue targeting and low transfection efficiencies. Nevertheless, new materials possessing enhanced properties have emerged. Lipid nanoparticles (LNPs), for example, have shown substantial promise in the delivery of nucleic acids as pharmaceuticals, as demonstrated by multiple preclinical and clinical investigations. The siRNA-LNP medication Onpattro® (patisiran) is one well-known example. The latest worldwide SARS-CoV-2 epidemic has led to extraordinary development of mRNA-based vaccinations against infectious illnesses [65].

Among these contenders, Moderna's mRNA-1273 (Spikevax®) and BioNTech/Pfizer's BNT162b2 (Comirnaty®) have shown excellent efficacy in preventing and managing SARS-CoV-2 infection. Owing to their excellent potency in clinical studies, mRNA vaccines have significant potential for both preventing and curing pandemics. China's first domestic COVID-19 mRNA vaccine for emergency use, SYS6006, was created by the CSPC Pharmaceuticals Group and was released in March 2023 [66]. According to a recent survey, approximately 20% of the 966 vaccine candidates under development were based on nucleic acids [67].

2.5.1 NANOMATERIALS FOR NUCLEIC ACID DELIVERY

Nucleic acid transfection frequently has to be encapsulated in safe material nanoparticles to ensure both safety and efficacy. Choosing appropriate materials is difficult because they need to properly convey genes to the desired place of action within the cell, be taken up by target cells, and have high biosafety and degradability qualities. For successful organ-targeted nucleic acid delivery, extracellular and intracellular obstacles must be overcome using nanomaterials. When it comes to delivery through the respiratory tract, it is difficult to overcome the obstacles caused by the highly branched respiratory tract, which is composed of different diameters and lengths. Owing to their small size, nanoparticles are rapidly expelled. To give particles inhaling properties, therefore, particular techniques, like combining nanoparticles with excipients, must be used. Drugs must pass through the vessel wall when injected intravenously for cells to endocytose them and release the nucleic acids that are encased in endosomes [68]. Therefore, nucleic acid delivery vehicles should have improved endosomal escape potentials. A thorough understanding of the chemical characteristics and uses of various nanomaterials is essential for the logical creation of more efficient and targeted nucleic acid delivery systems that target particular tissues and cells [69]. Nucleic acid delivery through nanoparticles is shown in Figure 2.2.

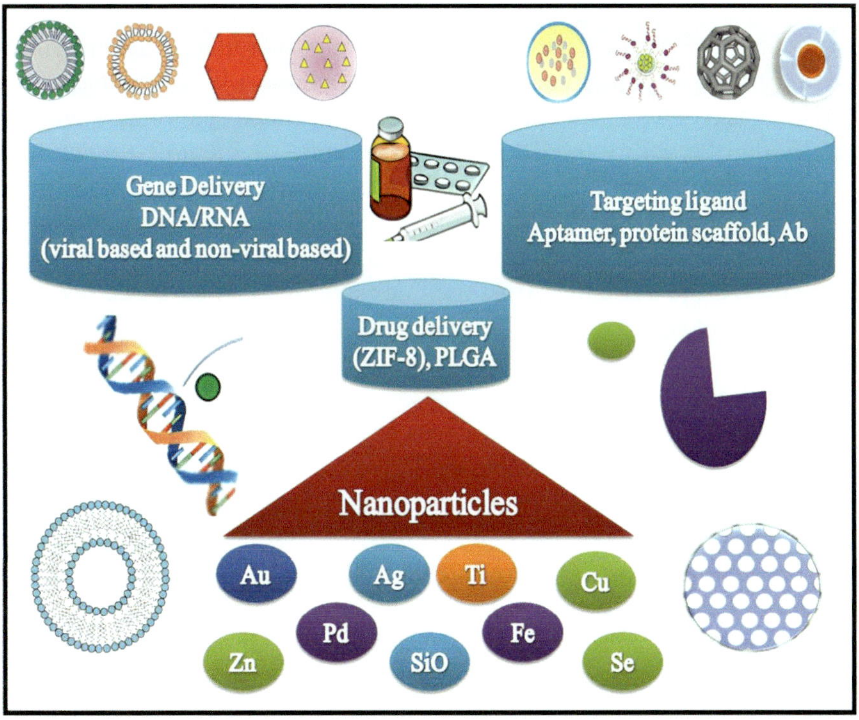

FIGURE 2.2 Nucleic acid delivery through nanoparticles.

2.5.2 POLYMER-BASED DELIVERY SYSTEM

2.5.2.1 POLYETHYLENEIMINE (PEI)

PEI can also be readily produced, which makes its physicochemical qualities easy to customize. This shows that transfection is a highly effective method for delivering nucleic acids *in vivo*. As a nucleic acid delivery medium, PEI's effective endosomal escape capacity is its primary benefit. The "proton sponge effect" is regarded as a fundamental idea. PEI is a multiproton capture device. Nevertheless, disruptive action is not restricted to endosomal membranes; cell membranes, mitochondria, and even necrosis can be caused by the uncontrollable proton sponge effect and high-density charge of the polymer [70]. Furthermore, PEI's cytotoxicity and challenging biodegradation have prevented its widespread use as a nucleic acid delivery medium. To overcome these constraints, efforts are being made to maintain PEI's distribution efficiency while enhancing its safety. Promising approaches include decreasing the molecular weight of PEI, conjugating with other polymers (such as PEG, chitosan, and hyaluronic acid) to produce nanoparticles, altering hydrophobicity, and minimizing branching structures (such as deacetylation). For instance, using PEGPEI as a delivery method for siRNA may reduce cytotoxicity without sacrificing the ability to silence the target gene. It should be mentioned that PEGylated alterations are usually insufficient to cause harm to lung tissue, but they can trigger inflammatory and immunological responses in the lungs. Another example revealed that, in comparison to naked 32P-siRNA, the 32P-siRNAPEI complex exhibited a negligible decrease in radiolucent signal detected following treatment [71].

There is a discernible change in the distribution of siRNA from the liver to the lungs as a consequence of fluorinated PEI. A further work by Fernando et al. showed that succinic acid-modified PEI was used to transfer pDNA into human hepatocellular carcinoma (HepG2) and retinal pigment epithelium (ARPE-19) cell lines. Researchers discovered that after intravenous injection of pDNA/PEI/DOPS ternary complex, the gene was substantially expressed in the spleen. In order to accomplish spleen targeting, Yang et al. developed a biocompatible biomimetic system based on black phosphorus nanosheets (BP) and nano-erythrocyte bodies (NER). PEI covalently altered BP, which then functioned as the center for effectively condensing mRNA via electrostatic interactions to create NER@BP mRNA [72].

2.5.2.2 CHITOSAN

The ability of chitosan to effectively encapsulate nucleic acids is facilitated by these characteristics, and because of its immunomodulatory qualities, it may be used as an adjuvant in nucleic acid vaccines. Chitosan's mucosal permeability and adhesion qualities facilitate the transport of nucleic acids to lungs through the respiratory system. Silva et al. demonstrated effective deposition of chitosan and siRNA powders in mouse lungs following the administration of carbon dioxide-assisted SASD. When delivered as a dry powder, chitosan was discovered by Okamoto et al. to result in a greater expression of pDNA than when administered intravenously or intratracheally. Chitosan was used as a carrier to transport the pDNA. In contrast to other polymeric materials, chitosan and nucleic acids have significant electrostatic interactions, which may make it difficult to achieve high transfection efficiency. Chitosan-derived nanocarriers with an improved N/P molar ratio, particle size, molecular weight, and degree of deacetylation must be created to achieve increased nucleic acid conveyance efficiency. Adding negatively charged substances to chitosan-nucleic acid complexes, including γ-polyglutamic acid (γ-PGA), is a potential solution to this problem [73]. Guanylated chitosan (GCS) increased the effectiveness of gene silencing by promoting the cellular absorption of siRNA. According to another study, SGCS-salbutamol chemical coupling enhanced the ability of siRNA nanoparticles to target lung cells with β2-adrenergic receptors. Capel and colleagues achieved enhanced siRNA-induced gene silencing in lung epithelial cells and efficient lung drug deposition through the substitution of piperazine with chitosan. Jin et al. explored the potential of utilizing chitosan modified with imidazole rings and allantoic acid as an aerosol delivery system, leading to a notable increase in gene transfection efficacy. In their gene delivery investigations, Klausner et al. employed NOVAFECT chitosan, a commercially available chitosan developed by Arthurson. The researchers found that NOVAFECT chitosan-DNA nanoparticles specifically expressed the luciferase gene in corneal fibroblasts, 5.4 times higher than when polyethyleneimine-DNA nanoparticles were administered. The researchers also engineered nanoparticles made of galactosylated chitosan, which encapsulated plasmids encoding interleukin (IL)-21 and macrophage colony-stimulating factor (GM-CSF). Similarly, Xiao and colleagues utilized galactosylated and quaternized chitosan to synthesize galactosylated chitosan-hydroxypropyl trimethylammonium (galHTCC).

In vitro gene transfection experiments demonstrated that, in contrast to chitosan and gal-chitosan, gal-HTCC exhibited significantly higher transfection efficiencies (7–32 times) when delivering a pGL3 luciferase plasmid targeting human hepatocellular carcinoma (HepG2) [74].

2.5.2.3 POLY-B-AMINO-ESTER (PBAE)

Because PEI is inherently cytotoxic, increasing attention is being paid to the development of polymers that have the benefits of PEI but are readily biodegradable. PBAE is a cationic polymer that has recently garnered interest owing to its potential for pulmonary nucleic acid delivery. PBAE is easily biodegradable and has a flexible chemical structure. Using the Michael addition process, it can be synthesized synthetically. The use of PBAE as a nucleic acid delivery vector has been attempted by Langer et al. They used PBAE to construct pDNA and discovered that the resultant complexes had minimal cytotoxicity and the desired nanosize. Subsequently, the physicochemical characteristics of the materials and the ability of pDNA-PBAE to overcome cellular barriers were investigated by Anderson et al. and Langer et al. They noted that improving the effectiveness of nucleic acid delivery requires the branching structure of the PBAE. In particular, because of their numerous end groups and three-dimensional (3D) spatial organization, branched polymers exhibit remarkable transfection efficiency. Specifically, they used hDD90-118 to transport mRNA expressing luciferase and observed that the nanoparticles were distributed evenly throughout both lung lobes [75]. They observed effective lung epithelial cell transfection in an Ai14 reporter mouse model. Santangelo et al. further examined the use of hDD90-118 in the nebulized transport of nucleic acids to the lungs. To transport mRNA expressing a membrane-anchored neutralizing antibody or a virus-specific CRISPR-Cas13a protein, hDD90-118 was used. In one study, mRNA expressing Cas13a was delivered to the respiratory tract of mice and hamsters via nebulization using hDD90-118. They discovered that P76 and at least five other polymers functioned better in influencing lung mRNA expression than hDD90-118 [76]. In hamster, ferret, cow, and non-human primate therapeutic models of viral infections, P76 demonstrated an enhanced pulmonary delivery efficiency of nucleic acids. Lung epithelial cells are the focus of most nebulized and other inhalation techniques. Alveolar capillary dysplasia and pulmonary hypertension are two acute and chronic lung disorders that can be greatly improved by targeting pulmonary vascular endothelial cells. By combining PBAE with lipids in the form of nanoparticles, Anderson et al. recently effectively delivered mRNA to lung endothelial cells on a targeted basis (detailed in the following section). The use of lysine/histidine oligopeptides to modify PBAE is another interesting strategy. Dosta et al. discovered that following intravenous injection of PBAE-siRNA nanocomplexes, large levels of gene silencing were seen in pulmonary vascular endothelium, significantly limiting featureless transport to tissues such as the liver. Through the use of the PBAE's special structural design, Kalinichenko's group was able to effectively accomplish endothelium targeting following intravenous injection, and it was discovered that after intravenous delivery, this modified PBAE could effectively transfer pDNA to lung microcapillaries [77]. They discovered that the newly created substance was minimally affected by freeze-drying and could be effectively collected in the spleen. They found that in comparison to polyethyleneimine (PEI), the chosen ternary polymer had a much higher transfection efficiency. The polymer had better biocompatibility and was mostly collected in the spleen. PBAE nanoparticles were injected into the hepatic arteries of rats in liver tumor models by Vaughan et al. They discovered that arterial injection of PBAEs, as opposed to intravenous delivery, enhanced targeted transfection of HCC tumors, suggesting that this approach might be used instead of transcatheter arterial chemotherapy (TACE) [78]. Green's team achieved targeted gene expression in mouse gliomas by intracranial administration of transgenes using PBAE. They observed that even after undergoing freeze-drying and storage for two years, the nanoparticles retained their efficacy. In a different study, Mastorakos et al. demonstrated how quickly DNA-delivering PEGylated PBAE nanoparticles entered both orthotopic brain tumor tissues and healthy brain parenchyma. The survival rates in the two aggressive orthotopic rat brain tumor models were significantly increased by nanoparticles [79].

2.5.3 LIPID-BASED DELIVERY SYSTEM

2.5.3.1 CATIONIC LIPIDS

Cationic lipids are characterized by a positively charged head group, which could be an amine, quaternary ammonium salt, or heterocyclic molecule, attached to a hydrophobic tail group through connecting chains, leading to a continuous positive charge. These lipids have been shown to enhance DNA loading capacity and effective gene expression, as demonstrated by DOTMA and DOPE, two cationic lipids synthesized by Felgner et al. in 1987. Cationic lipids have since become widely used as nucleic acid delivery vectors. Upon intravenous injection, electrostatic interactions between negatively charged erythrocytes and positively charged lipoplexes, composed of cationic lipids and siRNA, can occur [80]. These agglomerates facilitate lipoplex adsorption in the lung, where 60%–70% of the medication accumulates due to the greatly dilated pulmonary capillaries. In another study, 1,2-dioleoyl-3-trimethylammonium propane (DOTAP) was used to encapsulate complex formed between ichthyoglobulin and mRNA, resulting in strong cellular immune responses and a delayed tumor development. Researchers found that nanoparticles modified with LHRH peptide mostly targeted lung tumors. Aminoglycoside modified with cationic lipid (CLA) was used to transport mRNA to liver, with promising results. Researchers also synthesized a therapeutically viable LNP using T-junction and cationic amino-lipid KL52 [81].

In a study involving advanced hepatocellular carcinoma, investigators observed effective accumulation of LNP-delivered c-Jun N-terminal kinase-2 (Jnk2) siRNA in the liver, resulting in reduced carcinogenesis [82]. Another study illustrated that administering Rip2 siRNA intratracheally with Lipofectamine 2000 inhibited the accumulation and transcriptional activation of nuclear p65 in lung tissues, while also alleviating oxidative damage and inflammation caused by cigarette smoke (CS). Researchers first reported by Mo et al. that delivering siRNA by Lipofectamine 2000 increased autophagosome levels in hepatocellular carcinoma cell. The less hazardous monovalent cationic lipids, like DOTAP, have been found to be more preferable than multivalent lipids such as Lipofectamine®. GL67, recognized as the benchmark for non-viral respiratory gene delivery vectors, is a well-known cationic lipid initially characterized by a spermine head group and cholesterol arranged in a T-shaped structure. In a separate study, GL67A, which is a blend of GL67, DOPE, and DMPE-PEG5000, was employed to successfully deliver aerosolized plasmid DNA encoding the human cystic fibrosis transmembrane conductance regulator (CFTR) into the lungs of sheep [83]. A newer formulation called DACC consists of cholesterol, mPEG2000-DSPE, β-L-arginyl-2,3-L-diaminopropionic acid N-palmitoyl-N-oleyl-amide trihydrochloride (AtuFECT01), and other components. DACC has demonstrated a 50% reduction in VE-calmodulin mRNA expression in the lungs. Furthermore, a solitary administration of DACC lipid complexes has demonstrated the ability to suppress gene expression in pulmonary endothelial cells [84].

2.5.3.2 IONIZABLE LIPIDS

Ionizable lipids, characterized by their pH sensitivity, have been shown to enhance nucleic acid delivery *in vivo*. They are biocompatible under normal conditions as they remain electrically neutral, interacting less with negatively charged cell membranes. Within endosomes, which have a lower pH compared to the extracellular environment, ionizable lipids undergo ionization, resulting in a positive charge that aids in nanoparticle escape from endosomes. Generally, ionizable lipids exhibit superior endosomal escape efficiency and lower toxicity compared to cationic lipids. Noteworthy developments in the field of ionizable lipid molecules include the nucleic acid drug Onpattro®, which is based on DLinMC3-DMA. Furthermore, two mRNA vaccines based on ionizable lipids (mRNA-1273 and BNT162b2) were authorized for emergency use, showcasing their regulatory advantage [86]. AA-T3A-C12/siHSP47 LNP has been shown to effectively reduce collagen deposition and improve liver fibrosis without significantly increasing toxicity, according to a study. The liver is known to be the primary site of LNP accumulation after intravenous administration, making it challenging to create ionizable lipids for extrahepatic delivery. Nonetheless, scientists have achieved notable advancements in crafting new ionizable lipids tailored for the targeted delivery of mRNA to the spleen. These lipids carry a positive charge under physiological conditions but swiftly transition to a negative charge in the presence of esterases, facilitating effective mRNA release from the cytoplasm while preserving mRNA stability during storage and *in vivo* administration. Many acute and chronic lung diseases may benefit from therapy that targets pulmonary endothelial cells. Harashima's group altered a GALA peptide on the surface of MEND to achieve selective distribution to pulmonary endothelial cells. Subsequently, they engineered a GALA-MEND system that effectively transported siRNA to pulmonary endothelial cells, halting lung cancer metastases in mice. This was accomplished by employing a pH-sensitive lipid (YSK05) and a cell-penetrating R8 peptide to construct a dual-layer MEND delivery platform. This method delivered the splenic B cells and macrophages with pDNA selectively [86].

Xu and colleagues introduced an ionizable lipid named 113-O12B, designed to target lymph nodes and demonstrate robust gene expression within these organs. Directing mRNA to lymph nodes resulted in increased CD8+ T-cell responses to an antigen model encoding ovalbumin (OVA). Furthermore, the same team of researchers introduced a new ionizable lipid incorporating an amide bond in its tail, enabling the construction of a distinct lipid nanoparticle (LNP) that selectively transported mRNA to the lungs. Through a Michael addition technique, they identified the optimal lung-targeting lipid, 306-N16B, from a lipid library containing amide bonds. Notably, altering the head structure of the LNP allows for the targeting of specific lung cell types. Through proteomic analysis, the researchers identified the fibronectin beta chain as the predominant protein in the corona of 306-N16B. Subsequently, they encapsulated mRNA encoding mouse tuberous sclerosis complex 2 (*Tsc2*) using 306-N16B and successfully restored its expression in lung lymphangioleiomyomatosis (LAM) following intravenous administration of the resulting nanocomplex. In a separate investigation, Daniel [87]. Anderson and co-workers produced OF-Deg-Lin lipids, showing promise in regulating B cell function, achieving 85% protein expression in the spleen, and efficiently targeting B cells *in vivo* (approximately 7%). Subsequently, they synthesized 720 biodegradable lipids and identified the most effective ionizable lipid, RCB-4–8, utilizing a three-component reaction technique. RCB-4–8 demonstrated greater biodegradability compared to lipids containing ester groups, attributed to its carbonate groups. Observations revealed that RCB-4–8 LNPs were capable of transporting mRNA to club cells and ciliated cells, two important types of airway epithelial cells, following intratracheal injection [88]. To enhance intratracheal luciferase expression, cationic lipid DOTAP was incorporated into RCB-4–8 LNPs. LNPs containing DLin–MC3–DMA exhibited lower pulmonary transfection efficiency than those containing DOTAP. The research team also aimed to co-deliver SpCas9 and AAV with RCB-4–8 via intratracheal injection, with immunostaining of lung tissue sections revealing that $17.0 \pm 5.0\%$ of pulmonary cells activated the *tdTomato* fluorescent reporter gene [89].

2.5.4 OTHER LIPIDS

Researchers have investigated solid lipid nanoparticles (SLNs) for transporting nucleic acids to the lungs. Jacobson et al. found that a hydrophobic ion-pair technique effectively encapsulated small interfering RNA (siRNA)-DOTAP complexes within hydrophobic cores of SLNs [90]. Tey discovered that using 10%–40% of negatively charged 1,2-dioleoyl-sn-glycero3-phosphate (18PA) enhanced the production of proteins in the spleen when combined with SORT LNPs. Nevertheless, no expression of luciferase was detected in any other organ. Up to 50% more DOTAP was added to increase lung delivery, while 20% more DODAP allowed for liver targeting [91]. The vaccine shows strong DNAI1 protein expression, fast clearance of LNP in ciliated, rod, and basal cells, good tolerability, and the ability to be administered multiple times. The researchers also developed innovative phospholipids with endosomal escape features to create iPLNPs, a unique LNP delivery method. They found that supplementing high-performing iPhos 9A1P9 with DDAB effectively mediated CRISPR-Cas9 gene editing and improved mRNA delivery in lungs [92].

2.6 POLYMER–LIPID HYBRID DELIVERY SYSTEM

By capitalizing on the advantageous attributes of both polymer and lipid nanoparticles, polymer-lipid hybrid nanoparticles hold promise in augmenting the safety and sustained efficacy of a singular nanomaterial for delivering nucleic acids. Tanki et al. developed a lipid-polymer hybrid nanoparticle for administering siRNA, amalgamating DOTAP with poly(DL-lactic-co-glycolic acid) (PLGA). This hybrid nanoparticle significantly improved gene-silencing effect and efficiently boosted the siRNA payload when compared to DOTAP alone. Meyer and colleagues formulated PLGA nanoparticles containing MC3 or DOTAP, which were injected intravenously and primarily accumulated in the liver [93]. Santangelo's group used DOTAP and 7C1 to create NLD1, a hybrid nanoparticle that effectively prevented H1N1 influenza virus infection in mice. Anderson's team demonstrated substantial mRNA deposition in the lungs of mice administered with PBAE. Additionally, they discovered that PBAE's selectivity for the lungs was further enhanced, and the nanoparticle size was decreased by the addition of *PEGlipid*. The resultant nanoparticles effectively transported *Cre mRNA* to immunological and pulmonary endothelial cells [94].

2.7 CONCLUSION

This chapter discusses the challenges of delivering nucleic acids, such as enzymatic breakdown and off-target effects, and how nanotechnology-based methods can overcome these challenges by precisely controlling delivery mechanisms. The authors examine current advancements in the design of nanocarriers, particularly MNPs and their unique capabilities for the transport of nucleic acids. They also explore cutting-edge techniques like RNA aptamers and DNA origami, which have the potential to improve the efficiency and specificity of nucleic acid delivery. The authors also explore the feasibility of employing nanotechnology for precise administration to particular tissues or cells, underscoring the significance of functionalization and surface modification techniques in attaining targeted delivery to desired sites. The authors stress the importance of bridging the gap between preclinical research and clinical application to ensure the translational potential of these developments.

ACKNOWLEDGMENT

None

CONFLICT OF INTEREST

The authors declare no conflict of interest.

FUNDING

None

KEYWORDS

- **enzymatic degradation**
- **metal-based nanoparticles**
- **nanocarriers**
- **nanogels**
- **nanotechnology**
- **nanotubes**
- **nucleic acid delivery**
- **site-specific delivery**

REFERENCES

1. Zhang, L., Gu, F. X., Chan, J. M., Wang, A. Z., Langer, R. S., & Farokhzad, O. C. (2008). Nanoparticles in medicine: Therapeutic applications and developments. *Clinical Pharmacology & Therapeutics, 83*(5), 761–769. https://doi.org/10.1038/sj.clpt.6100400 (accessed on 23rd June 2025).
2. Shi, J., Votruba, A. R., Farokhzad, O. C., & Langer, R. (2010). Nanotechnology in drug delivery and tissue engineering: From discovery to applications. *Nano Letters, 10*(9), 3223–3230. https://doi.org/10.1021/nl102184c (accessed on 23rd June 2025).
3. Hoshyar, N., Gray, S., Han, H., & Bao, G. (2016). The effect of nanoparticle size on *in vivo* pharmacokinetics and cellular interaction. *Nanomedicine (London), 11*(6), 673–692. https://doi.org/10.2217/nnm.16.5 (accessed on 23rd June 2025).
4. Chenthamara, D., Subramaniam, S., Ramakrishnan, S. G., Krishnaswamy, S., Essa, M. M., Lin, F. H., & Qoronfleh, M. W. (2019). Therapeutic efficacy of nanoparticles and routes of administration. *Biomaterials Research, 23*, 20. https://doi.org/10.1186/s40824-019-0166-x (accessed on 23rd June 2025).
5. Gunasekaran, T., Haile, T., Nigusse, T., & Dhanaraju, M. D. (2014). Nanotechnology: An effective tool for enhancing bioavailability and bioactivity of phytomedicine. *Asian Pacific Journal of Tropical Biomedicine, 4*(Suppl 1), S1–S7. https://doi.org/10.12980/APJTB.4.2014C980 (accessed on 23rd June 2025).
6. Anselmo, A., Gokarn, Y., & Mitragotri, S. (2019). Non-invasive delivery strategies for biologics. *Nature Reviews Drug Discovery, 18*, 19–40. https://doi.org/10.1038/nrd.2018.183 (accessed on 23rd June 2025).
7. Shen, Z., Nieh, M. P., & Li, Y. (2016). Decorating nanoparticle surface for targeted drug delivery: Opportunities and challenges. *Polymers, 8*, 83. https://doi.org/10.3390/polym8030083 (accessed on 23rd June 2025).
8. Moher, D., Liberati, A., Tetzlaff, J., Altman, D. G., & PRISMA Group. (2009). Preferred reporting items for systematic reviews and meta-analyses: The PRISMA statement. *PLoS Medicine, 6*(7), e1000097. https://doi.org/10.1371/journal.pmed.1000097 (accessed on 23rd June 2025).
9. Li, F., Qin, Y., Lee, J., Liao, H., Wang, N., Davis, T. P., Qiao, R., & Ling, D. (2020). Stimuli-responsive nano-assemblies for remotely controlled drug delivery. *Journal of Controlled Release, 322*, 566–592. https://doi.org/10.1016/j.jconrel.2020.03.051 (accessed on 23rd June 2025).
10. Sercombe, L., Veerati, T., Moheimani, F., Wu, S. Y., Sood, A. K., & Hua, S. (2015). Advances and challenges of liposome assisted drug delivery. *Frontiers in Pharmacology, 6*, 286. https://doi.org/10.3389/fphar.2015.00286 (accessed on 23rd June 2025).
11. Al-Jamal, W. T., & Kostarelos, K. (2011). Liposomes: From a clinically established drug delivery system to a nanoparticle platform for theragnostic nanomedicine. *Accounts of Chemical Research, 44*(10), 1094–1104. https://doi.org/10.1021/ar200105p (accessed on 23rd June 2025).
12. Allen, T. M., & Cullis, P. R. (2013). Liposomal drug delivery systems: From concept to clinical applications. *Advanced Drug Delivery Reviews, 65*(1), 36–48. https://doi.org/10.1016/j.addr.2012.09.037 (accessed on 23rd June 2025).

13. Suk, J. S., Xu, Q., Kim, N., Hanes, J., & Ensign, L. M. (2016). Pegylation as a strategy for improving nanoparticle-based drug and gene delivery. *Advanced Drug Delivery Reviews, 99*(A), 28–51. https://doi.org/10.1016/j.addr.2015.09.012 (accessed on 23rd June 2025).
14. Tang, Y., Wang, X., Li, J., Nie, Y., Liao, G., Yu, Y., & Li, C. (2019). Overcoming the reticuloendothelial system barrier to drug delivery with a "don't-eat-us" strategy. *ACS Nano, 13*(11), 13015–13026. https://doi.org/10.1021/acsnano.9b05679 (accessed on 23rd June 2025).
15. Majeti, R., Chao, M. P., Alizadeh, A. A., Pang, W. W., Jaiswal, S., Gibbs, K. D., van Rooijen, N., & Weissman, I. L. (2009). CD47 is an adverse prognostic factor and therapeutic antibody target on human acute myeloid leukemia stem cells. *Cell, 138*(2), 286–299. https://doi.org/10.1016/j.cell.2009.05.045 (accessed on 23rd June 2025).
16. D'Mello, S. R., Cruz, C. N., Chen, M. L., Kapoor, M., Lee, S. L., & Tyner, K. M. (2017). The evolving landscape of drug products containing nanomaterials in the United States. *Nature Nanotechnology, 12*(6), 523–529. https://doi.org/10.1038/nnano.2017.67 (accessed on 23rd June 2025).
17. Naumenko, V. A., Vlasova, K. Y., Garanina, A. S., Melnikov, P. A., Potashnikova, D. M., Vishnevskiy, D. A., Vodopyanov, S. S., Chekhonin, V. P., Abakumov, M. A., & Majouga, A. G. (2019). Extravasating neutrophils open vascular barrier and improve liposomes delivery to tumors. *ACS Nano, 13*(11), 12599–12612. https://doi.org/10.3390/ph16111564 (accessed on 23rd June 2025).
18. MacLachlan, I. (n.d.). Antisense drug technology: Principles, strategies, and applications. In *Antisense Drug Technology* (pp. 237–270). CRC Press. https://doi.org/10.1201/9780849387951 (accessed on 23rd June 2025).
19. Barba, A. A., Bochicchio, S., Dalmoro, A., & Lamberti, G. (2019). Lipid delivery systems for nucleic-acid-based drugs: From production to clinical applications. *Pharmaceutics, 11*(8), 360. https://doi.org/10.3390/pharmaceutics11080360 (accessed on 23rd June 2025).
20. Xue, H. Y., Guo, P., Wen, W. C., & Wong, H. L. (2015). Lipid-based nanocarriers for RNA delivery. *Current Pharmaceutical Design, 21*(22), 3140–3147. https://doi.org/10.2174/1381612821666150531164540 (accessed on 23rd June 2025).
21. Parhiz, H., Shuvaev, V. V., Pardi, N., Khoshnejad, M., Kiseleva, R. Y., Brenner, J. S., Uhler, T., Tuyishime, S., Mui, B. L., Tam, Y. K., Madden, T. D., Hope, M. J., Weissman, D., & Muzykantov, V. R. (2018). PECAM-1 directed re-targeting of exogenous mRNA providing two orders of magnitude enhancement of vascular delivery and expression in lungs independent of apolipoprotein E-mediated uptake. *Journal of Controlled Release, 291*, 106–115. https://doi.org/10.1016/j.jconrel.2018.10.015 (accessed on 23rd June 2025).
22. Marcos-Contreras, O. A., Greineder, C. F., Kiseleva, R. Y., Parhiz, H., Walsh, L. R., Zuluaga-Ramirez, V., Myerson, J. W., Hood, E. D., Villa, C. H., Tombacz, I., Pardi, N., Seliga, A., Mui, B. L., Tam, Y. K., Glassman, P. M., Shuvaev, V. V., Nong, J., Brenner, J. S., Khoshnejad, M., & Muzykantov, V. R. (2020). Selective targeting of nanomedicine to inflamed cerebral vasculature to enhance the blood–brain barrier. *Proceedings of the National Academy of Sciences of the United States of America,*

117(7), 3405–3414. https://doi.org/10.1073/pnas.1912012117 (accessed on 23rd June 2025).
23. Mahapatro, A., & Singh, D. K. (2011). Biodegradable nanoparticles are excellent vehicle for site directed *in-vivo* delivery of drugs and vaccines. *Journal of Nanobiotechnology, 9*, 55. https://doi.org/10.1186/1477-3155-9-55 (accessed on 23rd June 2025).
24. Wiwanitkit, V. (2019). Biodegradable nanoparticles for drug delivery and targeting. In *Surface Modification of Nanoparticles for Targeted Drug Delivery* (pp. 167–181). https://doi.org/10.1007/978-3-030-06115-9_9 (accessed on 23rd June 2025).
25. Cabral, H., Miyata, K., Osada, K., & Kataoka, K. (2018). Block copolymer micelles in nanomedicine applications. *Chemical Reviews, 118*(14), 6844–6892. https://doi.org/10.1021/acs.chemrev.8b00199 (accessed on 23rd June 2025).
26. Batrakova, E. V., Bronich, T. K., Vetro, J. A., & Kabanov, A. V. (2006). Polymer micelles as drug carriers. In *Nanoparticulate as Drug Carriers* (pp. 57–93). https://doi.org/10.1142/9781860949074_0005 (accessed on 23rd June 2025).
27. Hussein, Y. H. A., & Youssry, M. (2018). Polymeric micelles of biodegradable deblock copolymers: Enhanced encapsulation of hydrophobic drugs. *Materials (Basel), 11*(5), 688. https://doi.org/10.3390/ma11050688 (accessed on 23rd June 2025).
28. Chen, W., Zhou, S., Ge, L., Wu, W., & Jiang, X. (2018). Translatable high drug loading drug delivery systems based on biocompatible polymer nanocarriers. *Biomacromolecules, 19*(6), 1732–1745. https://doi.org/10.1021/acs.biomac.8b00218 (accessed on 23rd June 2025).
29. Veiseh, O., Tang, B. C., Whitehead, K. A., Anderson, D. G., & Langer, R. (2015). Managing diabetes with nanomedicine: Challenges and opportunities. *Nature Reviews Drug Discovery, 14*(1), 45–57. https://doi.org/10.1038/nrd4477 (accessed on 23rd June 2025).
30. Han, X., Lu, Y., Xie, J., Zhang, E., Zhu, H., Du, H., Wang, K., Song, B., Yang, C., Shi, Y., & Cao, Z. (2020). Zwitterionic micelles efficiently deliver oral insulin without opening tight junctions. *Nature Nanotechnology, 15*(7), 605–614. https://doi.org/10.1038/s41565-020-0693-6 (accessed on 23rd June 2025).
31. Schudel, A., Chapman, A. P., Yau, M. K., Higginson, C. J., Francis, D. M., Manspeaker, M. P., Avecilla, A. R. C., Rohner, N. A., Finn, M. G., & Thomas, S. N. (2020). Programmable multistage drug delivery to lymph nodes. *Nature Nanotechnology, 15*(6), 491–499. https://doi.org/10.1038/s41565-020-0679-4 (accessed on 23rd June 2025).
32. Oltra, N. S., Swift, J., Mahmud, A., Rajagopal, K., Loverde, S. M., & Discher, D. E. (2013). Filo micelles in nanomedicine—from flexible, fragmentable, and ligand-targetable drug carrier designs to combination therapy for brain tumors. *Journal of Materials Chemistry B, 1*(39), 5177–5185. https://doi.org/10.1039/C3TB20431F (accessed on 23rd June 2025).
33. Shuvaev, V. V., Ilies, M. A., Simone, E., Zaitsev, S., Kim, Y., Cai, S., Mahmud, A., Dziubla, T., Muro, S., Discher, D. E., & Muzykantov, V. R. (2011). Endothelial targeting of antibody-decorated polymeric filo micelles. *ACS Nano, 5*(9), 6991–6999. https://doi.org/10.1021/nn2015453 (accessed on 23rd June 2025).
34. Yuan, Y., Guo, B., Hao, L., Liu, N., Lin, Y., Guo, W., Li, X., & Gu, B. (2017). Doxorubicin-loaded environmentally friendly carbon dots as a novel drug delivery

system for nucleus targeted cancer therapy. *Colloids and Surfaces B: Bio Interfaces, 159*, 349–359. https://doi.org/10.1016/j.colsurfb.2017.07.030 (accessed on 23rd June 2025).

35. Kong, T., Hao, L., Wei, Y., Cai, X., & Zhu, B. (2018). Doxorubicin conjugated carbon dots as a drug delivery system for human breast cancer therapy. *Cell Proliferation, 51*(5), e12488. https://doi.org/10.1111/cpr.12488 (accessed on 23rd June 2025).
36. Hettiarachchi, S. D., Graham, R. M., Mintz, K. J., Zhou, Y., Vanni, S., Peng, Z., & Leblanc, R. M. (2019). Triple conjugated carbon dots as a nano-drug delivery model for glioblastoma brain tumors. *Nanoscale, 11*(13), 6192–6205. https://doi.org/10.1039/c8nr08970a (accessed on 23rd June 2025).
37. Liyanage, P. Y., Zhou, Y., Al-Youbi, A. O., Bashammakh, A. S., El-Shahawi, M. S., Vanni, S., Graham, R. M., & Leblanc, R. M. (2020). Pediatric glioblastoma target-specific efficient delivery of gemcitabine across the blood–brain barrier via carbon nitride dots. *Nanoscale, 12*(14), 7927–7938. https://doi.org/10.1039/D0NR01647K (accessed on 23rd June 2025).
38. Pardo, J., Peng, Z., & Leblanc, R. M. (2018). Cancer targeting and drug delivery using carbon-based quantum dots and nanotubes. *Molecules, 23*(2), 378. https://doi.org/10.3390/molecules23020378 (accessed on 23rd June 2025).
39. Havrdova, M., Hola, K., Skopalik, J., Tomankova, K., Petr, M., Cepe, K., Polakova, K., Tucek, J., Bourlinos, A. B., & Zboril, R. (2016). Toxicity of carbon dots—effect of surface functionalization on the cell viability, reactive oxygen species generation and cell cycle. *Carbon, 99*, 238–248. https://doi.org/10.1016/j.carbon.2015.12.027 (accessed on 23rd June 2025).
40. Ali, A., Zafar, H., Zia, M., ul Haq, I., Phull, A. R., Ali, J. S., & Hussain, A. (2016). Synthesis, characterization, applications, and challenges of iron oxide nanoparticles. *Nanotechnology, Science and Applications, 9*, 49–67. https://doi.org/10.2147/NSA.S99986 (accessed on 23rd June 2025).
41. Vangijzegem, T., Stanicki, D., & Laurent, S. (2019). Magnetic iron oxide nanoparticles for drug delivery: Applications and characteristics. *Expert Opinion on Drug Delivery, 16*(1), 69–78. https://doi.org/10.1080/17425247.2019 (accessed on 23rd June 2025).
42. Zanganeh, S., Hutter, G., Spitler, R., Lenkov, O., Mahmoudi, M., Shaw, A., Pajarinen, J. S., Nejadnik, H., Goodman, S., Moseley, M., Coussens, L. M., & Daldrup-Link, H. E. (2016). Iron oxide nanoparticles inhibit tumor growth by inducing pro-inflammatory macrophage polarization in tumor tissues. *Nature Nanotechnology, 11*(11), 986–994. https://doi.org/10.1038/nnano.2016.168 (accessed on 23rd June 2025).
43. Wang, B., Yin, J. J., Zhou, X., Kurash, I., Chai, Z., Zhao, Y., & Feng, W. (2013). Physicochemical origin for free radical generation of iron oxide nanoparticles in bio microenvironment: Catalytic activities mediated by surface chemical states. *Journal of Physical Chemistry C, 117*(1), 383–392. https://doi.org/10.1021/jp3101392 (accessed on 23rd June 2025).
44. Vallabani, N. V. S., & Singh, S. (2018). Recent advances and future prospects of iron oxide nanoparticles in biomedicine and diagnostics. *3 Biotech, 8*(6), 279. https://doi.org/10.1007/s13205-018-1286-z (accessed on 23rd June 2025).
45. Arias, L. S., Pessan, J. P., Vieira, A. P. M., De Lima, T. M. T., Delbem, A. C. B., & Monteiro, D. R. (2018). Iron oxide nanoparticles for biomedical applications: A perspective on synthesis, drugs, antimicrobial activity, and toxicity. *Antibiotics*

(Basel), 7(2), 46. https://doi.org/10.3390/antibiotics7020046 (accessed on 23rd June 2025).

46. Oh, J. K., Drumright, R., Siegwart, D. J., & Matyjaszewski, K. (2008). The development of microgels/nanogels for drug delivery applications. *Progress in Polymer Science, 33*(4), 448–477. https://doi.org/10.1016/j.progpolymsci.2008.01.002 (accessed on 23rd June 2025).
47. Soni, K. S., Desale, S. S., & Bronich, T. K. (2016). Nanogels: An overview of properties, biomedical applications and obstacles to clinical translation. *Journal of Controlled Release, 240*, 109–126. https://doi.org/10.1016/j.jconrel.2015.11.009 (accessed on 23rd June 2025).
48. Neamtu, I., Rusu, A. G., Diaconu, A., Nita, L. E., & Chiriac, A. P. (2017). Basic concepts and recent advances in nanogels as carriers for medical applications. *Drug Delivery, 24*(1), 539–557. https://doi.org/10.1080/10717544.2016.1276232 (accessed on 23rd June 2025).
49. Eckmann, D. M., Composto, R. J., Tsourkas, A., & Muzykantov, V. R. (2014). Nanogel carrier design for targeted drug delivery. *Journal of Materials Chemistry B, 2*(46), 8085–8097. https://doi.org/10.1039/C4TB01141D (accessed on 23rd June 2025).
50. Glassman, P. M., Myerson, J. W., Ferguson, L. T., Kiseleva, R. Y., Shuvaev, V. V., Brenner, J. S., & Muzykantov, V. R. (2020). Targeting drug delivery in the vascular system: Focus on endothelium. *Advanced Drug Delivery Reviews, 157*, 96–117. https://doi.org/10.1016/j.addr.2020.06.013 (accessed on 23rd June 2025).
51. Gupta, U., & Perumal, O. (2014). Dendrimers and its biomedical applications. In *Natural and Synthetic Biomedical Polymers* (pp. 243–257). Elsevier. https://doi.org/10.1016/B978-0-12-396983-5.00016-8 (accessed on 23rd June 2025).
52. Madaan, K., Kumar, S., Poonia, N., Lather, V., & Pandita, D. (2014). Dendrimers in drug delivery and targeting: Drug-dendrimer interactions and toxicity issues. *Journal of Pharmacy and Bioallied Sciences, 6*(3), 139–150. https://doi.org/10.4103/0975-7406.130965 (accessed on 23rd June 2025).
53. Chauhan, A. S. (2018). Dendrimers for drug delivery. *Molecules, 23*(4), 938. https://doi.org/10.3390/molecules23040938 (accessed on 23rd June 2025).
54. Pan, J., Mendes, L. P., Yao, M., Filipczak, N., Garai, S., Thakur, G. A., Sarisozen, C., & Torchilin, V. P. (2019). Polyamidoamine dendrimers-based nanomedicine for combination therapy with siRNA and chemotherapeutics to overcome multidrug resistance. *European Journal of Pharmaceutics and Biopharmaceutics, 136*, 18–28. https://doi.org/10.1016/j.ejpb.2019.01.006 (accessed on 23rd June 2025).
55. Zhu, Y., Liu, C., & Pang, Z. (2019). Dendrimer-based drug delivery systems for brain targeting. *Biomolecules, 9*(12), 790. https://doi.org/10.3390/biom9120790 (accessed on 23rd June 2025).
56. Wang, H., Chen, Q., & Zhou, S. (2018). Carbon-based hybrid nanogels: A synergistic nanoplatform for combined biosensing, bioimaging, and responsive drug delivery. *Chemical Society Reviews, 47*(11), 4198–4232. https://doi.org/10.1039/C7CS00399D (accessed on 23rd June 2025).
57. Li, W., Liu, Q., Zhang, P., & Liu, L. (2016). Zwitterionic nanogels crosslinked by fluorescent carbon dots for targeted drug delivery and simultaneous bioimaging. *Acta*

Biomaterial, 40, 254–262. https://doi.org/10.1016/j.actbio.2016.04.006 (accessed on 23rd June 2025).

58. Eslami, P., Rossi, F., & Fedeli, S. (2019). Hybrid nanogels: Stealth and biocompatible structures for drug delivery applications. *Pharmaceutics, 11*(2), 71. https://doi.org/10.3390/pharmaceutics11020071 (accessed on 23rd June 2025).
59. Cao, S., Slack, S. D., Levy, C. N., Hughes, S. M., Jiang, Y., Yogodzinski, C., Roychoudhury, P., Jerome, K. R., Schiffer, J. T., Hladik, F., & Woodrow, K. A. (2019). Hybrid nanocarriers incorporating mechanistically distinct drugs for lymphatic CD4+ T cell activation and HIV-1 latency reversal. *Science Advances, 5*(3), eaav6322. https://doi.org/10.1126/sciadv.aav6322 (accessed on 23rd June 2025).
60. Blanco, E., Shen, H., & Ferrari, M. (2015). Principles of nanoparticle design for overcoming biological barriers to drug delivery. *Nature Biotechnology, 33*(9), 941–951. https://doi.org/10.1038/nbt.3330 (accessed on 23rd June 2025).
61. Ponce, A. M., Vujaskovic, Z., Yuan, F., Needham, D., & Dewhirst, M. W. (2006). Hyperthermia mediated liposomal drug delivery. *International Journal of Hyperthermia, 22*(3), 205–213. https://doi.org/10.1080/02656730600582956 (accessed on 23rd June 2025).
62. Rizvi, S. A. A., & Saleh, A. M. (2018). Applications of nanoparticle systems in drug delivery technology. *Saudi Pharmaceutical Journal, 26*(1), 64–70. https://doi.org/10.1016/j.jsps.2017.10.012 (accessed on 23rd June 2025).
63. Mura, S., Nicolas, J., & Couvreur, P. (2013). Stimuli-responsive nanocarriers for drug delivery. *Nature Materials, 12*(11), 991–1003. https://doi.org/10.1038/nmat3776 (accessed on 23rd June 2025).
64. Torchilin, V. P. (2014). Multifunctional, stimuli-sensitive nanoparticulate systems for drug delivery. *Nature Reviews Drug Discovery, 13*(11), 813–827. https://doi.org/10.1038/nrd4333 (accessed on 23rd June 2025).
65. Karimi, M., Ghasemi, A., Sahandi Zangabad, P., Rahighi, R., Moosavi Basri, S. M., Mirshekari, H., Amiri, M., Shafaei Pishabad, Z., Aslani, A., Bozorgomid, M., Ghosh, D., Beyzavi, A., Vaseghi, A., Aref, A. R., Haghani, L., Bahrami, S., & Hamblin, M. R. (2016). Smart micro/nanoparticles in stimulus-responsive drug/gene delivery systems. *Chemical Society Reviews, 45*(5), 1457–1501. https://doi.org/10.1016/j.mtbio.2022.100223 (accessed on 23rd June 2025).
66. Bordat, A., Boissenot, T., Nicolas, J., & Tsapis, N. (2019). Thermoresponsive polymer nanocarriers for biomedical applications. *Advanced Drug Delivery Reviews, 138*, 167–192. https://doi.org/10.1016/j.addr.2018.10.005 (accessed on 23rd June 2025).
67. Lin, S. Y. (2020). Thermoresponsive gating membranes embedded with liquid crystal(s) for pulsatile transdermal drug delivery: An overview and perspectives. *Journal of Controlled Release, 319*, 450–474. https://doi.org/10.1016/j.jconrel.2019.12.046 (accessed on 23rd June 2025).
68. Zhu, Y. J., & Chen, F. (2015). PH-responsive drug-delivery systems. *Chemistry – An Asian Journal, 10*(2), 284–305. https://doi.org/10.1002/asia.201402715 (accessed on 23rd June 2025).
69. Deirram, N., Zhang, C., Kermaniyan, S. S., Johnston, A. P. R., & Such, G. K. (2019). PH-responsive polymer nanoparticles for drug delivery. *Macromolecular Rapid Communications, 40*, 1800917. https://doi.org/10.1002/marc.201800917 (accessed on 23rd June 2025).

70. Xiong, H., Wu, Y., Jiang, Z., Zhou, J., Yang, M., Yao, J., & Yao. (2019). pH-activatable polymeric nanodrugs enhanced tumor chemo/antiangiogenic combination therapy through improving targeting drug release. *Journal of Colloid and Interface Science, 536*, 135–148. https://doi.org/10.1016/j.jcis.2018.10.039 (accessed on 23rd June 2025).
71. Wu, W., Luo, L., Wang, Y., Wu, Q., Dai, H. B., Li, J. S., Durkan, C., Wang, N., & Wang, G. X. (2018). Endogenous pH-responsive nanoparticles with programmable size changes for targeted tumor therapy and imaging applications. *Theragnostic, 8*(11), 3038–3058. https://doi.org/10.7150/thno.23459 (accessed on 23rd June 2025).
72. Goyal, A. K., Rath, G., Faujdar, C., & Malik, B. (2019). Application and perspective of pH-responsive nano drug delivery systems. In *Applications of Targeted Nano Drugs and Delivery Systems* (pp. 15–33). Elsevier. https://doi.org/10.1016/B978-0-12-814029-1.00002-8 (accessed on 23rd June 2025).
73. Hu, F., Yue, H., Lu, T., & Ma, G. (2020). Cytosolic delivery of HBsAg and enhanced cellular immunity by pH-responsive liposome. *Journal of Controlled Release, 324*, 460–470. https://doi.org/10.1016/j.jconrel.2020.05.042 (accessed on 23rd June 2025).
74. Liao, Z. S., Huang, S. Y., Huang, J. J., Chen, J. K., Lee, A. W., Lai, J. Y., Lee, D. J., & Cheng, C. C. (2018). Self-assembled pH-responsive polymeric micelles for highly efficient, noncytotoxic delivery of doxorubicin chemotherapy to inhibit macrophage activation: *In vitro* investigation. *Biomacromolecules, 19*(7), 2772–2781. https://doi.org/10.1021/acs.biomac.8b00380 (accessed on 23rd June 2025).
75. Zhou, X. X., Jin, L., Qi, R. Q., & Ma, T. (2018). pH-responsive polymeric micelles self-assembled from amphiphilic copolymer modified with lipid used as doxorubicin delivery carriers. *Royal Society Open Science, 5*(3), 171654. https://doi.org/10.1098/rsos.171654 (accessed on 23rd June 2025).
76. Seo, J., Lee, J., Lee, C. B., Bae, S. K., & Na, K. (2019). Nonpolymeric pH-sensitive carbon dots for treatment of tumor. *Bioconjugate Chemistry, 30*(3), 621–632. https://doi.org/10.1021/acs.bioconjchem.8b00813 (accessed on 23rd June 2025).
77. Cao, Y., Huang, H. Y., Chen, L. Q., Du, H. H., Cui, J. H., Zhang, L. W., Lee, B. J., & Cao, Q. R. (2019). Enhanced lysosomal escape of pH-responsive polyethyleneimine-betaine functionalized carbon nanotube for the codelivery of surviving small interfering RNA and doxorubicin. *ACS Applied Materials & Interfaces, 11*(10), 9763–9776. https://doi.org/10.1021/acsami.8b20810 (accessed on 23rd June 2025).
78. Prabhakar, A., & Banerjee, R. (2019). Nanobubble liposome complexes for diagnostic imaging and ultrasound-triggered drug delivery in cancers: A theragnostic approach. *ACS Omega, 4*(13), 15567–15580. https://doi.org/10.1021/acsomega.9b01924 (accessed on 23rd June 2025).
79. Canavese, G., Ancona, A., Racca, L., Canta, M., Dumontel, B., Barbaresco, F., Limongi, T., & Cauda, V. (2018). Nanoparticle-assisted ultrasound: A special focus on sonodynamic therapy against cancer. *Chemical Engineering Journal, 340*, 155–172. https://doi.org/10.1016/j.cej.2018.01.060 (accessed on 23rd June 2025).
80. Ekladious, I., Colson, Y. L., & Grinstaff, M. W. (2019). Polymer–drug conjugate therapeutics. *Nature Reviews Drug Discovery, 18*(4), 273–294. https://doi.org/10.1038/s41573-018-0005-0 (accessed on 23rd June 2025).

81. Hasnain, M. S., Ahmad, S. A., Hoda, M. N., Rishishwar, S., Rishishwar, P., & Nayak, A. K. (2018). Stimuli-responsive carbon nanotubes for targeted drug delivery. In *Stimuli Responsive Polymeric Nanocarriers for Drug Delivery Applications; Vol. 2: Advanced Nanocarriers for Therapeutics* (Woodhead Publishing). https://doi.org/10.1016/B978-0-08-101995-5.00015-5 (accessed on 23rd June 2025).
82. Tharkar, P., Varanasi, R., Wong, W. S. F., Jin, C. T., & Chrzanowski, W. (2019). Nano-enhanced drug delivery and therapeutic ultrasound for cancer treatment and beyond. *Frontiers in Bioengineering and Biotechnology, 7*, 324. https://doi.org/10.3389/fbioe.2019.00324 (accessed on 23rd June 2025).
83. Wang, Y., Deng, Y., Luo, H., Zhu, A., Ke, H., Yang, H., & Chen, H. (2017). Light-responsive nanoparticles for highly efficient cytoplasmic delivery of anticancer agents. *ACS Nano, 11*(12), 12134–12144. https://doi.org/10.1021/acsnano.7b05214 (accessed on 23rd June 2025).
84. Linsley, C. S., & Wu, B. M. (2017). Recent advances in light-responsive on-demand drug-delivery systems. *Therapeutic Delivery, 8*(2), 89–107. https://doi.org/10.4155/tde-2016-0060 (accessed on 23rd June 2025).
85. Raza, A., Hayat, U., Rasheed, T., Bilal, M., & Iqbal, H. M. N. (2019). 'Smart' materials-based near-infrared light-responsive drug delivery systems for cancer treatment: A review. *Journal of Materials Research and Technology, 8*(1), 1497–1509. https://doi.org/10.1016/j.jmrt.2018.03.007 (accessed on 23rd June 2025).
86. Liguori, I., Russo, G., Curcio, F., Bulli, G., Aran, L., Della-Morte, D., Gargiulo, G., Testa, G., Cacciatore, F., Bonaduce, D., & Abete, P. (2018). Oxidative stress, aging, and diseases. *Clinical Interventions in Aging, 13*, 757–772. https://doi.org/10.2147/CIA.S158513 (accessed on 23rd June 2025).
87. Huo, M., Yuan, J., Tao, L., & Wei, Y. (2014). Redox-responsive polymers for drug delivery: From molecular design to applications. *Polymer Chemistry, 5*(5), 1519–1528. https://doi.org/10.1039/C3PY01192E (accessed on 23rd June 2025).
88. Fang, T., Zhang, J., Zuo, T., Wu, G., Xu, Y., Yang, Y., Yang, J., & Shen, Q. (2020). Chemo-photothermal combination cancer therapy with ROS scavenging, extracellular matrix depletion and tumor immune activation by telmisartan and diselenide-paclitaxel prodrug loaded nanoparticles. *ACS Applied Materials & Interfaces, 12*(28), 31292–31308. https://doi.org/10.1021/acsami.0c10416 (accessed on 23rd June 2025).
89. Guo, X., Cheng, Y., Zhao, X., Luo, Y., Chen, J., & Yuan, W. E. (2018). Advances in redox-responsive drug delivery systems of tumor microenvironment. *Journal of Nanobiotechnology, 16*(1), 74. https://doi.org/10.1186/s12951-018-0398-2 (accessed on 23rd June 2025).
90. Kumari, R., Sunil, D., & Ningthoujam, R. S. (2020). Hypoxia-responsive nanoparticle-based drug delivery systems in cancer therapy: An up-to-date review. *Journal of Controlled Release, 319*, 135–156. https://doi.org/10.1016/j.jconrel.2019.12.041 (accessed on 23rd June 2025).
91. Sada, K., Nishikawa, T., Kukidome, D., Yoshinaga, T., Kajihara, N., Sonoda, K., Senokuchi, T., Motoshima, H., Matsumura, T., & Araki, E. (2016). Hyperglycemia induces cellular hypoxia through production of mitochondrial ROS followed by suppression of aquaporin-1. *PLOS ONE, 11*(7), e0158619. https://doi.org/10.1371/journal.pone.0158619 (accessed on 23rd June 2025).

92. Yu, J., Zhang, Y., Ye, Y., DiSanto, R., Sun, W., Ranson, D., Ligler, F. S., Buse, J. B., Gu, Z., & Ho, D. (2015). Microneedle-array patches loaded with hypoxia-sensitive vesicles provide fast glucose-responsive insulin delivery. *Proceedings of the National Academy of Sciences of the United States of America, 112*(27), 8260–8265. https://doi.org/10.1073/pnas.1505405112 (accessed on 23rd June 2025).
93. Hu, X., Yu, J., Qian, C., Lu, Y., Kahkoska, A. R., Xie, Z., Jing, X., Buse, J. B., & Gu, Z. (2017). H_2O_2-responsive vesicles integrated with transcutaneous patches for glucose-mediated insulin delivery. *ACS Nano, 11*(1), 613–620. https://doi.org/10.1021/acsnano.6b06892 (accessed on 23rd June 2025).
94. Yu, J., Qian, C., Zhang, Y., Cui, Z., Zhu, Y., Shen, Q., Ligler, F. S., Buse, J. B., & Gu, Z. (2017). Hypoxia and H_2O_2 dual-sensitive vesicles for enhanced glucose-responsive insulin delivery. *Nano Letters, 17*(2), 733–739. https://doi.org/10.1021/acs.nanolett.6b03848 (accessed on 23rd June 2025).

CHAPTER 3

Challenges in Nucleic Acid Delivery

SHRADHA DEVI DWIVEDI,[1] POOJA DESHPANDE,[2,*]
RAJESH CHOUDHARY,[3] and JAYA SHREE[3]

[1]University Institute of Pharmacy, Pandit Ravishankar Shukla University, Raipur, Chhattisgarh, India

[2]School of Pharmacy, Mody University of Science and Technology, Lakshmangarh, Sikar, Rajasthan, India

[3]Shri Shankaracharya College of Pharmaceutical Sciences, Junwani, Bhilai, Chhattisgarh, India

*Corresponding author

ABSTRACT

Nucleic acid delivery holds significant promise in transforming the treatment of different genetic abnormalities, infectious diseases, and malignancies. However, various obstacles have hampered its clinical application. This presentation presents a complete summary of the current challenges in nucleic acid delivery, including both viral and non-viral vectors. Key hurdles include obtaining effective cellular absorption, overcoming intracellular barriers such as endosomal entrapment and lysosomal degradation, minimizing off-target effects, ensuring enough payload delivery to target tissues, and dealing with immunogenicity concerns. Strategies for addressing these issues are presented, such as the creation of novel delivery vectors, formulation process optimization, and targeted delivery approaches. Furthermore, the significance of understanding the interaction between delivery mechanisms and biological obstacles for successful nucleic acid distribution is highlighted. Overcoming these hurdles is essential for unlocking the full therapeutic potential of nucleic acid-based therapies and advancing personalized medicine.

Nanotechnology for Nucleic Acid Delivery: Pankaj Sharma, Saloni Jain, and Vinay Jain (Eds.)

DOI: 10.1201/9781998511853-3

3.1 INTRODUCTION TO NUCLEIC ACID DELIVERY

Deoxyribonucleic acid (DNA) and ribonucleic acid (RNA) are the simple forms of nucleic acid, and early research on their functions was limited and restricted, but in a few decades, remarkable research on nucleic acid-based therapeutics and delivery [1] emerged. Presently, the use of nucleic acids as a drug is a promising new therapeutic strategy for a variety of diseases [2]. This is possible due to several discoveries in the last few decades, including decoding the human genome that postulates the variety of molecular pathways of human diseases; in addition to messenger RNA (mRNA) and transfer RNA (tRNA), finding several types of RNA such as microRNA (miRNA) and the short interfering RNA (siRNA) with complex biological and therapeutic functions [3]. Moreover, RNAs can act as enzymes, contributing to the formation of RNA analogs possessing useful or unusual therapeutic applications. And the major contribution is enhancing the bioavailability of nucleic acid-based drugs [1]. Nucleic acid delivery, a process of transportation of nucleic acids such as DNA, RNA, and analogs into the targeted cells or tissues, holds significant promise in transforming the treatment of different genetic abnormalities, infectious diseases, and malignancies. However, various obstacles have hampered its clinical application and safety. Nucleic acid therapy mainly depends on either viral or non-viral vectors. Viral vectors pose safety challenges because they may risk immune responses, mutagenesis, and carcinogenesis [4]. Therefore, in this chapter, we discuss nucleic acid therapy and current challenges in nucleic acid delivery.

3.1.1 OVERVIEW OF NUCLEIC ACID THERAPEUTICS

The use of nucleic acids as a medication to treat or manage a range of human illnesses is known as nucleic acid treatment. In 1972, over 50 years ago, Friedmann and Roblin proposed the theory that treating inherited genetic illnesses may be achieved with the introduction of a functioning gene copy [5]. Global efforts to combat the COVID-19 pandemic and other disorders are now centered on developing technologies and discoveries that enable nucleic acid delivery or therapy [6, 7]. Chemically edited lipid nanoparticles (LNPs), antisense oligonucleotides (ASOs), N-acetylgalactosamine (GalNAc)-ligand-modified small interfering RNA (siRNA) combines, and adeno-associated virus (AAV) vectors are the four primary methods that depend on nucleic acid treatments [7]. These technologies' specifics are covered in the section below.

ASO is a short synthetic nucleic acid having short single-stranded 13–30 mer DNA and is used to inhibit gene function by forming a DNA/RNA double-stranded structure at the target site. Besides the mRNA genes, it can also target the miRNA [8, 9]. ASO steric blocks by the formation of a stable double-stranded structure as well as induce the endogenous RNA degradation pathways, which are mediated by RNase H1 (recognized by DNA/RNA duplexes) and/or Argonaute 2 (Recognised by RNA/RNA duplexes) [10]. The complementarity between the target RNA and the whole ASO molecule, which normally comprises 13 to 30 nucleotides, precisely regulates how tightly ASO binds to RNA. The precise binding specificity directly influences ASO efficacy, but it can also amplify toxicity if off-target binding occurs [7].

GalNAc-siRNA Conjugates is a simple and efficient technique for delivering siRNA to the target site (liver-targeted delivery). These conjugates play an important role in cellular defenses that protect siRNA from entering cells. This chemical modification of siRNA ensures stability in blood circulation after parental administration in the absence of a protective delivery system [11]. To silence disease-causing genes in hepatocytes, these therapeutic agents consist of siRNA conjugated with triantennary GalNAc moiety, which selectively targets the asialoglycoprotein receptor (ASGPR) [12]. The ASGPR is highly expressed on hepatocytes and binds specifically to carbohydrates with terminal galactose and GalNAc residues. Additionally, clathrin-dependent receptor-mediated endocytosis internalizes the receptor-ligand complex. Moreover, its rapid internalization and efficient recycling (within minutes) enable a continuous uptake of siRNA molecules, leading to an increased concentration in target cells [13]. Biological membrane permeability is the main obstacle preventing big, charge-dense biomolecules like nucleic acids from passing through the plasma membrane. Lipid nanoparticles (LNPs) come in handy to get over this restriction by letting nucleic acid into the cells. A novel class of lipid-mediated methods for delivery achieved its breakthrough when Felgner et al. [14] experimented with cationic lipids. LNPs protect against serum nuclease and immune defense and allow for a drug-biodistribution profile dictated by the carrier. The LNPs are mainly developed for siRNA delivery to the hepatocyte. The finding of ionizable cationic lipids has played a crucial role in enabling the clinical application of LNP-based RNA therapeutics. This delivery system ensures the efficient encapsulation of siRNA (>85%), maintains neutral LNP surface charge at physiological pH, and plays a major part in endosomal escape [15]. Apolipoprotein E (ApoE) binds the LNP surface and facilitates their uptake by hepatocytes by low-density lipoprotein receptors. Consequently, more than 80% accumulation from systemic administered doses is achieved in the hepatocytes [16, 17].

AVV is another technology used in nucleic acid therapy. The creation of safe and effective eukaryotic infectious agents, such as retroviruses, adenoviruses, and adeno-associated viruses, has been crucial to clinical development since the proposal of gene therapies some decades back [7]. Early studies reported that the viral vectors could successfully used to deliver therapeutic transgenes, but clinical benefits were observed in a small number of research and immunotoxicity was observed significantly (even death in some cases) [18]. This ultimately led to the creation and clinical application of recombinant viral vectors, which exhibit enhanced effectiveness and reduced risk [19, 20]. The FDA and the EMA have currently approved several medications based on transgene delivery using recombinant viral vectors. These treatments utilize either *ex vivo* or *in vivo* approaches, where transgenes are directly administered to cells. This process is primarily facilitated by AAV vectors, following parenteral administration. Presently, recombinant AAVs (rAAVs) serve as the primary platform for *in vivo* gene therapy delivery. The AAVs are mainly used in retinal, liver, and central nervous disorders [7, 21].

3.12 THE NEED FOR AN EFFECTIVE DELIVERY SYSTEM

Nucleic acid as a drug therapy has its challenges, such as low solubility, rapid clearance from circulation, target cell delivery, improper cellular uptake, and immunogenicity of the nucleic acid [7]. The majority of drugs that are either approved or in the trial are administered either hepatically, delivered by systemic circulation, or locally given (including intrathecal delivery). Numerous investigations are still required to address the issue with the distribution system.

Enzymes may quickly digest nucleic acids, rendering them ineffective. Modified nucleic acids are being developed as a solution to this issue. A number of chemical changes have recently been made to improve ASO's suitability as a nucleic acid medication. A group is added to the nucleic acid at the sugar's 2' location during sugar alteration. Because of their high RNA binding strength, the sugar-modified nucleic acids form a robust double-strand [22]. Phosphorothioate alteration involves the conversion of a phosphate diester link to a phosphorothioate bond [23]. This results in an increase in the attraction to target RNA, nuclease stability, and blood protein binding. Phosphorothioate ASO enhances blood preservation, prolongs the half-life of plasma removal, and avoids glomerular filtration through serum protein binding [24, 25]. To improve selectivity to the target cell (hepatocyte), GalNAc-conjugated nucleic acids (GalNAc-siRNA) are more efficient, allowing increased bioavailability in hepatocytes at lower doses compared to unconjugated nucleic acids by increasing the cellular uptake. The conjugates decrease the plasma and extra-hepatic concentration. These results increase the plasma clearance and provide a wide margin of safety [26]. Nanoparticles are a new approach to help solve the different issues with nucleic acid medications, including better permeability and delivery method. Currently, nucleic acids may be delivered to target cells via a variety of nanoparticle forms, including polymer-based, lipid-based, inorganic-based, and nucleic acid-based ones. This technique offers protection against degradation and renal excretion, as well as penetration of the cellular barrier. As a result, this technique offers nucleic acid treatment an effective delivery method [9].

Moreover, exosomes are another efficient delivery system for cancer cells. A kind of extracellular tiny membranous vesicle known as an exosome gets released into the extracellular layer by many cells and may play a role in intercellular interaction [28]. Different nucleic acids (DNA, mRNA, miRNA, siRNA, and circRNA) can be delivered using it. It is regarded as a potential delivery method because of its nano size (40–150 nm), which offers various benefits over traditional LNPs, including improved drug protection, stability in bodily fluids, excellent biocompatibility, and decreased cytotoxicity and immunogenicity. Furthermore, it has the ability to transport both hydrophobic and hydrophilic molecules, traverse the blood-brain barrier, and readily adapt to its intended target [29]. Exosome nanovesicles, which have dimensions ranging from 30 to 120 nm, are secreted by several cell types, including mast cells, dendritic cells, cancerous cells, B cells, T cells, and epithelial cells. They are present in a variety of bodily fluids, including breast milk, bronchoalveolar drainage fluid, blood, feces, and neoplastic effusions [29, 30].

Exosome surfaces are found to include a range of proteins that can be utilized as biomarkers, including heat shock proteins, fusion proteins (flotillin), and tetraspanins (CD9, CD63, and CD81). According to certain research, the contact between the target cell's receptor molecules and surface proteins is what allows exosomes to go to their intended destination [31].

Additional strategies for effective nucleic acid delivery include polymeric micelles (PMs). PMs are composed of hydrophilic and hydrophobic copolymers and range in size from 10 to 100 nm. In order to generate stable nucleic acid–polymer complexes, which are often referred to as polyion structures, the nucleic acids must extensively engage positively charged electrostatically with micelle-forming charge polymers [32]. Their natural production in a solution of water under thermodynamic equilibrium circumstances is a significant advantage of polyion complex micelles [33]. In addition, PMs improve therapeutic efficacy, overcome the extracellular and intracellular barriers, provide protection and selective targeting, and can deliver both nucleic acids and chemotherapeutic agents simultaneously [32]. Currently, PMs are important tools for nucleic acid delivery. A class of positively charged peptides known as cell-penetrating peptides (CPPs) has made significant progress in the delivery of macromolecules. It serves as an efficient carrier for nucleic acid (DNA, RNA, miRNA, and siRNA) delivery. Presently, the use of peptides as a carrier for targeted delivery has been developed in the last few decades [35]. Low biodegradability, biocompatibility, and comparatively easy manufacture, standardization, and storage are the main benefits of CPPs over other vectors. These peptide vehicles do not induce mutations or elicit an immune response, in contrast to viral vectors [36].

3.2 CELLULAR UPTAKE AND INTRACELLULAR BARRIER

3.2.1 MECHANISM OF CELLULAR UPTAKE

The intracellular and extracellular barriers (Figure 3.1) are the important challenges to nucleic acid delivery. Extracellular barriers like nuclease degradation, immune clearance, extravasation, and non-specific biodistribution are the major limitations of nucleic acid therapy [37]. For overcoming the extracellular barrier, chemical modification and conjugation are effective approaches to nucleic acid drug delivery systems. It can provide stability against degradation [32].

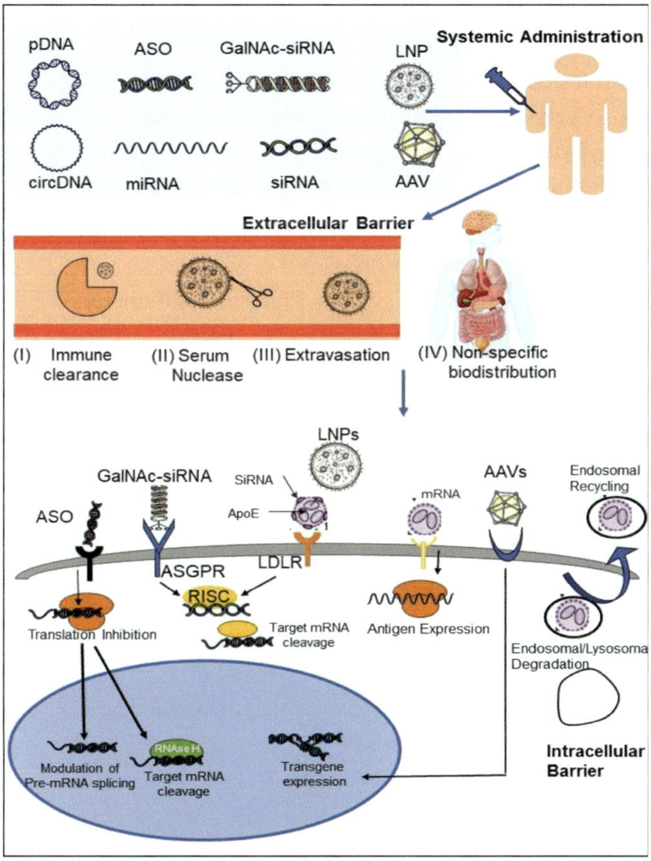

FIGURE 3.1 Extracellular and intracellular barriers, and mechanism of action of nucleic acid therapeutics.

After overcoming the extracellular barriers, the nucleic acid should reach the target site to overcome the intracellular barrier. The cellular uptake mechanism is an important part of this therapy. The mechanism of the cellular uptake system depends on the nucleic acid therapy techniques. Some important cellular uptake systems or delivery systems are discussed above. Phagocytosis, micropinocytosis, and endocytosis/pinocytosis are the major mechanisms of the cellular uptake system (Figure 3.2). White blood cells are the primary initiators of the adaptive immune response through the actin-dependent route of phagocytosis. Magnetic nanoparticles have been targeted to macrophages and delivered via phagocytosis. Larger particles, around

5–10 μm in size, can be internalized by macrophages, with an enhanced preference for ellipsoid-shaped particles over spherical ones. Notwithstanding this capability, it is not a universal method that can be relied upon to transport medications to cells other than these particular kinds. Another mechanism is micropinocytosis, which encapsulates the extracellular fluids in a vesicle (150–5000 nm diameter size). This pathway is actin-driven, characterized by outward-directed actin polymerization [38].

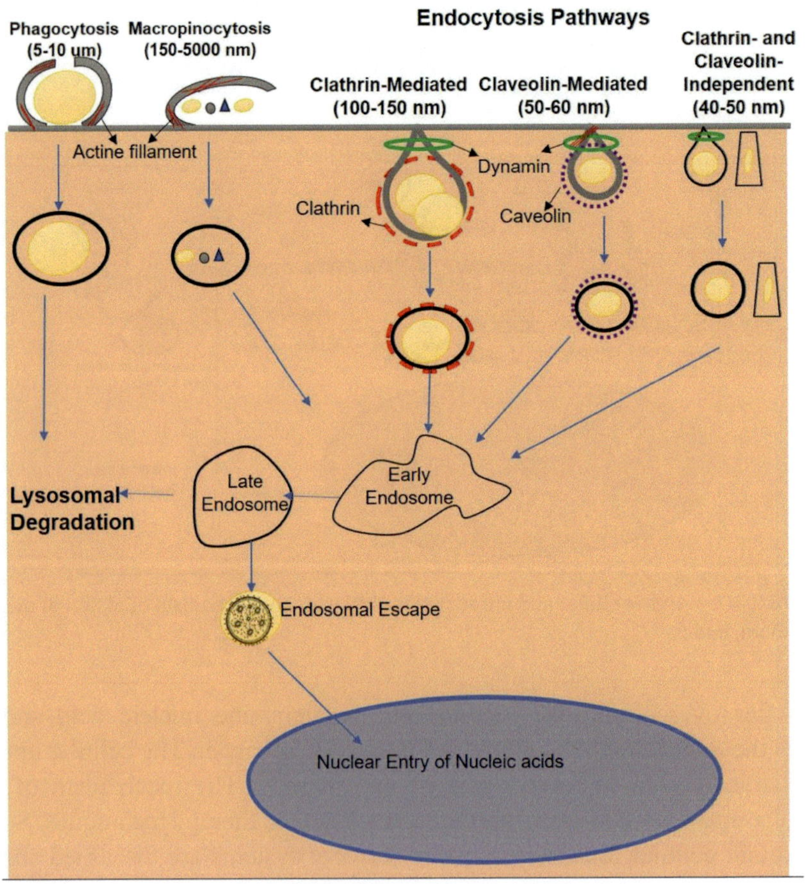

FIGURE 3.2 Mechanisms of Intracellular uptake system.

Endocytosis pathways are the primary route of cellular absorption. Substances are taken in by cells through a process called endocytosis.

The physiochemical characteristics of nanocarriers, such as their size, shape, charge, stiffness, lipophilicity, and so forth, and their cell types, influence the endocytosis pathways [39]. Clathrin-dependent, caveolae-dependent, and clathrin- and caveolae-independent endocytosis techniques (Figure 3.2) are further subclassified [38]. The two processes mentioned above, the caveolae-dependent and clathrin-dependent pathways, are reliant on size. Cells absorb things, including nucleic acids, by clathrin-mediated endocytosis, which is the inner bursting of plasma membrane compartments carrying molecules with receptor sites unique to those molecules being absorbed [40]. The presence of clathrin protein depths, which create a polygonal lattice structure around a section of the cell membrane and pinch it off to produce an internalized vesicle, is a characteristic of clathrin-mediated endocytosis. It takes up 100–150 nm diameter of size. However, transferrin and low-density lipoprotein (LDL) receptors also concentrate within these organelles besides clathrin-mediated endocytosis [41].

A second kind of protein-coated endocytosis is caveolae-mediated, and these vesicles have a diameter of around 50–60 nm. They have hydrophobic domains termed lipid rafts that are rich in glycosphingolipids and cholesterol. These domains usually form a flask, although they can also take the form of flat or tubular structures (Khalil et al., 2006; Kirkham and Parton, 2005). Activation of these pathways is both dynamin and actin-dependent [42, 43]. Some other pathways involve the formation of lipid rafts but are independent of clathrin and caveolin protein; they are called clathrin- and caveolin-independent pathways. They may produce 40–50 nm-sized, cholesterol-rich structures that are either dynamin- and actin-dependent or independent. These autonomous vesicles are thought to be able to combine with other pathways as endosomes mature [38, 41].

3.2.2 ENDOSOMAL ENTRAPMENT AND LYSOSOMAL DEGRADATION

Endocytosis is the major pathway of cellular uptake of nucleic acids. During the intracellular delivery by endocytosis, biological molecules like nucleic acids are trapped by endosomes and lysosomes and further go for degradation. Mechanisms such as the proton sponge effect and osmotic lysis, membrane fusion, pore creation, membrane destabilization/disturbance, and vesicle budding and collapse can all result in endosomal entrapment. The endosome–lysosome pathway is considered a degradative transport pathway because biomolecules are further degraded by enzymes and acids, and these become a problem for drug delivery [44].

The cell first uses one or more endocytic mechanisms to swallow a cargo of nucleic acids, which is then subsequently confined into a young endosome (Figure 3.2). Protons are forcefully transported into the endosome by vacuolar ATPase proton pumps, decreasing the luminal pH to around 5.5 whilst the initial endosome (that has an alkaline pH of approximately 6.3) gradually transforms into the late endosome. The intraluminal enzymes are eventually broken down by lysosomal enzymes when the late endosome fuses into the lysosome (pH 4–5) [45].

Consequently, cargo cannot be reduced apart within the lysosome until it reaches the cytosol and escapes from endosomal/lysosomal capture, which is necessary for cargo to initiate a biological process. Unfortunately, for the majority of non-viral vectors, endosomal escape is inadequate. Furthermore, exocytosis by endocytic recycling (by evacuation from the later endosome/lysosome) might further lower the efficacy of cytosolic transport [45]. Consequently, in order to enhance the therapeutic benefits and nucleic acid delivery system, it is imperative to comprehend the endosomal escape process. In order to stop endosomal-lysosomal destruction and endosomal recycling, endosomal escape is essential. Endosomal evacuation is explained by several mechanisms, the best-known ones being particle swelling, membrane instability, and the proton sponge mechanism [32].

3.2.3 STRATEGY TO ENHANCE INTRACELLULAR DELIVERY

To efficiently deliver nucleic acids into the cytosol is to enhance endosomal leakage or escape. These can be achieved by membrane-active agents. For example, small molecules like Amphotericin B and Triton X-100 monomer work by directly disrupting membranes and increasing endosomal leakage [46]. While cationic amphiphilic medications like bafilomycin, siramesine, and chloroquine disrupt endosomal maturation because they increase nonspecific escape and prevent acidification [44]. Moreover, several techniques have been developed for endosomal escape, such as cell-penetrating peptides (CPPs) or endosomal escape peptides (EEPs), which effectively disrupt membranes and are usually cationic or amphipathic [44]. There are several mechanisms and strategies proposed to explain the cytoplasmic release of nucleic acids from endosomal vesicles. These are as follows:

Osmotic lysis and pH buffering mechanisms provide an explanation for the "proton sponge" theory. Such agents are used to moderate it; they have a large capacity for buffering and the ability to expand upon protonation. Protonation causes the endosomal membrane to break, releasing nucleic acids that had been trapped and measuring osmotic pressure. Polyethyleneimine and poly(amidoamine) polymers are a couple of such agents. Moreover, histidine-rich compounds produce endosomal release and have a buffering function upon protonation [45, 47]. Destabilization of the endosomal membrane by fusogenic peptides (haemagglutinin, L-lysine) and endosomal membrane pore formation are additional mechanisms involved in the liposomal transport system. The force responsible for pore growth is the combination of a membrane tension that expands the pore and a line tension that closes it. Certain substances, such as peptides, exhibit a strong attraction to the pore's rim [47].

3.3 OFF-TARGET EFFECTS AND IMMUNOGENICITY

Considerations about off-target effects and immunogenicity are of utmost importance in the development and implementation of drugs and therapies. Off-target effects refer to the unintentional interactions of a medicine with non-intended targets in the body, resulting in side effects or undesirable responses. Pharmacology involves the creation of medications that are intended to selectively attach to certain molecular targets, such as proteins or receptors, in order to achieve a desired therapeutic outcome. Nevertheless, owing to the intricate nature of biological systems, medications can potentially engage with additional molecules, leading to unintended effects on non-targeted areas. The range of symptoms can vary from minor to severe and might potentially affect the safety and effectiveness of the medicine. Gaining comprehension and reducing unintended impacts are crucial for the advancement of safer and more efficacious pharmaceuticals [48].

The ability of a medicinal material, such as a biologic or drug, to elicit an immune response in the body is known as immunogenicity. On rare occasions, the therapeutic agent may be recognized by the immune system as an outside invader, prompting an immunological response against it.

This may lead to the generation of antibodies that oppose the therapeutic intervention, reduce its effectiveness, or cause adverse reactions. For biologic drugs, such therapeutic proteins or monoclonal antibodies, which are derived from living things and may be seen as foreign by the immune system, immunogenicity is particularly crucial. Ensuring the safety and efficacy of biologic therapies requires an efficient management of their immunogenicity [48].

Both the unintended effects on non-target molecules and the potential to provoke an immune response are important obstacles in the process of creating drugs. The preclinical and clinical phases of drug development must thoroughly address these issues. Methods like structure-activity relationship investigations, computational modeling, and immunogenicity evaluation assays are used to anticipate and reduce these hazards. Furthermore, post-marketing surveillance and pharmacovigilance initiatives help to monitor and control unintended effects and immunogenicity in real-life scenarios [48].

3.3.1 CAUSES AND CONSEQUENCES OF OFF-TARGET EFFECTS

Off-target effects in nucleic acid delivery can occur for a variety of reasons related to the design, distribution, and interaction of nucleic acids with biological systems.

Nucleic acid sequences can exhibit similarities with unintended destinations in the genome, resulting in off-target interactions. This can lead to inadvertent suppression or stimulation of gene expression. This can lead to non-specific binding. Nucleic acids, like siRNA or ASOs, can attach to proteins or other molecules in the cell in a way that isn't specific, which can change how they work or how stable they are. Immunological activation can occur when nucleic acids, particularly those with specific sequences or changes, stimulate innate immunological responses, resulting in inflammation or other undesirable effects associated with the immune system. Another challenge: the vehicles or carriers used to move nucleic acids into cells may interact with biological parts, causing effects that were not intended on the intended areas. When cationic lipids or polymers are used in delivery systems, for example, they might break down cell membranes or cause immune responses. Intracellular trafficking refers to the movement of nucleic acids carried by viral vectors or nanoparticles within a cell. Improper execution of this trafficking could potentially release or localize the nucleic acids in unexpected areas of the cell, leading to off-target consequences [48].

3.3.2 IMMUNOGENECITY CONCERNS IN NUCLEIC ACID DELIVERY

The implications of targeting nucleic acids involve toxicity, lack of specificity, immunogenicity, and altered gene expression. Non-specific effects can lead to cellular toxicity or harm, affecting cell survival and operation. This can lead to detrimental effects on tissues or organs and jeopardize the safety of nucleic acid treatments. Loss of specificity means that nucleic acid-based therapies might have effects that aren't supposed to happen. This could lead to changes in gene expression or function that aren't wanted. This can diminish the therapeutic effectiveness and precision of the treatment. Non-specific interactions can trigger the immune system, leading to inflammation, immune cell activation, or antibody formation against the administered nucleic acids or delivery vehicles. This can undermine the safety and effectiveness of the treatment intervention. Off-target effects may cause unexpected alterations in gene expression patterns, resulting in physiological disturbances or disruptions in cellular processes. This can have cascading impacts on biological pathways and functions [48].

It's crucial to comprehend how nucleic acids function completely and to carefully enhance delivery methods, nucleic acid design, and delivery vehicle features in order to minimize unintended impacts during nucleic acid distribution. To improve the safety and specificity of nucleic acid-based therapeutics while minimizing off-target effects, we employ high-throughput screening, targeted delivery strategies, and computational modeling [48].

3.3.3 APPROACHES TO MINIMIZE OFF-TARGET EFFECTS AND IMMUNOGENICITY

Ensuring minimal off-target effects and immunogenicity during nucleic acid delivery is essential for the advancement of safe and efficient therapies. Here are several methodologies that have been substantiated by academic research:

1. **Nucleic Acid Design:** The deliberate creation of nucleic acids using well-selected sequences and chemical alterations might decrease unintended consequences and improve durability. Introducing alterations such as 2'-O-methyl, 2'-fluoro, or locked nucleic acids (LNAs) can enhance precision and decrease immunological activation [48]. Applying bioinformatics tools and algorithms to forecast possible unintended interactions and create nucleic acids that have minimal unintended effects [49].

2. **Delivery Vehicle Optimization:** It involves the modification of delivery vehicles, such as LNPs, polymeric nanoparticles, or viral vectors, to enhance their ability to target specific areas and reduce unintended interactions with non-target areas [16].

3. **Intracellular Trafficking Control:** The process of modifying the surface of delivery vehicles by attaching targeting ligands or shielding agents is done to improve specificity and decrease the likelihood of an immune response [50]. Intracellular trafficking control involves the manipulation of routes within cells to enhance the delivery of substances and reduce unintended effects. This can be achieved by utilizing cell-penetrating peptides or endosomal escape enhancers [51]. The objective is to create delivery systems that are sensitive to stimuli and can selectively release nucleic acids in the desired cellular compartment, hence minimizing interactions with unintended targets [41].

4. **Immunomodulatory Strategies:** It involves the use of immunomodulatory agents, such as Toll-like receptor (TLR) antagonists or immunosuppressive medicines, in delivery systems. The purpose is to decrease immune responses and minimize immunogenicity [52]. Modifying nucleic acids to possess immune-evasive characteristics, such as suppressing CpG or avoiding immunostimulatory motifs, in order to reduce immunological activation [53].

5. **Targeted Delivery Approaches:** By employing ligand-mediated targeting or cell-specific promoters, nucleic acids can be delivered to certain cell types or tissues, resulting in reduced off-target effects [54]. By utilizing tissue-specific delivery methods, such as ultrasound-mediated delivery or local injection techniques, the aim is to restrict the exposure of the treatment to certain tissues and

minimize any unintended effects on other parts of the body [55]. These approaches are now being studied to enhance the precision and safety of nucleic acid delivery systems. Although every technique has displayed potential in preclinical investigations, more verification via clinical trials and real-world implementations is required to establish their effectiveness in reducing off-target effects and immunogenicity [55].

3.4 TARGETED DELIVERY APPROACHES

3.4.1 RATIONALE FOR TARGETED DELIVERY

1. Targeted delivery in nucleic acid delivery is focused on providing precise administration to specific cells or tissues, while reducing unintended effects and enhancing the effectiveness of the therapy. By utilizing targeted delivery, nucleic acids can be carefully directed towards cells that express the desired antigen or receptor. This approach minimizes exposure to non-target cells and decreases the occurrence of off-target effects [54].
2. Targeted delivery methods can improve the specificity of nucleic acid distribution by using ligands or antibodies that detect cell surface markers or receptors specific to the target cells [50].
3. Targeted delivery of nucleic acids can decrease systemic exposure, therefore limiting the potential toxicity and deleterious consequences that may arise from off-target interactions [51].
4. Targeted delivery methods can enhance safety profiles by localizing nucleic acid distribution to specific tissues or organs, thus avoiding exposure to healthy tissues to therapeutic drugs [50].
5. Targeted delivery enables the administration of larger concentrations of nucleic acids directly, resulting in improved therapeutic results [40].
6. Targeted delivery systems can improve the effectiveness of gene silencing, gene editing, or gene expression modulation by raising the concentration of therapeutic nucleic acids in certain cells [57]. Tailored medicine refers to the use of targeted delivery methods to customize treatment tactics based on the molecular characteristics of specific patients or their diseases. This approach to affected cells or tissues allows for tailored therapeutic interventions [58].

7. Targeted techniques can enhance treatment responses and patient outcomes by customizing delivery systems to biomarkers or genetic signatures linked to certain disease subtypes [59]. Specialized delivery methods can be engineered to overcome biological obstacles like the blood-brain barrier or tumor microenvironment, allowing efficient transportation of nucleic acids to locations that are normally unreachable [60].
8. Targeted delivery techniques can improve the distribution and accumulation of nucleic acids at specific locations of action by using strategies to bypass or penetrate biological barriers [61]. These considerations emphasize the significance of focused delivery strategies in transporting nucleic acids to achieve heightened specificity, less toxicity, enhanced effectiveness, and tailored treatment methods [61].

3.4.2 STRATEGIES FOR TISSUE-SPECIFIC TARGETING

Precise targeting of certain tissues in the delivery of nucleic acids is essential to optimize the effectiveness of therapy while avoiding any unintended effects on non-targeted tissues. A strategy for tissue-specific targeting involves ligand-mediated targeting, cell-specific promoters, physical targeting methods, pH-responsive delivery systems, and tumor-targeting strategies.

3.4.3 LIGAND MEDIATED AND STIMULUS RESPONSIVE TARGETING

Ligand-mediated targeting involves the use of ligands that selectively attach to receptors or antigens that are excessively present on the outer surface of desired cells or tissues. This method allows for targeted delivery of nucleic acids to specific areas [51]. An instance of this is the frequent overexpression of folate receptors in cancer cells, leading to the development of folate-conjugated nanoparticles for the specific transport of nucleic acids to tumor tissues [63].

Cell-specific promoters are used to selectively activate the transcription and expression of therapeutic nucleic acids in target cells. This is achieved by including these promoters into viral vectors or expression cassettes [63]. This approach guarantees that the therapeutic impact is limited to particular cell types, while simultaneously reducing any unintended effects on non-target cells [64].

Physical targeting approaches involve the use of techniques such as ultrasound, magnetic targeting, or photoactivation to direct the delivery of nucleic acids to particular tissues or organs [65]. The aforementioned methods can optimize the gathering of nucleic acids at specific locations and boost the effectiveness of treatments, while reducing the overall exposure to the body and avoiding unintended effects on non-target areas [66]. pH-responsive delivery systems have the objective of creating delivery systems that are sensitive to changes in pH and can release nucleic acids specifically in acidic microenvironments of certain tissues or intracellular compartments [67].

This method allows for precise delivery to acidic environments, such as tumor tissues or endosomes, which improves the effectiveness of therapy and reduces unintended effects on other areas [68]. Utilizing the distinct features of tumor microenvironments, such as the presence of leaky blood vessels and the increased permeability and retention (EPR) effect, to passively accumulate nucleic acid delivery systems in tumor tissues [69]. The specificity and therapeutic results of delivery vehicles can be improved by modifying their surface with tumor-homing peptides or antibodies, which enhances tumor targeting [70]. These methodologies provide different methods for delivering targeted distribution of nucleic acids to specific tissues, each with its own benefits and applications in different disease scenarios [70].

3.5 NOVEL DELIVERY VECTORS AND FORMULATIONS TECHNIQUES

3.5.1 VIRAL VECTORS: ADVANTAGES, LIMITATIONS, AND ADVANCEMENTS

Vectors are safe variations of viruses that are employed in the production of vaccinations, medicinal therapies, and the transfer of genetic material to cells. To transfer genetic information to cells, vectors are employed. In gene therapy and medication delivery, vectors and carriers are essential components. There are two different kinds of vectors: non-viral and viral.

The most significant method of transferring genes to modify a particular cell type or tissue and express therapeutic genes is using viral vectors. RNA and DNA viruses with single-stranded (ss) or double-stranded (ds) genomes are the two types of viral vectors [71]. Herpes simplex viruses, baculoviruses, adeno-associated viruses, poxviruses, γ-retroviruses, lentiviruses, and adenoviruses (Ads) are a few examples of different vectors. Some of the viral vectors have been discussed in subsections.

3.5.1.1 ADENOVIRUS

Uncovered dsDNA Adenoviruses have the ability to package up to 7.5 kilobases of foreign DNA, which allows them to temporarily express the target gene episomally in a wide variety of host cells. While improved second and third generation vectors with deletions have been shown to cause significantly reduced immunogenicity, the exclusive adenovirus vectors elicit robust immune responses. Adenoviruses are a group of viruses that may infect the brain, intestines, eyes, lungs, and respiratory system. In addition to pink eye, they can induce fever, coughing, sore throats, and diarrhea [71].

3.5.1.2 RETROVIRUSES

The genetic substance of these viruses is RNA. They are retroviruses and are members of the order Retroviridae. By use of reverse transcription, it transforms the RNA-infected cells into DNA. The virus then begins to replicate when its DNA is introduced into the host cell. For instance, HIV stands for human immunodeficiency virus. Replication-defective retroviral vectors are more frequently designed by replacing retroviral sequences; however, replication-competent vectors can also be created by appending sequences to pre-existing viruses. Furthermore, in comparison to replication-defective vectors, replication-competent vectors can tolerate far less foreign DNA than can failure-prone vectors. A single regulator located in the 5′ long terminal repetition (LTR) drives the development of retroviral proteins in the majority of naturally generated oncogenic retroviruses. Several viral coding areas are expressed by alternatively splicing the genome. Vector design, nevertheless, is not restricted to employing an individual retroviral promoter with different splicing techniques. Other tactics include using internal ribosome entry sites (IRESs), reversing the position of genes, and utilizing numerous promoters [71].

3.5.1.3 POXVIRUS

Since poxvirus vector interventions may have a permanent effect on the host's immune system, they have been thoroughly researched for both curative purposes and the creation of vaccines. More significantly, poxviruses have been developed as cancer therapies thanks to their oncolytic qualities. With encouraging outcomes, two poxviruses—vaccinia virus (VACV) and myxoma virus (MYXV)—have been thoroughly investigated as virotherapeutics. Following achievement in phase I/II clinical trials, vaccine viral vectors have made their way into the clinic where they are being investigated as oncolytic therapies for several cancer types [72].

3.5.1.4 ADENO ASSOCIATED VIRUSES (AAV)

AAV vectors are the most popular method of delivering genes to treat a wide range of human illnesses. Gene therapy has grown significantly as a result of recent developments in creating therapeutically appealing AAV capsids, refining genome designs, and utilizing cutting-edge biotechnologies [21]. One of the gene therapy vehicles that is being researched the most is the AAV. It was first identified as an adenovirus preparatory contamination.

3.5.1.5 BACULOVIRUSES

The baculovirus is a commonly used and very efficient way to produce recombinant protein in insect cells. Synthetic baculoviruses are a desirable option for producing big eukaryotic protein molecules at a high scale. Large DNA inserts may be handled in the AcNPV genome due to the elasticity of its sheath. In contrast to alternative systems, the baculovirus production technique demonstrates substantial yields together with appropriate glycosylation and further changes crucial to its immunogenic capability. Therefore, a large number of recombinant proteins and commercialized vaccines have been produced using the baculovirus–insect cell transcription method. Recombinant baculovirus production is done in two stages. Prior to being introduced into the baculovirus genome by identical recombination in insect cells to produce recombinant offspring, foreign genes have to be subcloned onto an exchange vehicle and maintained in *E. coli* [74].

3.5.1.6 HERPES SIMPLEX VIRUS (HSV)

HSV is an extremely cytotoxic human infection with a big and complicated genome that encodes at least 80 DNA products. At first glance, HSV is not the best vector for delivering genes. The human herpesvirus group is a significant group of viruses that install themselves in different tissues during the course of the host's life. HSV is a complicated human neurotrophic virus which enters the sensory nerve ends supplying the location of addition and is retrogradely shipped to the nucleus of sensory neurons following the initial infection and lytic multiplication at the human perimeter, usually at oral or sexually transmitted epithelial cells [75].

3.5.2 NON-VIRAL VECTORS: LIPOSOMES, NANOPARTICLES, AND POLYMERS

Gene therapy uses non-viral vectors, which can be chemical or particle-based, to introduce genetic material into a range of cells, tissues, and entire organs with the purpose of healing or enhancing disease. Polymers, lipids, inorganic particles, or mixtures of other kinds are examples of non-viral vectors. Non-viral vectors have lower cytotoxicity, immunogenicity, and mutagenesis than viral vectors, which has led scientists to find a unique delivery method and advance the area of gene therapy [76]. Furthermore, there are several non-viral vectors which are reported in the subsections below.

3.5.2.1 POLYMERS

The utilization of polymers as a non-viral vector presents several advantages: (i) facile and affordable synthesis; (ii) biodegradability of diverse polymers; (iii) non-immunogenicity; (iv) extensibility; and (v) ability to form polyelectrolyte complexes that protect nucleic acid compounds from distinct proteins. The four main kinds of production procedures are monomer polymerization, evaporated solvent emulsification–solvent dispersion, and solvent relocation. Many polymers have found broad application in delivery systems, such as dendrimers, polylactic acids (PLA), polyethylene (PEI), and chitosan, or CS [76].

3.5.2.2 DENDRIMERS

With a hyperbranched, three-dimensional framework, dendrimers are linear polymer chains that have a dendron on each repeated unit. By using synthetic techniques, their functioning, size, and level of branching may all be modified and regulated [77]. Conversely, dendrimers have a range of peripheral groups with functions, including peptides, antibodies, transferrin, biotin, folic acid, and galactose, that may be effectively altered using surface modification techniques.

3.5.2.3 GOLD NANOPARTICLES (AUNPS)

Their biocompatibility and stability are good. AuNPs exhibit a high drug loading due to the quantum effect of size and a high surface area-to-volume ratios [78]. In the meantime, gold nanoparticles are often utilized in immunological analysis, drug administration, and the identification of tumor cells and microbes due to their ease of modification and ability to enhance the pharmacokinetics of numerous medications.

3.5.2.4 MESOPOROUS SILICA NANOPARTICLES

1992 saw the Mobile Device Science and Technology Company create the first organized mesoporous silica (MCM type). Later, a range of enhanced techniques were used to manufacture several different forms of mesoporous silica nanomaterials (MSNs) [79].

3.5.2.5 CARBON NANOTUBES

CNTs have a significant aspect ratio and an enormous surface area since their dimensions and length are in the range of microns and nano, respectively [27]. CNTs have been applied in many biological domains, including drug transport and cancer therapy, because of their exceptional qualities, which include tremendous electrical and thermal efficiency, outstanding tear strength, remarkable chemical stability, and excellent adsorption capacity.

3.6 INTERPLAY BETWEEN DELIVERY SYSTEMS AND BIOLOGICAL BARRIERS

The delivery of drugs to a target site involves crossing various biological barriers, which depends upon the degree and nature of the obstruction to flux, and potential approaches, which depend on the tissue, the drug, and a number of factors. Biological barriers are present throughout the body, and various approaches, like chemical, physical, and biomolecule-mediated approaches, to overcome biological barriers have been developed for a variety of anatomic locations [34].

3.6.1 ENGINEERING DELIVERY SYSTEMS TO OVERCOME BIOLOGICAL BARRIERS

By overcoming different biological barriers, engineered delivery mechanisms like nanoparticles (ENPs) have the potential to be harmful. They may also alter the physicochemical characteristics of biofluid and the physiological and medical conditions of the human organism. Because people are being exposed to different synthetic nanoparticles (ENPs), which can be hazardous if they traverse biological obstacles and gather in critical organs, the use of nanoparticle-based goods and techniques is growing quickly. ENPs can be toxic when they enter the human body. To cause adverse outcomes, ENPs must cross biological barriers that protect human organs from invasion by harmful agents such as viruses and bacteria. ENPs exposed via dermal contact, inhalation, or oral administration need to pass through the skin, the alveolar air–blood barrier, or the intestinal barrier to enter the blood circulation because these biological barriers are our first line of defense [74].

3.6.2 ENGINEERING DELIVERY SYSTEM TO OVERCOME BIOLOGICAL BARRIERS

There are two possible pathways to cross a biological barrier. Firstly, ENPs can cross the barrier via a receptor; for example, lactoferrin receptor-mediated transcytosis was involved in the translocation of both PEG-coated Fe_3O_4 NPs and carboxylated polystyrene NPs across the *in vitro* BBB models and rat BBB. Secondly, ENPs can cross the biological barrier via paracellular pathways by inducing dysfunction of tight junctions. ENPs, such as gold NPs, silver NPs, TiO_2, NPs, ZnO NPs, and Al_2O_3 NPs, are reported to increase the permeability of the BBB, BPB by reducing the expression of various tight junction-related genes or proteins, including *Zonula occludens*-1 (ZO-1), claudin-5, and occludin. Loss of tight junctions may result in shedding of epithelial/endothelial cells of biological barriers [56].

3.6.3 IMPORTANCE OF IN VITRO AND IN VIVO MODELS FOR EVALUATING DELIVERY EFFICACY

The structural integrity and functions of biological barriers can vary under different physiological and pathological conditions. ENPs cross the barriers by exhibiting different efficiency; the immature barriers have higher permeability than the mature ones, and ENPs may cross the immature barriers more easily. For example, the translocation of gold NPs from lungs to the rest of the body is significantly higher in infants than that in adults. During pregnancy, formation of mature placenta occurs at gestational day; the gold NPs exposed prior to embryonic day 11.5 crossed the placental barriers and entered the fetuses, while after this gestational timepoint, fewer gold NPs transferred to fetus were found. As an example, the trans-intestinal efficiency of silver NPs was significantly reduced in overweight mice compared to normal mice, as most of the NPs were trapped in the fat surrounding the intestine. More susceptible animal models as well as suitable *ex vivo* or *in vitro* models should be developed for a better understanding on how physiological and pathological conditions affect the crossing efficiency of ENPs through various biological barriers [56].

3.7 CLINICAL TRANSLATION AND FUTURE PERSPECTIVES

3.7.1 CURRENT STATUS OF NUCLEIC ACID BASED THERAPIES IN CLINICAL TRIALS

ENPs are known to cause toxicity by crossing biological barriers via both transcellular and paracellular pathways. Various experimental data shows that activation of various signaling pathways and down regulation of tight junction proteins, various factors that affect the crossing efficiency includes physicochemical properties of ENPs, bio- modification of ENPs during their translocation in the body, and physiological and pathological conditions of the animal body. The complexity of *in vivo* animal models and the development of advanced *in vitro* or *ex vivo* models, improved *in vivo* models, such as susceptible animal models, is necessary. High-throughput screening assays are highly valuable. Table 3.1 indicates a list of FDA-approved nucleic acid therapeutics. Applications of machine learning for a better understanding of barrier crossing efficiency and development of "safe-by-design" are expected with recent technical advantages in big data and artificial intelligence [56].

3.7.2 REGULATORY CHALLENGES AND CONSIDERATIONS

Nucleic acid (NA) treatments have been increasingly popular over the past 10 years, yet there remain several clinical problems, including inadequate kinetics and pharmaceutical dynamics. One important way to keep NA treatments from becoming very popular is to ensure that they are delivered to the intended organs. Off-target adverse reactions need to be closely watched since negative charges, a hydrophilic nature, and sensitivity to enzyme breakdown can all affect how well NA medicines are delivered. In order for the product to be developed on time, several problems must be resolved. Frequently suggested actions to increase NA delivery include chemical, sugar ribose, and terminal alterations, including moieties that penetrate cells [56].

3.7.3 FUTURE DIRECTIONS AND EMERGING TECHNOLOGIES IN NUCLEIC ACID (NA) DELIVERY

Over the last few decades, the influence of NA therapies in the pharmaceutical industry has been linked to premium production and drug delivery. Even though NA delivery has advanced significantly, there are still important factors to take into account when analyzing new excipients and their role in NA therapies. As of right now, 23 nucleic acid therapies have received approval; Table 3.2 lists those that are still undergoing phase 3 trials. Scientists advise closely evaluating stability at all phases of the

TABLE 3.1 List of FDA Approved Nucleic Acid Therapeutics

Product	Gene target	Indication	Route	Approval year	Company
		Antisense Oligonucleotides (ASOs)			
Vitravene, fomivirsen	Cytomegalovirus gene (UL123)	Cytomegalovirus infection	Intravitreal	1998 (withdrawn 2002/2006)	Ionis Pharmaceuticals
Exondys 51, eteplirsen	Dystrophin (exon 51)	Duchenne muscular dystrophy	Intrathecal	2016	Sarepta Therapeutics
Tegsedi, inotersen	Transthyretin (TTR)	TTR-mediated amyloidosis	Subcutaneous	2018	Ionis Pharmaceuticals
Spinraza, nusinersen	Survival of motor neuron 2 (SMN2)	Spinal muscular atrophy	Intrathecal	2016	Ionis Pharmaceuticals
Kynamro, mipomersen	Apolipoprotein B-100	Hypercholesterolemia	Subcutaneous	2013	Ionis Pharmaceuticals
Waylivra, Volanesoren	Apolipoprotein CIII	Familial chylomicronemia syndrome	Subcutaneous	2019	Ionis Pharmaceuticals/ Akcea
Vyondys 53, golodirsen	Dystrophin (exon 53)	Duchenne muscular dystrophy	Subcutaneous	2019 (confirmatory trial required)	Sarepta Therapeutics
Amondys 45, casimersen	Dystrophin (exon 45)	Duchenne muscular dystrophy	Subcutaneous	2021	Sarepta Therapeutics
		GalNAc–siRNA Conjugates			
Givlaari, Givosiran	ALAS1	Acute hepatic porphyrias	Subcutaneous	2019	Alnylam Pharmaceuticals
Leqvio, inclisiran	PCSK9	Hypercholesterolemia	Subcutaneous	2020	Novartis/Alnylam Pharmaceuticals
Oxlum, lumasiran	Glycolate oxidase	Primary hyperoxaluria type 1	Subcutaneous	2020	Alnylam Pharmaceuticals

TABLE 3.1 *(Continued)*

Product	Gene target	Indication	Route	Approval year	Company
		LNP-RNA			
Onpattro, patisiran	TTR siRNA	TTR-mediated amyloidosis	Intravenous	2018	Alnylam Pharmaceuticals
Comirnaty, tozinameran	SARS-CoV-2 spike protein mRNA	COVID-19 (FDA, emergency use; Switzerland, full approval)	Intramuscular	2020	BioNTech/Pfizer
mRNA-1273	SARS-CoV-2 spike protein mRNA	COVID-19 (FDA, emergency use)	Intramuscular	2020	Moderna/NIAID/BARDA
		AAV Vectors			
Glybera, alipogene tiparvovec	Lipoprotein lipase (LPL) (AAV1)	LPL deficiency	Intramuscular	2012 (withdrawn 2017)	uniQure
Luxturna, voretigene neparvovec-rzyl	RPE65 (AAV2)	Leber congenital amaurosis	Subretinal	2017	Spark Therapeutics
Zolgensma, onasemnogene abeparvovec	SMN1 (AAV9)	Spinal muscular atrophy	Intravenous	2019	AveXis/Novartis
Vaxzevria, AZD1222, ChAdOx1 nCoV-19	SARS-CoV-2 spike protein DNA (ChAdOx1)	COVID-19 (FDA and EMA emergency use)	Intramuscular	2021	AstraZeneca
Ad26.COV2.S	SARS-CoV-2 spike protein DNA (Ad26)	COVID-19 (FDA and EMA emergency use)	Intramuscular	2021	Johnson and Johnson
Convidecia, Ad5-nCoV	SARS-CoV-2 spike protein DNA (Ad5)	COVID-19 (Approved in China)	Intramuscular	2021	CanSinoBIO

TABLE 3.2 List of Under Trial (Phase-3) Nucleic Acid Therapeutics

Product	Gene target	Indication	Route	Clinical trial identifier(s)	Company
			ASOs		
Tominersen	Huntingtin	Huntington's disease	Intrathecal	NCT03761849	Ionis Pharmaceuticals/Roche
Tofersen, BIIB067	SOD-1	Amyotrophic lateral sclerosis	Intrathecal	NCT02623699	Ionis Pharmaceuticals/Biogen
			GalNAc–siRNA Conjugates		
Fitusiran, ALN-AT3sc	SERPINC1	Hemophilia and rare bleeding disorders	Subcutaneous	NCT03417102, NCT03417245, NCT03549871, NCT03754790	Sanofi/Alnylam Pharmaceuticals
Vutrisiran, ALN-TTRsc02	TTR	TTR-mediated amyloidosis	Subcutaneous	NCT03759379	Alnylam Pharmaceuticals
Nedosiran, DCR-PHXC	Lactate dehydrogenase	Primary hyperoxaluria	Subcutaneous	NCT04042402	Dicerna Pharmaceuticals
			GalNAc–ASO Conjugates		
AKCEA-TTR-LRx	TTR	TTR-mediated amyloid polyneuropathy or cardiomyopathy	Subcutaneous	NCT04136184, NCT04136171	Akcea/ Ionis Pharmaceuticals
Pelacarsen, AKCEA-APO(a)-LRx	Apoliprotein A1	Cardiovascular disease	Subcutaneous	NCT04023552	Akcea/ Ionis Pharmaceuticals
			LNPs		
Onpattro, patisiran	TTR siRNA	Cardiomyopathy-associated TTR-mediated amyloidosis	Intravenous	NCT03997383	Alnylam Pharmaceuticals
			AAV Vectors		
Lumevoq, lenadogene Nolparvovec, GS010	ND4 (AAV2)	Leber hereditary optic neuropathy	Intravitreal	NCT03293524, NCT02652767, NCT02652780, NCT03153293	GenSight Biologics

TABLE 3.2 *(Continued)*

Product	Gene target	Indication	Route	Clinical trial identifier(s)	Company
AVXS-101	SMN2 (AAV9)	Spinal muscular atrophy	Intrathecal	NCT03505099, NCT03461289, NCT03306277, NCT03837184	Novartis
Valoctocogene roxaparvovec, BMN 270	FVIII (AAV5)	Hemophilia A	Intravenous	NCT03370913, NCT04323098, NCT03392974	BioMarin Pharmaceutical
Etranacogene dezaparvovec AMT-061	FIX-Padua (AAV5)	Hemophilia B	Intravenous	NCT03569891	uniQure
Fidanacogene elaparvovec, SPK-9001,	FIX-Padua (AAV100)	Hemophilia B	Intravenous	NCT03587116	Pfizer, Spark Therapeutics
Timrepigene emparvovec, NSR-REP1	REP1 (AAV2)	Chloridemia	Subretinal	NCT03496012	Biogen/Nightstar Therapeutics
Olenasufligene relduparvovec, LYS-SAF302	SGSH (AAVrh10)	MPS-IIIA	Intracerebral	NCT03612869	Lysogene
NSR-RPGR	RPGR (AAV8)	X-linked retinitis pigmentosa	Subretinal	NCT03116113	Biogen/ Nightstar Therapeutics
FLT180a	FIX (AAVs3)	Hemophilia B	Intravenous	NCT03641703	Freeline Therapeutics
Adenovirus Serotype Vectors					
Sputnik V, Gam-COVID-Vac	SARS-CoV-2 spike protein (Ad26/Ad5)	COVID-19	Intramuscular	NCT04530396	Gamaleya Research Institute

creation of NA therapies, especially for extremely diluted NA medicines. The supply of vitamin A supplementation is a main issue throughout the medical use of vutrisiran because it is crucial for tracking deficits induced by the use of different NA therapies, such as vutrisiran, which has created vitamin A insufficiency in patients. Monitoring of the side effects and preventative measures is necessary for NA therapies treatment [73].

ACKNOWLEDGMENT

None

CONFLICT OF INTEREST

The authors declare no conflict of interest.

FUNDING

None

KEYWORDS

- **advancing personalized medicines.**
- **cellular uptake**
- **genetic abnormalities**
- **immunogenicity**
- **intracellular barriers**
- **macrophages**
- **nucleic acid delivery**
- **targeted delivery**
- **viral vectors**

REFERENCES

1. Sridharan, K., & Gogtay, N. J. (2016). Therapeutic nucleic acids: Current clinical status. *British Journal of Clinical Pharmacology, 82*, 659–672.
2. Busignies, V., Charrueau, C., Tchoreloff, P., & Escriou, V. (2017). Chapter 6–Nanostructures for oral delivery of therapeutic nucleic acids. In E. Andronescu & A. M. Grumezescu (Eds.), *Nanostructures for Oral Medicine* (pp. 147–172). Elsevier.
3. Breaker, R. R., & Joyce, G. F. (2014). The expanding view of RNA and DNA function. *Chemistry & Biology, 21*, 1059–1065.
4. Nguyen, J., & Szoka, F. C. (2012). Nucleic acid delivery: The missing pieces of the puzzle? *Accounts of Chemical Research, 45*, 1153–1162.
5. Friedmann, T., & Roblin, R. (1972). Gene therapy for human genetic disease? *Science, 175*, 949–955.
6. Anderson, E. J., Rouphael, N. G., Widge, A. T., Jackson, L. A., Roberts, P. C., Makhene, M., Chappell, J. D., Denison, M. R., Stevens, L. J., Pruijssers, A. J., McDermott, A. B., Flach, B., Lin, B. C., Doria-Rose, N. A., O'Dell, S., Schmidt, S. D., Corbett, K. S., Swanson, P. A., 2nd, Padilla, M., & Beigel, J. H. (2020). Safety and immunogenicity of SARS-CoV-2 mRNA-1273 vaccine in older adults. *The New England Journal of Medicine, 383*, 2427–2438.
7. Kulkarni, J. A., Witzigmann, D., Thomson, S. B., Chen, S., Leavitt, B. R., Cullis, P. R., & van der Meel, R. (2021). The current landscape of nucleic acid therapeutics. *Nature Nanotechnology, 16*, 630–643.
8. Krützfeldt, J., Rajewsky, N., Braich, R., Rajeev, K. G., Tuschl, T., Manoharan, M., & Stoffel, M. (2005). Silencing of microRNAs *in vivo* with 'antagomirs.' *Nature, 438*, 685–689.
9. Yamada, Y. (2021). Nucleic acid drugs—Current status, issues, and expectations for exosomes. *Cancers, 13*.
10. Hammond, S. M., Bernstein, E., Beach, D., & Hannon, G. J. (2000). An RNA-directed nuclease mediates post-transcriptional gene silencing in Drosophila cells. *Nature, 404*, 293–296.
11. Springer, A. D., & Dowdy, S. F. (2018). GalNAc-siRNA conjugates: Leading the way for delivery of RNAi therapeutics. *Nucleic Acid Therapeutics, 28*, 109–118.
12. Nair, J. K., Willoughby, J. L. S., Chan, A., Charisse, K., Alam, M. R., Wang, Q., Hoekstra, M., Kandasamy, P., Kel'in, A. V., Milstein, S., Taneja, N., O'Shea, J., Shaikh, S., Zhang, L., van der Sluis, R. J., Jung, M. E., Akinc, A., Hutabarat, R., Kuchimanchi, S., & Manoharan, M. (2014). Multivalent N-acetyl galactosamine-conjugated siRNA localizes in hepatocytes and elicits robust RNAi-mediated gene silencing. *Journal of the American Chemical Society, 136*, 16958–16961.
13. Stockert, R. J. (1995). The asialoglycoprotein receptor: Relationships between structure, function, and expression. *Physiological Reviews, 75*, 591–609.
14. Felgner, P. L., Gadek, T. R., Holm, M., Roman, R., Chan, H. W., Wenz, M., Northrop, J. P., Ringold, G. M., & Danielsen, M. (1987). Lipofection: A highly efficient, lipid-mediated DNA-transfection procedure. *Proceedings of the National Academy of Sciences of the United States of America, 84*, 7413–7417.

15. Jayaraman, M., Ansell, S. M., Mui, B. L., Tam, Y. K., Chen, J., Du, X., Butler, D., Eltepu, L., Matsuda, S., Narayanannair, J. K., Rajeev, K. G., Hafez, I. M., Akinc, A., Maier, M. A., Tracy, M. A., Cullis, P. R., Madden, T. D., Manoharan, M., & Hope, M. J. (2012). Maximizing the potency of siRNA lipid nanoparticles for hepatic gene silencing *in vivo*. *Angewandte Chemise International Edition, 51*, 8529–8533.
16. Akinc, A., Querbes, W., De, S., Qin, J., Frank-Kamenetsky, M., Jayaprakash, K. N., Jayaraman, M., Rajeev, K. G., Cantley, W. L., Dorkin, J. R., Butler, J. S., Qin, L., Racie, T., Sprague, A., Fava, E., Zeigerer, A., Hope, M. J., Zerial, M., Sah, D. W., & Maier, M. A. (2010). Targeted delivery of RNAi therapeutics with endogenous and exogenous ligand-based mechanisms. *Molecular Therapy, 18*, 1357–1364.
17. Chen, S., Tam, Y. Y. C., Lin, P. J. C., Sung, M. M. H., Tam, Y. K., & Cullis, P. R. (2016). Influence of particle size on the *in vivo* potency of lipid nanoparticle formulations of siRNA. *Journal of Controlled Release, 235*, 236–244.
18. Wilson, J. M. (2009). Lessons learned from the gene therapy trial for ornithine transcarboxylase deficiency. *Molecular Genetics and Metabolism, 96*, 151–157.
19. Dunbar, C. E., High, K. A., Joung, J. K., Kohn, D. B., Ozawa, K., & Sadelain, M. (2018). Gene therapy comes of age. *Science, 359*.
20. Naldini, L. (2015). Gene therapy returns to center stage. *Nature, 526*, 351–360.
21. Wang, D., Tai, P. W. L., & Gao, G. (2019). Adeno-associated virus vector as a platform for gene therapy delivery. *Nature Reviews Drug Discovery, 18*(5), 358–378. https://doi.org/10.1038/s41573-019-0012-9 (accessed on 23rd June 2025).
22. Prakash, T. P. (2011). An overview of sugar-modified oligonucleotides for antisense therapeutics. *Chemistry & Biodiversity, 8*, 1616–1641.
23. Eckstein, F. (2014). Phosphorothioates, essential components of therapeutic oligonucleotides. *Nucleic Acid Therapeutics, 24*, 374–387.
24. Geary, R. S., Norris, D., Yu, R., & Bennett, C. F. (2015). Pharmacokinetics, biodistribution and cell uptake of antisense oligonucleotides. *Advanced Drug Delivery Reviews, 87*, 46–51.
25. Yu, R. Z., Grundy, J. S., & Geary, R. S. (2013). Clinical pharmacokinetics of second-generation antisense oligonucleotides. *Expert Opinion on Drug Metabolism & Toxicology, 9*, 169–182.
26. Crooke, S. T., Baker, B. F., Xia, S., Yu, R. Z., Viney, N. J., Wang, Y., Tsimikas, S., & Geary, R. S. (2019). Integrated assessment of the clinical performance of GalNAc (3)-conjugated 2′-O-methoxyethyl chimeric antisense oligonucleotides: I. Human volunteer experience. *Nucleic Acid Therapeutics, 29*, 16–32.
27. Liu, X., Tao, H., Yang, K., Zhang, S., Lee, S. T., & Liu, Z. (2011). Optimization of surface chemistry on single-walled carbon nanotubes for *in vivo* photothermal ablation of tumors. *Biomaterials, 32*(1), 144–151. https://doi.org/10.1016/j.biomaterials.2010.08.096 (accessed on 23rd June 2025).
28. Balaphas, A., Meyer, J., Sadoul, R., Morel, P., Gonelle-Gispert, C., & Bühler, L. H. (2019). Extracellular vesicles: Future diagnostic and therapeutic tools for liver disease and regeneration. *Journal of Hepatology, 39*, 1801–1817.
29. Zhang, Y., Liu, Q., Zhang, X., Huang, H., Tang, S., Chai, Y., Xu, Z., Li, M., Chen, X., Liu, J., & Yang, C. (2022). Recent advances in exosome-mediated nucleic acid delivery for cancer therapy. *Journal of Nanobiotechnology, 20*, 279.

30. Gurunathan, S., Kang, M. H., Jeyaraj, M., Qasim, M., & Kim, J. H. (2019). Review of the isolation, characterization, biological function, and multifarious therapeutic approaches of exosomes. *Cells, 8*, 307.
31. Vyas, N., & Dhawan, J. (2017). Exosomes: Mobile platforms for targeted and synergistic signaling across cell boundaries. *Cellular and Molecular Life Sciences, 74*, 1567–1576.
32. Sinani, G., Durgun, M. E., Cevher, E., & Özsoy, Y. (2023). Polymeric-micelle-based delivery systems for nucleic acids. *Pharmaceutics, 15*, 2021.
33. Harada, A., & Kataoka, K. (2018). Polyion complex micelle formation from double-hydrophilic block copolymers composed of charged and non-charged segments in aqueous media. *Polymer Journal, 50*, 95–100.
34. Yang, R., Wei, T., Goldberg, H., Wang, W., Cullion, K., & Kohane, D. S. (2017). Getting drugs across biological barriers. *Advanced Materials, 29*(37), 1606596.
35. Timotievich, E. D., Shilovskiy, I. P., & Khaitov, M. R. (2023). Cell-penetrating peptides as vehicles for delivery of therapeutic nucleic acids: Mechanisms and application in medicine. *Biochemistry (Moscow), 88*, 1800–1817.
36. Jiang, J. (2021). Cell-penetrating peptide-mediated nano vaccine delivery. *Current Drug Targets, 22*, 896–912.
37. Hamilton, A. G., Swingle, K. L., & Mitchell, M. J. (2023). Biotechnology: Overcoming biological barriers to nucleic acid delivery using lipid nanoparticles. *PLOS Biology, 21*, e3002105.
38. Malefyt, A. P., Walton, S. P., & Chan, C. (2012). Endocytosis pathways for nucleic acid therapeutics. *Nano LIFE, 2*, 1241005.
39. Manzanares, D., & Ceña, V. (2020). Endocytosis: The nanoparticle and submicron nano compounds gateway into the cell. *Pharmaceutics, 12*.
40. Li, J., Xu, J., Yan, C., Wang, J., & Zhang, Y. (2018). Engineering targeted mRNA nanoparticles for cancer therapy. *Advanced Science, 5*, 1–11.
41. Conner, S. D., & Schmid, S. L. (2003). Regulated portals of entry into the cell. *Nature, 422*, 37–44.
42. Khalil, I. A., Kogure, K., Akita, H., & Harashima, H. (2006). Uptake pathways and subsequent intracellular trafficking in nonviral gene delivery. *Pharmacological Reviews, 58*, 32–45.
43. Kirkham, M., & Parton, R. G. (2005). Clathrin-independent endocytosis: New insights into caveolae and non-caveolar lipid raft carriers. *Biochemical et Biophysical Acta, 1745*, 273–286.
44. Narum, S., Deal, B., Ogasawara, H., Mancuso, J. N., Zhang, J., & Salaita, K. (2024). An endosomal escape Trojan horse platform to improve cytosolic delivery of nucleic acids. *ACS Nano, 18*, 6186–6201.
45. Pei, D., & Buyanova, M. (2019). Overcoming endosomal entrapment in drug delivery. *Bioconjugate Chemistry, 30*, 273–283.
46. Regen, S. L. (2021). Membrane-disrupting molecules as therapeutic agents: A cautionary note. *JACS Au, 1*, 3–7.
47. Varkouhi, A. K., Scholte, M., Storm, G., & Haisma, H. J. (2011). Endosomal escape pathways for delivery of biologicals. *Journal of Controlled Release, 151*, 220–228.

48. Swayze, E. E., Bhat, B., Vickers, T. A., Crooke, S. T., Lima, W. F., & Griffey, R. H. (2007). Antisense oligonucleotides containing locked nucleic acid improve potency but cause significant hepatotoxicity in animals. *Nucleic Acids Research, 35*, 687–700.
49. Birmingham, A., Anderson, E. M., Reynolds, A., Ilsley-Tyree, D., Leake, D., Fedorov, Y., Baskerville, S., Maksimova, E., Robinson, K., Karpilow, J., & Hannon, G. J. (2006). 3′ UTR seed matches, but not overall identity, are associated with RNAi off-targets. *Nature Methods, 3*, 199–204.
50. Lee, H., Lytton-Jean, A. K. R., Chen, Y., Love, K. T., Park, A. I., Karagiannis, E. D., Sehgal, A., Yen, Y. C., Fire, A. Z., & Anderson, D. G. (2013). Principles and applications of mRNA delivery systems. *Advanced Drug Delivery Reviews, 65*, 499–509.
51. Wang, J., Lu, Z., Wientjes, M. G., & Au, J. L. S. (2018). Mechanisms of cell-penetrating peptides for intracellular delivery of nucleic acids. *Frontiers in Pharmacology, 9*, 1–9.
52. Kranz, L. M., Diken, M., Haas, H., Kreiter, S., Loquai, C., Reuter, K. C., Meng, M., Fritz, D., Vascotto, F., Hefesha, H., Grunwitz, C., Vormehr, M., Hüsemann, Y., Selmi, A., Kuhn, A. N., Buck, J., Derhovanessian, E., Rae, R., Attig, S., & Sahin, U. (2016). Systemic RNA delivery to dendritic cells exploits antiviral defense for cancer immunotherapy. *Nature, 534*, 396–401.
53. Judge, A. D., Sood, V., Shaw, J. R., Fang, D., McClintock, K., & MacLachlan, I. (2005). Sequence-dependent stimulation of the mammalian innate immune response by synthetic siRNA. *Nature Biotechnology, 23*, 457–462.
54. Davis, M. E., Zuckerman, J. E., Choi, C. H. J., Seligson, D., Tolcher, A., Alabi, C. A., Yen, Y., Heidel, J. D., & Ribas, A. (2010). Evidence of RNAi in humans from systemically administered siRNA via targeted nanoparticles. *Nature, 464*, 1067–1070.
55. Tachibana, R., Uchida, S., Ogino, K., Ishihara, T., & Kanazawa, T. (2016). Ultrasound-mediated delivery of siRNA and a chemotherapeutic drug by using microbubble technology. *Biomaterials, 82*, 176–185.
56. Jia, J., Wang, Z., Yue, T., Su, G., Teng, C., & Yan, B. (2020). Crossing biological barriers by engineered nanoparticles. *Chemical Research in Toxicology, 33*(5), 1055–1060.
57. Peer, D., Karp, J. M., Hong, S., Farokhzad, O. C., Margalit, R., & Langer, R. (2007). Nanocarriers as an emerging platform for cancer therapy. *Nature Nanotechnology, 2*, 751–760.
58. Bobbin, M. L., & Rossi, J. J. (2016). RNA interference (RNAi)-based therapeutics: Delivering on the promise? *Annual Review of Pharmacology and Toxicology, 56*, 103–122.
59. Guo, S., Lin, C., Xu, Z., Zhang, X., & Zhang, Y. (2019). Targeted delivery of therapeutic nucleic acids to subcellular compartments for precision medicine. *Advanced Drug Delivery Reviews, 134*, 83–101.
60. Hrkach, J., Von Hoff, D., Ali, M. M., Andrianova, E., Auer, J., Campbell, T., De Witt, D., Figa, M., Figueiredo, M., Horhota, A., Low, S., McDonnell, K., Peeke, E., Retnarajan, B., Sabnis, A., Schnipper, E., Song, J. J., Song, Y. H., Summa, J., & Zale, S. (2012). Preclinical development and clinical translation of a PSMA-targeted docetaxel nanoparticle with a differentiated pharmacological profile. *Science Translational Medicine, 4*, 128ra39.

61. Xiong, Q., Li, Y., Fan, J., Chen, H., & Zhang, Y. (2016). A versatile click chemistry strategy for facile synthesis of targeted stealth polymer-coated iron oxide nanoparticles. *Chemical Communications, 52*, 6462–6465.
62. Gabizon, A., Shmeeda, H., Horowitz, A. T., Zalipsky, S., & Barenholz, Y. (2003). Targeting folate receptor with folate linked to extremities of poly (ethylene glycol)-grafted liposomes: *In vitro* studies. *Bioconjugate Chemistry, 14*, 563–574.
63. Thomas, M., Klibanov, A. M., & Zintchenko, A. (2005). Full diacylation of polyethyleneimine dramatically boosts its gene delivery efficiency and specificity to mouse lung. *Proceedings of the National Academy of Sciences of the United States of America, 102*, 5679–5684.
64. Felgner, P. L., Gao, X., & Cheng, H. (2003). Enhanced gene delivery and mechanism studies with a novel series of cationic lipid formulations. *Journal of Biological Chemistry, 278*, 44826–44835.
65. Chen, Y., Yang, F., & Xia, W. (2018). Recent advances in the use of ultrasound to promote gene therapy. *Journal of Ultrasound in Medicine, 37*, 2677–2687.
66. Lentacker, I., Geers, B., Demeester, J., De Smedt, S. C., & Sanders, N. N. (2010). Ultrasound-responsive polymer-coated microbubbles that bind and protect DNA. *Langmuir, 26*, 17624–17628.
67. Zhou, K., Liu, H., Zhang, S., & Liu, J. (2016). Multicolored pH-tunable and activatable fluorescence nanoplatform responsive to physiologic pH stimuli. *Journal of the American Chemical Society, 138*, 10–13.
68. Bae, Y., Fukushima, S., Harada, A., & Kataoka, K. (2003). A novel pH-sensitive poly (ethylene glycol)–poly(L-lysine)–DNA complex for efficient gene delivery. *Journal of Controlled Release, 82*, 323–334.
69. Maeda, H., Wu, J., Sawa, T., Matsumura, Y., & Hori, K. (2000). Tumor vascular permeability and the EPR effect in macromolecular therapeutics: A review. *Journal of Controlled Release, 65*, 271–284.
70. Torchilin, V. (2011). Tumor delivery of macromolecular drugs based on the EPR effect. *Advanced Drug Delivery Reviews, 63*, 131–135.
71. Warnock, J. N., Daigre, C., & Al-Rubeai, M. (2011). Introduction to viral vectors. *Methods in Molecular Biology, 737*, 1–25. https://doi.org/10.1007/978-1-61779-095-9_1 (accessed on 23rd June 2025).
72. Conrad, S. J., & Liu, J. (2019). Poxviruses as gene therapy vectors: Generating poxviral vectors expressing therapeutic transgenes. *Methods in Molecular Biology, 1937*, 189–209. https://doi.org/10.1007/978-1-4939-9065-8_11 (accessed on 23rd June 2025).
73. Ingle, R. G., & Fang, W. J. (2023). An overview of the stability and delivery challenges of commercial nucleic acid therapeutics. *Pharmaceutics, 15*(4), 1158.
74. Hassan, S. S., & Roy, P. (1999). Expression and functional characterization of bluetongue virus VP2 protein: Role in cell entry. *Journal of Virology, 73*(12), 9832–9842. https://doi.org/10.1128/jvi.73.12.9832-9842.1999 (accessed on 23rd June 2025).
75. Roizman, B., & Baines, J. (1991). The diversity and unity of Herpesviridae. *Comparative Immunology, Microbiology and Infectious Diseases, 14*(2), 63–79. https://doi.org/10.1016/0147-9571(91)90122-t (accessed on 23rd June 2025).

76. Zu, H., & Gao, D. (2021). Non-viral vectors in gene therapy: Recent development, challenges, and prospects. *AAPS Journal, 23*(4), 78. https://doi.org/10.1208/s12248-021-00608-7 (accessed on 23rd June 2025).
77. Sharma, A. K., Gothwal, A., Kesharwani, P., Alsaab, H., Iyer, A. K., & Gupta, U. (2017). Dendrimer nanoarchitectures for cancer diagnosis and anticancer drug delivery. *Drug Discovery Today, 22*(2), 314–326. https://doi.org/10.1016/j.drudis.2016.09.013 (accessed on 23rd June 2025).
78. Daniel, M. C., & Astruc, D. (2004). Gold nanoparticles: Assembly, supramolecular chemistry, quantum-size-related properties, and applications toward biology, catalysis, and nanotechnology. *Chemical Reviews, 104*(1), 293–346. https://doi.org/10.1021/cr030698+ (accessed on 23rd June 2025).
79. Beck, J. S., Vartuli, J. C., Roth, W. J., Leonowicz, M. E., Kresge, C. T., Schmitt, K. D., & Schlenker, J. L. (1992). A new family of mesoporous molecular sieves prepared with liquid crystal templates. *Journal of the American Chemical Society, 114*(27), 10834–10843. https://doi.org/10.1021/ja00053a020 (accessed on 23rd June 2025).

CHAPTER 4

Role of Polymers in Nucleic Acid Delivery

NIMISHA JAIN,[1,2] AVINASH SINGH MANDALOI,[2] ANKIT MISHRA,[2,*] PRANALI MISHRA,[3] and PANKAJ SHARMA[2,4]

[1]*Institute of Pharmacy, Rabindranath Tagore University, Bhopal, Madhya Pradesh, India*

[2]*VNS Group of Institutions, Faculty of Pharmacy, Bhopal, Madhya Pradesh, India*

[3]*Swami Vivekananda College of Pharmacy, Bhopal, Madhya Pradesh, India*

[4]*Shri Ram College of Pharmacy, Banmore, Morena, Madhya Pradesh, India*

*Corresponding author

ABSTRACT

Thanks to newer technologies, innovative therapies are accessible to treat previously untreatable diseases. Nucleic acid-based gene therapy is one such innovative therapy that has numerous clinical uses in treating genetically based disorders. These nucleic acid-based gene therapies are also helpful in creating novel vaccine formulations. Nucleic acids can alter protein synthesis by blocking gene expression or restoring functionally deficient protein production. Research is being carried out to increase the effectiveness of nucleic acid deliveries by reducing their degradation by enzyme nucleases, excretion or uptake by non-target tissues, and immunological activation by binding to other receptors. The topic of interest

Nanotechnology for Nucleic Acid Delivery: Pankaj Sharma, Saloni Jain, and Vinay Jain (Eds.)

DOI: 10.1201/9781998511853-4

for further research in nucleic acid delivery is ineffective cellular uptake owing to its large size and hydrophilic nature. Various scientists suggest one prominent method: to use carrier systems to deliver nucleic acid, which will facilitate intracellular trafficking, guide nucleic acid to tissue distribution, and provide protection. Numerous nano-carrier systems, such as synthetic and natural lipids, polymers, and viral vectors, have been investigated. Developing the best possible nucleic acid carrier system requires understanding the polymer chemistry that permits nucleic acid transport. This chapter focuses on various polymers investigated as a material for the carrier system of nucleic acid. This chapter concludes with the various uses and needs of further polymer development for specific drug therapies.

4.1 INTRODUCTION

We have seen throughout history how disease outbreaks have raised health concerns, many of which had the potential to become pandemics and resulted in the deaths of millions of people globally. The advent of novel ailments concomitant with population expansion and worldwide integration suggests the desire to acquire novel tools to mitigate the dissemination of infectious agents and the likelihood of subsequent pandemics [1, 2]. Nucleic acid therapies, which take advantage of the genetic code, offer a promising novel perspective in medicine that can prevent or treat human disease at its source [3, 4]. Nucleic acid medications have several advantages over traditional small-molecule and antibody drugs, including a rapid development cycle, a wide range of targets, and a notable ability to cure patients. Moreover, nucleic acid medications provide a way through limitations related to undruggable targets [5, 6]. Nucleic acids can suppress protein synthesis by blocking gene expression or restoring functionally deficient protein production [7, 8]. When delivering nucleic acids *in vivo*, many obstacles exist, like quick degradation by nucleases, excretion or uptake by non-target tissues, immunological activation by binding to Toll-like receptors, and ineffective cellular uptake because of their comparatively large size and hydrophilic nature [9]. This nucleic acid delivery is presented in Figure 4.1. Numerous carrier systems, such as synthetic and natural lipids, polymers, and viral vectors, have been investigated to overcome and achieve nucleic acid's complete functions

[10, 11]. Developing the best possible nucleic acid carrier system requires understanding the polymer chemistry that permits nucleic acid transport [12, 13]. This chapter focuses on various polymers investigated as a material for the carrier system of nucleic acid.

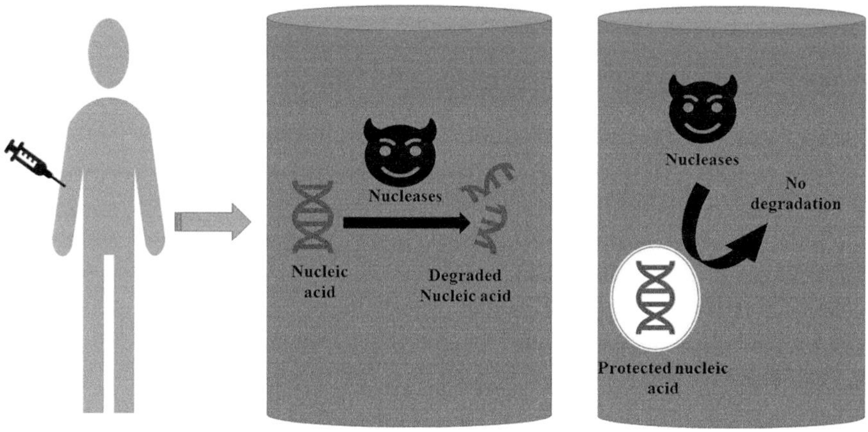

FIGURE 4.1 Representing fate of nucleic acid, unprotected and protected, in systemic circulation by nuclease enzyme.

4.2 THERAPEUTIC NUCLEIC ACIDS

Nucleic acids themselves or compounds closely linked to them are employed as therapeutic nucleic acids (TNAs) to treat various diseases [14]. Despite the fact that TNAs come in many forms, they all function similarly due to the Watson-Crick base pairing, which allows for the sequence-specific identification of endogenous nucleic acids [15]. TNAs are charged, significant molecular weight substances that are unstable in a biological environment and have different physicochemical characteristics from small molecule medications [16]. TNAs must also be administered to the appropriate intracellular compartment. Regulators regarded them as novel chemical entities (NCEs) due to their chemical synthesis, but the qualities listed above bring them closer to new biological entities (NBEs). Nucleic acid treatments are classified into two main categories: DNA therapeutics (which includes gene therapy, antisense oligonucleotides (ASOs), DNA aptamers) and RNA therapeutics (which include RNA decoys, micro RNAs (miRNAs), short interfering RNAs (siRNAs), ribozymes, and circular RNAs) [15].

4.2.1 GENE THERAPY AND NUCLEIC ACID DELIVERY

4.2.1.1 GENE THERAPY

The idea of gene therapy was first put forth 30 years ago, but advancements in delivery techniques have only been made in the last 10 years. Gene therapy involves the replacement of a defective or non-functional gene with a functional one. Gene therapy mainly covers the treatment of genetic disorders like adenosine deaminase deficiency, α-1-antitrypsin deficiency, cystic fibrosis, familial hypercholesterolemia, Gaucher's disease, and hemophilia B [17]. In gene therapy, a vector (typically a virus, most frequently a retrovirus or less commonly an adenovirus) transfers the desired gene through a therapeutic gene expression cassette. Typically, a therapeutic gene expression cassette consists of the target transgene, a promoter that initiates gene transcription, and a termination signal to stop gene transcription [18]. There are two gene delivery methods: somatic gene therapy and germ-line gene therapy. Somatic gene therapy generally involves the transmission of the desired gene to the non-heritable somatic cells, whereas in the case of germ-line therapy, the desired gene transfers into germ cells, which can be passed down to the next generations [5]. *Genecidine* and *Alipogene tiparvovec* are the only gene treatments approved in humans, although many ongoing clinical trials exist [15, 20].

4.2.1.2 NUCLEIC ACID DELIVERY

In contrast to treatments that target downstream processes, the antisense oligonucleotides (ASOs) field is an emerging drug discovery field that targets the disease's RNA level as its source. Short-stranded, single-stranded sequences, ASOs, range from 8–50 base pairs and bind to the target mRNA by the conventional Watson–Crick base pairing mechanism. ASOs control protein production via various methods by binding precisely to the target RNA. Prior research has employed unmodified ASOs, or ASOs containing a phosphodiester backbone [21], to target RNA with varying degrees of effectiveness. Nevertheless, unaltered ASOs are susceptible to nuclease degradation because they include a phosphodiester bond. Furthermore, the large size and charge of unaltered ASOs limit their passive diffusion into the cell [22]. Therefore, efforts have been made to explore more recent, chemically modified ASOs to improve their enzymatic stability, efficacy, and reduce off-target toxicity and immune response.

DNA aptamers are short, single-stranded oligonucleotide sequences that structurally recognize target nucleic acids with a high affinity, similar to ASO. A method known as Systematic Evolution of Ligands by Exponential Enrichment, or SELEX, is used to separate aptamers from an extensive collection of nucleic acids [15].

4.2.2 VACCINE DELIVERY

Using DNA or RNA plasmids as antigen precursors, genetic vaccines are comprised of immunization or immunotherapeutic strategies. The sequence of a gene, or genes, that code for the target antigen is taken in by host cells and translated into a protein. These so-called third-generation vaccine technologies, also known as synthetic antigen vaccines, have the ability to elicit humoral and cellular responses. They can also be enhanced by using *in silico* technologies that enable the selection of antigenic epitopes. As for their capacity to elicit $CD4^+$ and $CD8^+$ T cell responses, nucleic acid vaccines show notable advantages over conventional vaccinations [23].

4.3 CHALLENGES IN NUCLEIC ACID DELIVERY:

One of the primary challenges in the nucleic acid delivery sector is designing delivery vehicles with features that make them both safe and effective in transfection. Protein medications may face unique stability issues due to the complex and delicate nature of NAs. Naked or unmodified NAs have extremely short half-lives in circulation due to enzymatic (e.g., nucleases, which can destroy ribonucleases and deoxyribonucleases) and chemical (e.g., oxidation, hydrolysis, deamidation, depurination, and strand cleavage) degradation. Therefore, chemical modifications are usually necessary to improve NA stability [24]. Nowadays, the most effective way to combat coronavirus is with messenger RNA (mRNA) vaccines (COVID-19). However, mRNAs are susceptible to phosphate backbone hydrolysis and nuclease degradation due to the intramolecular attack of the 2′-hydroxyl group in physiological fluids. Therefore, lipid nanoparticles (LNPs) are used in COVID-19 mRNA vaccinations and kept under (ultra) cold storage conditions; thus, drug delivery systems, such as LNPs, act as a shield for mRNA to prevent degradation and assure its potency [25, 26].

4.4 DELIVERY ROUTES FOR NUCLEIC ACIDS

Scientists have tried numerous routes for *in vivo* drug delivery of nucleic acids, two of which have been found to be successful and used for commercial use, and these are discussed here.

4.4.1 SYSTEMIC ROUTES

Subcutaneous injection (SC), intramuscular injection (IM), intradermal injection (ID), and intravenous injection (IV) are the principal forms of systemic delivery. Among these, the nanoparticles delivered by SC, IM, and ID are absorbed by antigen-presenting cells (APCs) in the subcutaneous or muscle tissue rather than going directly into the bloodstream [27]. Subcutaneous injections are often thought to have a lower capillary density, permitting a steady antigen release at a predetermined pace following SC [28]. It is challenging to accomplish targeted delivery to central immune organs or other specified tissues to date, even though nucleic acid medications or vaccines delivered by SC, IM, and ID mainly activate immune cells in peripheral lymph nodes. These methods are still the cornerstone of preventive immunization because of their increased safety and patient compliance over IV. The majority of nanoparticles that are effective at reaching a particular tissue often use the IV route. In this instance, nanoparticles reach the bloodstream as quickly as possible after injection and participate in blood circulation. IV is an excellent delivery method, particularly for nucleic acid medications that target the liver. Even with the development of different material-based nucleic acid delivery systems, it is still difficult to effectively transport nucleic acid-nanocarrier complexes to extrahepatic regions through systemic injection. When nucleic acid nano-carrier complexes are administered intravenously, a significant portion of the complex is primarily retrieved by hepatocytes because the drug must be transported via the circulatory system from the injection site to the target cells, leading to a larger-than-expected release of nucleic acids from the liver and, as a result, a lower-than-expected concentration of the medication entering the target tissues.

LNP-RNA approaches attempt to overcome the difficulties involved in systemic administration while enhancing the targeted delivery of nucleic acid-nanocarrier complexes to the target tissues and improving their therapeutic efficacy [29].

4.4.2 RESPIRATORY ROUTES

The respiratory pathway is the most effective in reaching lung epithelial cells [30]. With this method, viral infections and respiratory illnesses have been successfully treated and prevented [31]. In contrast to other organs, the respiratory system's mucosa offers a large absorptive surface area, and the lungs are immediately exposed to the outside world through the respiratory tract. Due to its exceptional quality, nebulization and intratracheal/intranasal drops are up-and-coming methods for delivering nucleic acid-nanocarrier complexes to the lungs [32, 33]. Without relying on systemic circulation, complexes can directly reach cells, such as alveolar epithelial cells, in the pulmonary airways and alveoli employing the respiratory tract. This method reduces drug loss and delivers drugs effectively. Usually, this technique requires the use of specialist equipment. Earlier equipment consisted of metered-dose inhalers (MDIs), which provide quick and easy drug delivery by dissolving or suspending medications in a liquid propellant (such as hydro-fluoro-alkanes). The issue of restricted drug deposition in the lower respiratory tract caused by MDIs was resolved by the administration of dry powder inhalers (DPIs). The patient's respiratory function plays a significant role in the effectiveness of dry powder inhalers, which presents significant difficulties for quality control stability [34].

Afterward, nebulization devices were developed that can cover almost all areas of the lungs with the liquid aerosols generated by nebulizers, which have the capacity to deliver hundreds of nanoparticles per drop. Philip et al. explained the uses of devices such as small animal vibrating sieve mesh nebulizers and nebulizing towers, which delivered the nucleic acids to counter respiratory pathogens. Persistently rising levels of environmental contamination and pandemic outbreaks, including COVID-19, influenza, and respiratory syncytial virus (RSV) infections, have caused a noticeable rise in the prevalence of lung illnesses. Nucleic acid drugs are involved in the extraordinary treatment of inherited lung diseases like lung cancer, asthma, infectious pneumonia, and so forth [35].

4.5 BIOLOGICAL BARRIERS

Three biological barriers affect nucleic acid delivery to the cells: systemic, organ, and cellular. These barriers are discussed in subsequent points and represented in Figure 4.2.

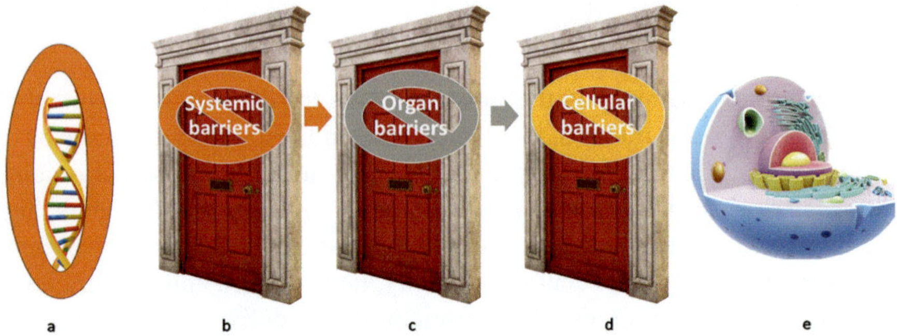

FIGURE 4.2 Symbolic barriers to the entrapped nucleic acid entry to the cell. (a). nucleic acid entrapped in carrier; (b). systemic barrier; (c). organ barrier; (d). cellular barrier; and (e). target cell.

4.5.1 SYSTEMIC BARRIERS

The extracellular barrier, which is present in the bloodstream and intercellular matrix, prevents nanoparticles from entering target cells. The complex substances found in blood are the main components of this barrier. Several nucleases, including endonucleases and exonucleases, are present in blood serum and can hydrolyze and inactivate the phosphodiester bonds of exposed nucleic acids [36]. In early nucleic acid delivery research, nucleic acids were chemically or strongly bonded to carrier materials to avoid nuclease-induced degradation. Once detected by the mononuclear phagocyte system (MPS), nanoparticles, like all foreign compounds, can undergo disintegration and unintentionally elicit unwanted immune reactions at inappropriate places [37]. Once within the bloodstream, the surface of the nanoparticles rapidly adsorbs a layer of proteins known as the "protein corona," which includes complement, serum albumin, opsonins, and other proteins. In addition to increasing phagocytic cells' ability to phagocytose nanoparticles, the protein corona can mask ligands on the surface of the particle that are necessary for active targeting, reducing the specificity of the nanoparticles. It has been discovered that modification of polyethylene glycol (PEG) inhibits MPS clearance and stops the creation of protein corona [38].

4.5.2 ORGAN BARRIERS

Because of the characteristics of the nanoparticles (size, surface charge, etc.), there is a chance that the liver and kidneys will clear them, but not other organs. Once in the bloodstream, the kidneys quickly eliminate nanoparticles with a diameter of less than 5 nm. On the other hand, the liver's reticuloendothelial system (RES) eliminates larger nanoparticles. Furthermore, the ability of nanoparticles to enter structures unique to a given tissue is correlated with their size. For example, after the nanoparticles escape from the blood vessels, they must cross the splenic barrier to reach the spleen [39]. Only nanoparticles of the right size can pass through the bridging channel and cross the marginal zone to reach the white medulla's T-cell and B-cell zones, which are densely populated with lymphocytes capable of quickly and successfully triggering an adaptive immune response against particular antigens. In addition, the human body contains several organs with strong defenses, like the brain and placenta. Transporting nanoparticles to these organs requires overcoming additional barriers, such as the blood-brain barrier for delivering nucleic acids to the brain and the blood-labyrinth barrier for the inner ear [40]. For the lungs, there is an even more particular situation in which the inhalation of nanoparticles into the lungs must pass through a highly intricate respiratory barrier. The first obstacle to be overcome is the mucus-cilia clearance system (MC) on the airway epithelium. Through electrostatic interactions, the mucus layer immobilizes inhaled foreign substances, such as nucleic acid-nanocarrier complexes, and removes them from binding sites. Research has indicated that particles smaller than 40 nm can only efficiently penetrate the mucus layer via passive Brownian motion [41, 42]. In order to facilitate prolonged siRNA release within the mucus layer, Angelo et al. have created mucus-inert nanomaterials that take advantage of the natural characteristics of the mucus layer [43].

4.5.3 CELLULAR BARRIERS

The cell membrane is the first barrier encountered during cellular absorption after overcoming the aforementioned barriers and approaching the target cells. In contrast to small molecule medications, nanoparticles enter cells through active uptake processes such as receptor-mediated endocytosis, macropinocytosis, and caveolae-mediated endocytosis. Two general categories can be used to describe how cells absorb nanoparticles:

pinocytosis and phagocytosis. Pinocytosis is generally seen in many cell types, whereas phagocytosis can only occur in phagocytic cells like monocytes, neutrophils, and macrophages [44]. Distinct nanoparticles use different methods to breach the cell membrane. Kubota et al. discovered that caveolae-mediated endocytosis is primarily responsible for the cellular uptake of lipid nanoparticles (LNPs) after treating HeLa cells with specific inhibitors targeting various uptake mechanisms. The cellular uptake efficiency of nanoparticles can be influenced by their composition, size, surface charge, and shape [45]. According to Suberi et al., [46] PEG's content on the surface of polymers influences their cellular uptake efficiency. Extensive research has demonstrated that elevated PEG density can modify polymer peripheral conformation, affecting how target cells interact with nucleic acid-loaded nanoparticles. Hatakeyama et al. also came to a related conclusion by using a dissimilar material to deliver siRNA [47]. Acidic organelles in cells with a firm acidity are called lysosomes (pH near 5) [48]. Because of this, in the harsh lysosome environment, the nano-carrier and its payload will be killed if the nano-carriers containing nucleic acids cannot escape quickly. Notably, specific helper lipids can also undergo protonation in acidic situations. For instance, in the endosome, membrane phospholipids and 1,2-dioleoyl-sn-glycero-3-phosphoethanolamine (DOPE), which has a hexagonal inverted cone structure, can generate ion pairs, thereby promoting the process of endosomal escape [49].

4.6 POLYMERIC DELIVERY SYSTEMS AND NANOPARTICLE-BASED GENE DELIVERY SYSTEM

As discussed earlier, nucleic acid-based gene therapy can be utilized to treat various diseases of genetic origin. This therapy can also be exceptionally advantageous for vaccine delivery. Due to extracellular nuclease enzymes, nude nucleic acids degrade immediately, have poor distribution in the body, and cannot cross the cell membranes to reach inside the cell. Therefore, carrier systems are compulsorily required to deliver these nucleic acids. Developing ideal carriers for nucleic acids, which can protect them against enzymatic attack, increase their circulation half-lives after systemic availability, and help cell binding and internalization of nucleic acids, is today's demand and is of interest to biomedical researchers. These carriers can be broadly divided into viral vectors, polymeric, and lipid-based carriers. Viral vectors are clinically used and have high efficiency in intracellular delivery of such nucleic acid delivery, but due to their limitations, polymeric and lipid-based drug delivery systems are of interest to scientists. This section will discuss polymeric carriers for nucleic acids, also called polyplexes [50].

4.6.1 CATIONIC POLYMERS

Cationic-charged polymers and lipids are most efficient for drug delivery of nucleic acids, owing to their electrostatic interactions or complexation with anionic nucleic acids. This interaction is presented in Figure 4.3. These polyplexes are sufficiently nanosized to allow cellular entry and guide the path intracellularly to the nucleic acids of exogenous origin. Due to the advantages of scientific methodologies, scientists have developed various cationic polymers to develop polyplexes. These cationic polymers can be altered in properties by changing their molecular weights, branching of polymers, dissociation constants of cationic groups, charge density, and nature of biodegrading, and therefore, the scope of developing an ideal dosage form is of interest [51].

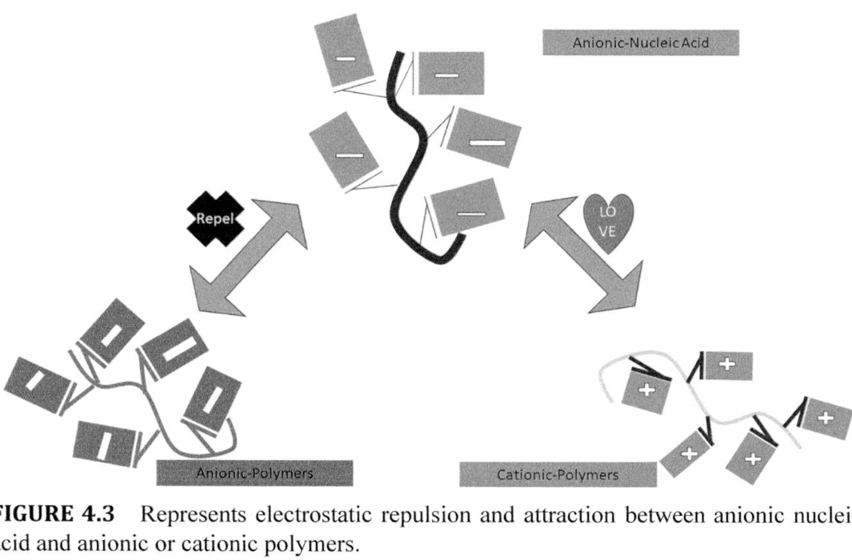

FIGURE 4.3 Represents electrostatic repulsion and attraction between anionic nucleic acid and anionic or cationic polymers.

Based on the era of development, these cationic polymers can be divided into two Generation first and generation second polyplexes.

4.6.1.1 GENERATION-FIRST POLYCATIONIC POLYMERS

Generation-first polycationic polymers are homopolymers, which are permanently charged. Various polymers studied by scientists are presented in Table 4.1.

Out of the generation-first polymers, poly-l-ornithine was optimized in various aspects, which were finalized and presented in the literature by Farber and Butel [52]. They proposed a strong shielding interaction between positive charges on PLO and negative charges between DNA; this shielding protects DNA from exocytic attack of nuclease. This shielding also protects DNA from target cell rejection. The researchers also proposed similar mechanisms for all the polymers. Later, detailed structural analysis provided the stereostructural basis for better effectiveness of polyornithine [53].

Approaches are continuously studied to improve transfection with polyplex, and several approaches have demonstrated enhanced cellular uptake and specificity for the receptors. One of the prominent approaches was the covalent bonding of ligands with PLL, studied by Wu et al. and Schreiber et al., which is summarized in Table 4.1 [54, 55].

The use of other excipients is another approach to increase transfection by these polyplexes; this method was studied by Luthman and Magnusson [56] and Cotten and Birnstiel [57] and presented again in Table 4.1. In both studies, researchers proposed that chloroquine accumulation in lysosomes protected the lysis of pDNA by lysosomal nucleases [58]. Some reports suggest chloroquine may enhance DNA release from polyplexes inside the cell [59].

TABLE 4.1 Summarizing Cationic Polymers and Their Uses in Nucleic Acid Delivery System

Sl. No.	Name of the Generation First Polymer	Common Abbreviation	Used for	References
1	Diethyl aminoethyl Dextran	DEAE-Dextran	Transfection of infectious viral nucleic acid	60
2	Diethyl aminoethyl Dextran	DEAE-Dextran	Chloroquine significantly enhanced pDNA/DEAE-dextran transfection	56
3	poly-L-lysine	PLL	nuclease resistance of plasmid DNA	61
4	poly-L-lysine	PLL	Receptor-mediated gene by covalently coupling with ligands for asialoglycoprotein receptor expressed on hepatic cells	54
5	Poly-L-lysine	PLL	Polylysine-transferrin-based gene transfer into K562 cells enhanced by chloroquine therapy	57

TABLE 4.1 *(Continued)*

Sl. No.	Name of the Generation First Polymer	Common Abbreviation	Used for	References
6	poly-L-lysine	PLL	First human clinical gene therapy studies with pDNA polyplexes	55
7	poly-L-lysine	PLL	human melanoma vaccine consisting of irradiated autologous tumor cells transfected with a human IL-2 gene construct	62
8	poly-L-ornithine	PLO	Plasmid DNA And exogenous DNA transfection	63
9	poly-L-arginine	PLR	cancer gene therapy	64
10	amphipathic peptide KALA	KALA	binds to DNA, causes membrane disruption	65
11	GALA peptide	GALA	conjugated to positively charged polymers for DNA delivery	66

4.6.1.2 GENERATION SECOND POLYPLEX

Polymers with improved transfection were developed later by various scientists. Polycationic dendrimers prepared by Polyamidoamine (PAMAM) were game-changing and highly efficient. The effectiveness of this polymer was irrespective of chloroquine or any other attached protein fragment. The charge density of these dendrimers is high, and the dissociation constant is near 6. Higher transfection is suggested to be achieved by the enhanced escape of polyplex complexes by either of the two mechanisms: the proton sponge effect and the destabilization of the endothelial membrane. The proton sponge effect suggests that this dissociation constant favors intracellular DNA release by a more significant influx of anionic chloride ions, thereby rupturing the endosome due to higher osmotic pressure. Another mechanism suggests the destabilization of the endosomal membrane due to the cationic polymer domain [67, 68].

Polyethylenimine (PEI) was the leading generation-second transfusion polymer working with a proton sponge mechanism [69]. PEI was found to be effective both *in vitro* and *in vivo*. However, few reported some cellular toxicity, depending on its molecular weight and cationic charge density. Few researchers reported this toxicity to be *in vitro* only [70]. Lower cellular toxicity was reported by lower molecular weight PEI and other cationic polymers; these low molecular weight cationic polymers show better complexation with nucleic acids when compared to higher molecular weight ones. These cationic polymers showed reduced toxicity when combined with cholesterol and if coated with polyethylene glycol [71].

A wide range of branched and linear PEI are available commercially and show different levels of transfection, cellular toxicities, and stability of polyplexes [72]. However, the higher stability of polyplexes cannot be correlated with effectiveness, as the release of nucleic acid is required intracellularly.

Itaka et al. concluded through their studies that linear PEI provides better transfection than branched PEI owing to lesser stability. Their studies also demonstrated that both linear and branched PEI show transfection better than PLL [73]. Research findings showed that nuclear delivery of pDNA was higher through linear PEI in nondividing cells; however, branched PEI showed enhanced delivery of the same pDNA in cells undergoing or preparing for mitosis. LPEI-based polyplexes can be transported in intact nuclei, whereas BPEI relies on nuclear envelope breakdown [74]. Generation first and second polymers have limitations on their biological degradation, therefore exerting tissue toxicities. This toxicity is correlative to the molecular weight of the polymer.

The mechanism of narcosis and apoptosis of the cells is reportedly triggered by PEI, which is found to be the generation of defects in the cell surface or surface of cell-organelles like the nucleus or mitochondria. Synthesis of ATP in mitochondria is found in PEI cytotoxic. In *in vitro* studies, innate immune systems can recognize these cationic polymers [75]. However, this activation can be minimized by layering it with polyethylene glycol. These polycations show promising transfection but show toxicity, too. Therefore, searching for a successful polymer with minimum toxicity is interesting for biotechnological scientists.

4.7 SPECIFIC DELIVERY THROUGH THE PROTON SPONGE EFFECT

The Proton Sponge Effect is observed in some polymers, particularly PEI, used in gene delivery. When these polymers are introduced into cells, they effectively buffer the acidic environment within endosomes.

This buffering capacity leads to an influx of protons into the endosome, causing it to swell and eventually burst, releasing the contents, such as nucleic acids (like DNA or RNA), into the cytoplasm [76–78].

This mechanism is utilized in nucleic acid delivery because it enhances the escape of nucleic acids from endosomes, a critical step for their successful delivery into the cell's cytoplasm. Once in the cytoplasm, nucleic acids can exert their therapeutic effects, such as gene expression or silencing [76]. So, specific delivery through the Proton Sponge Effect for nucleic acid delivery involves using polymers that exploit this effect to facilitate the release of nucleic acids from endosomes, thereby improving their delivery and efficacy in gene therapy or other nucleic acid-based therapies [79].

The Proton Sponge Effect, utilized in gene delivery via dendrimers, involves buffering endosomal acidification and promoting nucleic acid release. Computational models suggest it enhances intracellular gene delivery by inducing osmotic pressure, rupturing endosomes, and releasing nucleic acids, offering promise for improving delivery efficiency [77].

In summary, the Proton Sponge Effect is a mechanism for enhancing intracellular gene delivery that relies on the ability of certain weakly basic molecules to induce an endosome to burst, releasing the nucleic acids they contain. The properties of the dendrimers used influence this effect, and computational modeling has provided valuable insights into optimizing dendrimer design for gene therapy applications.

4.8 BIODEGRADABLE POLYMERS

Many polymers that cannot biodegrade lack a defined mechanism to exit cells and tissues post-administration [80]. Prolonged exposure to these foreign materials and the potential build-up within the body can lead to toxicity. Using biodegradable polymers as carriers enhances biocompatibility, especially when the polymer breaks into non-toxic, natural byproducts [81]. Naturally derived and synthetic polymers can be biodegradable [82], offering potentially safer options for systemic gene delivery. It is commonly believed that natural polymers have a lower cytotoxicity profile and better biodegradability; however, this is not always the case because synthetic polymers have also been developed with good biocompatibility and customizable biodegradability [83].

Developing and applying biodegradable synthetic polymers can improve polyplex biocompatibility, reduce cytotoxicity, and prevent body accumulation. Crucially, degradability can also induce the cytosolic release of siRNA or pDNA following the cell's internalization of polyplexes based on these polymers. PLL and PEI are examples of polycations whose molecular weight strongly influences cytotoxicity.

While high molecular weight (HMW) PEI 22 kDa or BPEI 25 kDa are more potent but noticeably more hazardous, PEI with a low molecular weight (LMW) of 800 (less than 20 monomer units) exhibits low cellular toxicity but also low transfection effectiveness. Thus, new approaches were developed to combine the benefits of HMW polymers' high transfection efficiency with LMW polymers' low cytotoxicity. It has proven possible to create a variety of biodegradable PEI-based polymers using amides such as polyglutamic acid amide and others, as well as ester linkages, disulfides, ketals, and imines, and including hydrolyzable ester links, endosomally degradable acetal or imine bonds, or bio-reducible disulfide bonds into the cationic polymer backbone significantly decreased cytotoxicity and preserved or even increased nucleic acid transfection efficiency. Kim et al. [64] reported the synthesis of biodegradable poly(alpha-(4-aminobutyl)-L-glycolic acid) through ester bond replacement of the amide bonds in polylysine. Because there was no efficient endosomal escape, transfection activity increased but remained moderate compared to PLL. Compared to pLys, poly(alpha-(4-aminobutyl)-L-glycolic acid) was significantly less toxic. Subsequently, Michael added amines to acrylate esters to create more potent hyperbranched network-type poly (amino esters) known as n-PAE. N-PAE demonstrated significantly higher biocompatibility than PEI regarding transfection efficiency and endosomal escape characteristics. By reacting several primary amines and secondary diamines by Michael's addition with a range of bis-acrylates, Langer and colleagues created a library of more than 2000 biodegradable cationic polymers. Through high throughput screening for transfection efficiency, promising candidates were found. Other teams generated biodegradable polymers based on disulfides using the Michael addition technique. In several publications, Engbersen and associates demonstrated that polyplexes built on these polymers exhibited low cytotoxicity and high pDNA and siRNA transfection efficiency. Cationic-charged groups within the nanogel core effectively load nucleic acids into aqueous solutions through electrostatic interactions. Following cellular uptake, the nanogel's proton buffering properties facilitate endosomal escape. Due to the cytoplasm's comparatively high glutathione concentration, the thiol-disulfide exchange reaction quickly cleaves the disulfide bonds in the nanogel network. This exchange causes the nanogel cage to disassemble quickly and releases the free payload. Cysteine bis-acrylamide was reacted with tiny oligoethylenimines to create bioreducible PEI oligoamines. These polymers exhibited no or minimal cytotoxicity along with increased gene expression levels. These findings show that bio-reducible polymers have great promise for effective and secure gene delivery [84, 85].

4.9 NATURAL POLYMERS

Chitosan, collagen, gelatin, and their modified derivatives are examples of natural polymers being researched for gene therapy applications [86]. In addition to collagen and gelatin, various protein-based carriers have been utilized for nucleic acid transfection, including histones and the chromosomal protein HMG1. These carriers may have changed. It has been demonstrated that cationized gelatin can help transfer siRNA into the kidney when administered through the ureter. After systemic treatment, soluble collagen, known as Atelocollagen, was helpful in siRNA transport into bone metastatic cancers. Chitosan and its derivatives, poly-D-glucosamines generated from the natural polymer chitin via acetylation, are some of the most studied naturally occurring polymeric gene carriers. The degree of deacetylation and molecular weight of the Chitosan, the concentration of plasmids, the charge ratio of amine (Chitosan) to phosphate (DNA), serum concentration, pH, and cell type are some of the variables that affect how well chitosan/DNA complexes transfect. Chitosan is also particularly effective in the oral and nasal delivery of medications based on nucleic acids because of its mucoadhesive properties. The creation and colloidal stability of pDNA/chitosan polyplexes have been demonstrated to be enhanced by methylation and PEGylation of Chitosan. Other advantageous changes include histidinylation for better endosomal escape and targeting ligands or thiolation for more excellent cellular absorption. Cyclodextrin (CD) conjugates are cyclic oligosaccharides that can form host-guest complexes with hydrophobic molecules. These conjugates can be alpha, beta, or gamma forms [87].

The toxicity of pDNA polyplexes was decreased by covalent conjugation of beta-CD, which can form complexes with the conjugate of cholesterol with LPEI and BPEI without compromising transfection efficacy. These PEI polyplexes were incubated with adamantane-PEG, which produced PEGylated PEI polyplexes that were effectively utilized for systemic gene transfer into the liver. In a different work, pDNA polyplexes were created using low molecular weight PEICD conjugates, and then they were modified using an adamantane peptide ligand that was specific for the fibroblast growth factor (FGF) receptor and an adamantane disulfide-linked PEG for shielding. Hwang and Davis produced β-cyclodextrin-based linear cationic polymers (β-CDPs) that exhibited superior biocompatibility compared to the unaltered polycations. Furthermore, the CD groups on these polycations introduced transferrin via adamantane host-guest interaction. Clinical investigations involving these polyplexes assessed them and showed that gene silencing in metastatic cancers was mediated by intravenous siRNA delivery. It was demonstrated that the degree of cationic modification can be adjusted and is crucial for creating nucleic acid polyplexes. Synthesized polycationic poly-rotaxane polymers exhibiting enhanced DNA transfection were created by assembling mono-cationic CDs into degradable linear polymer chains [88].

Within naturally derived polymers, structural proteins and polysaccharides like cationic collagen derivatives and Chitosan have been explored as gene-delivery vehicles. Cationic collagenous proteins have been utilized to deliver nucleic acids to articular cartilage bone for regenerative medicine and treating metastatic tumors. Chitosan, a linear cationic polysaccharide derived from chitin, is non-toxic even at high concentrations and can form polyplexes to protect and transfect nucleic acid cargos effectively. Chitosan has been used in various applications, such as delivering miR-124 to rat microglia, osteopathic tumors, multiple myeloma tumors, and bone regeneration. Compared to other cationic polymers like PEI, Chitosan readily dissociates from nucleic acid cargo upon internalization, leading to more efficient gene transfection. Combining Chitosan with PEI can leverage the stronger nucleic acid association with PEI while minimizing negative consequences from charge density [89].

Due to their favorable physicochemical properties, cyclodextrins (CDs) are another group of naturally derived carbohydrate-based polymers suitable for gene delivery. CDs in various forms can be used alone or in combination with other cationic polymers such as PEI. For instance, β-CD can interact with adamantane, supporting the formulation of blends with PEI and other materials, leading to high transfection efficiency in different tissues and via various administration routes [90].

4.10 SYNTHETIC POLYMERS

Synthetic biodegradable polymers are created by assembling low molecular weight monomers into polymers through reversible linkages like sulfide or ester bonds. Examples include poly(lactic acid) (PLA), poly(glycolic acid) (PGA), and copolymers like poly(lactic-co-glycolic acid) (PLGA). These materials degrade slowly via bulk hydrolysis, allowing for sustained cargo release. PLGA-based systems have been used to deliver therapeutic agents, including nucleic acids such as siRNA, miRNA, and PNAs. Despite being FDA-approved for certain applications, PLGA has challenges in nucleic acid delivery due to low loading efficiency. Strategies like precomplexation with spermidine or blending with cationic polymers like PEI have enhanced loading and transfection efficiency [91].

Poly(beta-amino esters) (PBAEs) are a class of degradable cationic polymers effective in encapsulating nucleic acids, promoting cellular uptake, and facilitating endosomal escape. They are synthesized relatively quickly and can be customized for specific applications. However, their high density of amine groups can lead to aggregation with anionic serum molecules and increased toxicity. Blending PBAEs with PLGA can reduce cytotoxicity, with toxicity decreasing as the ratio of PBAE to PLGA decreases [92].

Poly(amine-co-esters) (PACEs) are designed to have lower charge densities to minimize toxicity. These polymers, synthesized via copolymerization of hydrophobic and amine-containing monomers, can be controlled in terms of physical properties and formulated into various delivery vehicles. Although they tend to aggregate in serum like other cationic polymers, this can be mitigated through coatings or surface modifications [92].

Recent advancements in polymerization techniques allow for precise control over polymer sequence and structure, enabling systematic evaluation of their effects on nucleic acid delivery. Techniques like reversible addition-fragmentation chain transfer (RAFT) polymerization and ligase-based polymerization offer high chemical precision and flexible design, leading to the identification of polymers optimized for specific applications through structure-function relationships. Despite being time-consuming, these methods control properties like hydrophilicity/hydrophobicity, charge density, and architecture, offering promising avenues for tailored nucleic acid delivery systems [93].

4.11 CONJUGATE DELIVERY SYSTEMS

Gene delivery vectors frequently utilize surface modifications to target specific cells or sites and enhance nucleic acid cargo's stability. For instance, when cationic polymers coat negatively charged nanoparticles, their delivery into the cytosol is enhanced. Lee et al. demonstrated that gold nanoparticles coated with PBAE and conjugated with siRNA targeting luciferase expression achieved over 90% silencing of the luciferase gene in HeLa cells compared to control groups [92].

Antibody-based therapy has undergone a significant transformation with the advent of polyspecific monoclonal antibodies capable of targeting multiple tumor antigens without affecting normal cells. Over 60 antibody-drug conjugates are undergoing clinical trials; six have received FDA approval for cancer therapy. Similarly, antibody-conjugated nanoparticles carrying nucleic acids have been investigated for site-specific targeting. Okamoto et al. recently developed anti-HB-EGF antibody-conjugated LNPs containing siRNA targeting PLK-1 for triple-negative breast cancer therapy, resulting in enhanced tumor accumulation and reduced tumor growth in xenografted mice [94].

In addition to surface coating, direct conjugation with chemical scaffolds such as cholesterol to synthetic nucleic acid mimics like siRNAs is also employed to enhance specificity and decrease enzymatic degradation after delivery. Covalently linked ligands facilitate receptor uptake and nucleic acid delivery to target tissues. The most explored conjugate delivery systems include N-acetylgalactosamine (GalNAc) conjugates and dynamic polyconjugate (DPC) technologies, which have been clinically utilized for siRNA delivery. GalNAc conjugates have successfully treated liver diseases, targeting liver hepatocytes via the asialoglycoprotein receptor. Several GalNAc-conjugated siRNA drug candidates have entered clinical trials for various conditions.

The first-generation DPC technology utilized PBAVE polymer with GalNAc and PEG conjugates for hepatocyte uptake and enzymatic stability. The second generation improved upon this by co-injecting cholesterol-siRNA and PBAVE polymer linked with PEG and GalNAc, resulting in significantly enhanced efficacy. This technology has been optimized for delivering ARC-520, a lead candidate for hepatitis B virus (HBV) treatment, by Arrowhead Research Corporation [95].

4.12 LIPID-BASED DELIVERY SYSTEM

Lipid-based polymeric systems are like versatile couriers, blending the best lipids and polymers to deliver genetic materials such as DNA, RNA, and siRNA to where they are needed in the body. Picture them as tiny molecular delivery trucks comprising lipids and polymers working together to package and transport genetic cargo to specific cells [96].

Their significance in gene delivery is enormous because they tackle many of the formidable challenges of gene therapy [97]. Think of it like this: genetic materials are delicate packages, easily damaged or lost in the bloodstream. However, these lipid-based polymeric systems act like sturdy shields, shielding genetic cargo from being broken down by enzymes outside cells [79]. Plus, they are smart—they know how to sneak genetic payloads into cells by hitching a ride through cellular gateways called endocytosis or even bypassing those gateways altogether and delivering directly into the cell's inner space [98]. However, their magic does not stop there. These systems can also be personalized for specific destinations within the body. By dressing up the surface of their delivery trucks with particular targeting molecules, it is possible to steer them straight to the suitable cells or tissues, minimizing unintended side effects and maximizing their healing power [99]. Moreover, the best part is that they are safe for the body. The lipids and polymers they are made from are friendly to our biology, breaking down harmlessly once they are done their job, reducing the risk of unwanted effects [100]. So, these lipid-based polymeric systems are not just delivery systems; they are like superheroes, swooping in to rescue genetic therapies from their most demanding challenges and bringing hope for a healthier future.

4.12.1 CATIONIC LIPID

Cationic lipids are like molecular magnets, drawn to the negatively charged backbone of nucleic acids like DNA, RNA, and siRNA. Think of them as tiny delivery vessels with a positive charge attracted to the negative charge of genetic material. This attraction allows them to form stable complexes or nanoparticles with nucleic acids, creating protective bubbles around them [97].

Once these protective bubbles are formed, cationic lipids can navigate through the body's terrain, guided by the currents of the bloodstream. When they encounter target cells, they slip through the cell's outer membrane, like an essential fitting into a lock. These lipid-based delivery vessels release their genetic cargo inside the cell, like a package opened at its destination [101]. However, it is not just about getting through the cell's front door. Cationic lipids have another trick: they know how to navigate the cell's inner landscape. Once inside, they can send genetic material to the cell's nucleus, which can integrate with the cell's DNA, or they can release it directly into its cytoplasm, where it can start its work without delay [102].

Cationic lipids are not just delivery systems; they are like expert navigators, guiding genetic therapies safely to their targets within the body and unlocking the door to a world of potential treatments. Various cationic lipids have been used for nucleic acid delivery; some are discussed below.

4.12.1.1 LIPOFECTAMINE

Lipofectamine is a well-known commercial cationic lipid-based transfection reagent that delivers nucleic acids into cells in research and therapeutic applications. It consists of a mixture of cationic lipids, such as DOTAP (1,2-dioleoyl-3-trimethylammonium-propane) or DMRIE (1,2-dimyristyloxypropyl-3-dimethyl-hydroxy ethyl ammonium bromide), and neutral lipids. Lipofectamine forms complexes with nucleic acids through electrostatic interactions, protecting them from degradation and facilitating cell uptake. Once inside the cells, these complexes release the nucleic acids, allowing them to exert their therapeutic effects or be integrated into the cell's genome [103, 104].

4.12.1.2 DOTAP/DOPE LIPOSOMES

Another example is the formulation of liposomes composed of the cationic lipid DOTAP (1,2-dioleoyl-3-trimethylammonium-propane) and the neutral lipid DOPE (dioleoyl phosphatidyl ethanolamine).

These liposomes have been widely used in research and clinical trials to deliver nucleic acids, including mRNA and siRNA. DOTAP/DOPE liposomes form stable complexes with nucleic acids, protecting them during delivery. The positive charge of DOTAP facilitates the interaction with the negatively charged nucleic acids, while DOPE helps to stabilize the liposome structure. These liposomes can efficiently deliver nucleic acids to target cells, where they can exert their therapeutic effects [96].

4.12.1.3 DMRIE (1,2-DIMYRISTYLOXYPROPYL-3-DIMETHYL-HYDROXY ETHYL AMMONIUM BROMIDE)

DMRIE is another cationic lipid commonly used in nucleic acid delivery systems. Like DOTAP, DMRIE forms stable complexes with nucleic acids, enabling efficient cell delivery. DMRIE lipoplexes have been employed in gene therapy applications to deliver various types of nucleic acids, including plasmid DNA and siRNA. The positive charge of DMRIE facilitates electrostatic interactions with nucleic acids, promoting their cellular uptake and intracellular release.

4.12.1.4 DLIN-KC2-DMA

A potent cationic lipid creates lipid nanoparticles to deliver nucleic acids into cells. Its unique structure allows it to form stable complexes with nucleic acids, safeguarding them during delivery. One of its standout features is its pH-sensitive behavior, crucial for releasing nucleic acids into the cell's cytoplasm. DLin-KC2-DMA LNPs have shown promise in various diseases, making them a valuable tool for gene-based therapies [105]. DLin-KC2-DMA has been extensively studied and optimized for lipid nanoparticles, and it is considered a promising delivery vehicle for nucleic acid therapeutics. Lipid nanoparticles containing DLin-KC2-DMA have been used in various preclinical and clinical studies to treat various diseases, including cancer, genetic disorders, and infectious diseases [106].

Overall, DLin-KC2-DMA represents a significant advancement in nucleic acid delivery, offering a highly efficient and versatile platform for developing novel therapeutics. Its unique properties make it a valuable tool for researchers and clinicians developing gene-based treatments.

4.12.2 IONIZABLE LIPIDS

Ionizable lipids are a specialized type of lipid used in nucleic acid delivery systems, particularly in developing lipid nanoparticles (LNPs). Unlike traditional cationic lipids, ionizable lipids possess a unique property: they can change their charge in response to the pH environment [107–109].

In a neutral or slightly basic environment, ionizable lipids carry no net charge. However, in the acidic environment of endosomes, which are cellular compartments involved in intracellular trafficking, these lipids become positively charged. This pH-dependent charge conversion is crucial for facilitating the release of nucleic acids from the LNPs into the cell's cytoplasm, where they can exert their therapeutic effects [110].

DLin-MC3-DMA is a well-known ionizable lipid extensively used in developing LNPs for nucleic acid delivery. In its neutral state, DLin-MC3-DMA has a neutral charge. However, when exposed to the acidic environment of endosomes, it becomes positively charged, facilitating the release of nucleic acids from the LNPs into the cytoplasm of target cells. DLin-MC3-DMA LNPs have been utilized in various preclinical and clinical studies for delivering mRNA, siRNA, and other nucleic acid therapeutics.

C12-200: C12-200 is another example of an ionizable lipid used in nucleic acid delivery. Like DLin-MC3-DMA, C12-200 undergoes a pH-dependent charge conversion, transitioning from neutral to positively charged in acidic environments. This property enables the efficient release of nucleic acids from LNPs into target cells. C12-200 LNPs have been investigated for delivering mRNA vaccines and siRNA therapeutics in preclinical studies.

4.12.2.1 FUSOGENIC LIPIDS

Fusogenic lipids are a class of lipids that can promote fusion between lipid bilayers. In nucleic acid delivery, fusogenic lipids play a crucial role in facilitating the release of nucleic acids from delivery vehicles into the target cells. When incorporated into lipid-based delivery systems such as liposomes or lipid nanoparticles, fusogenic lipids can enhance the endosomal escape of nucleic acids, which is a critical step for efficient gene delivery [111].

4.12.2.2 DIOLEOYLPHOSPHATIDYLETHANOLAMINE (DOPE)

DOPE is a commonly used fusogenic lipid due to its ability to destabilize lipid bilayers at acidic pH, such as those found within endosomes. It can promote membrane fusion and facilitate the release of nucleic acids from endosomes into the cytoplasm [112].

4.12.2.3 DIOLEOYLPHOSPHATIDYLSERINE (DOPS)

DOPS is another fusogenic lipid that can destabilize membranes under acidic conditions [113]. Liposomal formulations have been utilized to enhance endosomal escape and improve transfection efficiency.

4.12.2.4 CHOLESTEROL HEMISUCCINATE (CHEMS)

CHEMS is a pH-sensitive fusogenic lipid commonly used in liposome formulations. It can destabilize endosomal membranes and facilitate cargo release into the cytoplasm [114].

4.12.3 LIPIDS WITH IMIDAZOLE MOIETY

Lipids containing an imidazole moiety can be crucial in nucleic acid delivery systems. Imidazole is a five-membered aromatic ring containing two non-adjacent nitrogen atoms, making it a versatile functional group for molecular interactions. When incorporated into lipid structures, it imparts unique properties that can enhance the efficiency and specificity of nucleic acid delivery [115]. These lipids possess hydrophilic and hydrophobic regions, allowing them to interact with cell membranes and nucleic acids. Imidazole's pH-responsive behavior facilitates membrane fusion, aiding in intracellular nucleic acid delivery. Imidazole-containing lipids destabilize endosomal membranes in response to pH changes. Protonation of imidazole groups triggers lipid structure alteration, promoting membrane disruption. This protonation allows nucleic acids to escape endosomes and exert therapeutic effects in the cytoplasm [116].

Modification of imidazole-containing lipids enables targeting of specific cell types or tissues. Functional groups attached to the imidazole moiety allow ligand conjugation or surface modification, enhancing delivery specificity and reducing off-target effects. These lipids are synthesized to be biocompatible and stable in physiological conditions. This ensures minimal cytotoxicity and degradation during delivery, preserving nucleic acid integrity and maximizing therapeutic potential [115]. Incorporating imidazole-modified lipids into LNPs has enhanced mRNA-LNP stability and improved immunization properties in mice and non-human primates. These lipids can also confer enhanced stability and strong immunization properties to mRNA-LNPs, making them promising candidates for vaccine development [115]. Further, imidazole-based synthetic lipidoids are effective for *in vivo* mRNA delivery into primary T lymphocytes, indicating their potential for therapeutic applications [117].

In summary, imidazole-containing lipids have shown great promise in enhancing nucleic acid delivery systems' stability, efficiency, and specificity, particularly in mRNA LNP delivery.

4.12.3.1 CATIONIC LIPIDS WITH IMIDAZOLINIUM OR IMIDAZOLIUM POLAR HEAD

Cationic lipids with imidazolinium or imidazolium polar heads are a class of lipids commonly used in nucleic acid delivery systems. These lipids typically comprise a hydrophobic tail region and a cationic polar head group containing an imidazolinium or imidazolium moiety. The imidazolinium or imidazolium groups confer a positive charge to the lipid molecule, allowing electrostatic interaction with negatively charged nucleic acids such as DNA or RNA. This electrostatic interaction forms nanoparticles or complexes where the nucleic acids are encapsulated or complexed with the cationic lipids, protecting them from degradation and facilitating their delivery into target cells [109, 118].

Dobbs et al. underscore the potential of amphiphilic imidazolium salts as a promising new generation of transfection reagents for RNA interference applications [119]. Further, including the imidazolium salt group in the novel macrocyclic polyamine cationic lipid significantly enhances its interaction with DNA and transfection activity as a gene delivery vector. This addition underscores the importance of imidazoline in facilitating efficient nucleic acid delivery for potential therapeutic applications [120].

4.12.3.2 POLYMER–LIPID HYBRID DELIVERY SYSTEM

Polymer-lipid hybrid delivery systems are innovative nanostructures designed to efficiently deliver various therapeutic agents, including nucleic acids like DNA, RNA, and siRNA. They combine the unique properties of both polymers and lipids to create versatile platforms for targeted drug delivery [121]. Polymer–lipid hybrid delivery systems, also known as lipid–polymer hybrid nanoparticles (LPHNPs), are next-generation core-shell nanostructures that combine the benefits of both liposomes and polymeric nanoparticles [122]. The system comprises a polymeric core surrounded by a lipid layer, forming a lipid shell. The therapeutic agents are loaded inside the polymer core, while the lipid layer ensures the system's biocompatibility. An aqueous layer of water fills the space between the lipid and polymeric core. The polymer influences drug release, improving the lipid layer's stability [123].

The core of the LPHNPs could be made up of polymeric biomaterial like polylactic acid (PLA), polycaprolactone (PCL), pluronic F-68, chitosan, and so forth, to attain biodegradability and biocompatibility [122].

The construction of LPHNPs involves three segments: the polymer core, the lipid shell, and the junction where the polymer and lipid components meet. The polymer core is a sturdy foundation for loading drugs, while the lipid shell improves compatibility with biological systems and facilitates drug passage through membranes. The interaction at the interface between the polymer and lipid components is pivotal for the stability and drug-release characteristics of LPHNPs [121,123].

These systems have shown great potential in cancer treatment, where low aqueous solubility, strong toxic reactions affecting multiple organs, non-targeted delivery, cancer cell heterogeneity, and drug degradation are common challenges. LPHNPs offer several advantages as a delivery system, including uniform release of drugs, stability, acceptable size, and, importantly, enhanced encapsulation efficiency [123].

In summary, polymer–lipid hybrid delivery systems offer a promising approach to drug delivery, combining the benefits of liposomes and polymeric nanoparticles. These systems have shown potential in cancer treatment, where they can improve drug solubility, stability, and targeted delivery.

4.12.4 HELPER-LIPIDS

Helper lipids are pivotal in crafting lipid nanoparticles (LNPs) to deliver nucleic acids like siRNA, mRNA, and plasmid DNA. They are strategically arranged to form a lipid bilayer structure, bolstering LNP stability, biocompatibility, and the ability to traverse cell membranes [124, 125]. Various types of helper lipids are employed in LNP formulations. One example is di-stearoyl phosphocholine (DSPC), often combined with cholesterol and other lipids to establish a robust lipid bilayer crucial for nucleic acid delivery. DSPC, being a neutral lipid, fortifies bilayer stability, a critical factor in nucleic acid delivery [124, 126].

Another helper lipid category includes ionizable lipids, which become positively charged in acidic conditions, like those found in endosomes. This property aids mRNA delivery *in vivo* by minimizing interactions with blood cell membranes and enhancing biocompatibility. Additionally, ionizable lipids promote endosomal escape by destabilizing endosomal membranes [99].

Ethylphosphatidylcholine (ePC) and BHEM-Cholesterol are other helper lipids engineered to augment LNP fusion with cellular membranes, thereby enhancing the delivery of mRNA-based cancer immunotherapies and protein replacement therapies [99, 107, 126]. These lipids are also crucial in DNA delivery formulations, particularly for plasmid DNA encoding short hairpin RNA or CRISPR/Cas9. Typically cationic, these helper lipids form stable nanoparticles by complexing with negatively charged DNA, facilitating delivery to target cells [124, 127].

In essence, helper lipids are indispensable in LNPs for nucleic acid delivery, playing a vital role in bolstering stability, biocompatibility, and drug permeation, ensuring successful delivery to target cells.

4.13 CLINICAL STATUS

Polymers have shown promising progress in nucleic acid delivery, especially in preclinical studies. However, their clinical status varies on safety, efficacy, and scalability. Some polymers have advanced to clinical trials, while others are still preclinical. Delivery systems used in various clinical trials are summarized in Table 4.2.

TABLE 4.2 Delivery System Used in Various Clinical Trials

SL. No.	Treatment	Delivery System	Target/ Disease	References
1	HLA-B7	DNA-liposome	Melanoma	[131]
2	Cystic Fibrosis transmembrane conductance regulator (CFTR)	Cationic liposome	Cystic fibrosis	[132]
3	mRNA	Lipid nanoparticle	Solid tumor or lymphoma	[133]
4	siRNA	Cationic lipid Nanoparticle	Solid tumor	[134]
5	mRNA	Lipid nanoparticle	Zika virus	[19]
6	mRNA	Lipid nanoparticle	Influenza	[19]
7	mRNA	Lipid nanoparticle	COVID-19	[19]

Polymeric delivery systems such as liposomes, polyethyleneimine (PEI), polyamidoamine (PAMAM) dendrimers, and poly(lactic-co-glycolic acid) (PLGA) nanoparticles have been investigated for their ability to protect nucleic acids, enhance cellular uptake, and facilitate endosomal escape [128]. Specific polymer-based delivery systems have been evaluated in clinical trials for their potential in gene therapy and nucleic acid-based vaccines. For example, LNPs, composed of lipid-based polymers, have been utilized in mRNA-based COVID-19 vaccines, demonstrating their clinical viability and effectiveness on a large scale [129, 130].

4.14 CONCLUSION

Overall, while polymers hold significant promise for nucleic acid delivery, continued research is needed to address challenges such as toxicity, immunogenicity, and achieving targeted delivery to specific cells or tissues. Clinical translation will depend on successfully resolving these issues and demonstrating safety and efficacy in human trials.

ACKNOWLEDGMENT

The author acknowledges the management of VNS Group of Institutions Faculty of Pharmacy, Swami Vivakand College, and Ravindranath Tagore University for providing essential support for literature and time for writing the chapter.

CONFLICT OF INTEREST

The authors declare no conflict of interest.

FUNDING

None

KEYWORDS

- **antibody drug**
- **gene therapy**
- **nanomedicine**
- **nucleic acids**
- **polyethyleneimine**
- **polymers**
- **vaccine delivery**

REFERENCES

1. Jocelyne, P., & Guy, B. (2020). Pandemics throughout history. *Frontiers in Microbiology, 11*, 631736. https://doi.org/10.3389/fmicb.2020.631736 (accessed on 23rd June 2025).
2. Baker, R. E., Mahmud, A. S., Miller, I. F., Rajeev, M., Rasambainarivo, F., Rice, B. L., Takahashi, S., Tatem, A. J., Wagner, C. E., Wang, L. F., Wesolowski, A., & Metcalf, C. J. E. (2022). Infectious disease in an era of global change. *Nature Reviews Microbiology, 20*(4), 193–205. https://doi.org/10.1038/s41579-021-00639-z (accessed on 23rd June 2025).
3. Kulkarni, J. A., Witzigmann, D., Thomson, S. B., Chen, S., Leavitt, B. R., Cullis, P. R., & van der Meel, R. (2021). The current landscape of nucleic acid therapeutics. *Nature Nanotechnology, 16*, 630–643. https://doi.org/10.1038/s41565-021-00937-w (accessed on 23rd June 2025).
4. Rao, V. A., Kim, J. J., Patel, D. S., Rains, K., & Estoll, C. R. (2020). A comprehensive scientific survey of excipients used in currently marketed, therapeutic biological drug products. *Pharmaceutical Research, 37*(200), 1–13.

5. Nayerossadat, N., Ali, P. A., & Maedeh, T. (2012). Viral and nonviral delivery systems for gene delivery. *Advanced Biomedical Research, 1*(27), 1–11.
6. Yamada, Y. (2021). Nucleic acid drugs—Current status, issues, and expectations for exosomes. *Cancers (Basel), 13*(19), 5002. https://doi.org/10.3390/cancers13195002 (accessed on 23rd June 2025).
7. Hüttenhofer, A., Schattner, P., & Polacek, N. (2005). Non-coding RNAs: Hope or hype? *Trends in Genetics, 21*(5), 289–297. https://doi.org/10.1016/j.tig.2005.03.007 (accessed on 23rd June 2025).
8. Moccia, M., Pascucci, B., Saviano, M., Cerasa, T., Terzidis, M. A., Chatgilialoglu, C., & Masi, A. (2024). Advances in nucleic acid research: Exploring the potential of oligonucleotides for therapeutic applications and biological studies. *International Journal of Molecular Sciences, 25*(1), 146.
9. Chen, G., Ruiz, B. Z. E. F., & Zhang, F. (2022). Advances in the polymeric delivery of nucleic acid vaccines. *Theragnostic, 12*(9), 4081–4109. https://doi.org/10.7150/thno.70853 (accessed on 23rd June 2025).
10. Huang, P., Deng, H., Zhou, Y., & Chen, X. (2022). The roles of polymers in mRNA delivery. *Matter, 5*(6), 1670–1699. https://doi.org/10.1016/j.matt.2022.03.006 (accessed on 23rd June 2025).
11. Karpenko, L. I., Apartsin, E. K., Dudko, S. G., Starostina, E. V., Kaplina, O. N., & Antonets, D. V. (2020). Cationic polymers for the delivery of the Ebola DNA vaccine encoding artificial T-cell immunogen. *Vaccines, 8*(4), 718. https://doi.org/10.3390/vaccines8040718 (accessed on 23rd June 2025).
12. Bishop, C. J., Kozielski, K. L., & Green, J. J. (2015). Exploring the role of polymer structure on intracellular nucleic acid delivery via polymeric nanoparticles. *Journal of Controlled Release, 219*, 488–499. https://doi.org/10.1016/j.jconrel.2015.09.046 (accessed on 23rd June 2025).
13. Fenton, O. S., Olafson, K. N., Pillai, P. S., Mitchell, M. J., & Langer, R. (2018). Advances in biomaterials for drug delivery. *Advanced Materials, 30*(29). https://doi.org/10.1002/adma.201705328 (accessed on 23rd June 2025).
14. Le, T. K., Paris, C., Khan, K. S., Robson, F., Ng, W. L., & Rocchi, P. (2021). Nucleic acid-based technologies targeting coronaviruses. *Trends in Biochemical Sciences, 46*(5), 351–365. https://doi.org/10.1016/j.tibs.2020.11.010 (accessed on 23rd June 2025).
15. Sridharan, K., & Gogtay, N. J. (2016). Therapeutic nucleic acids: Current clinical status. *British Journal of Clinical Pharmacology, 82*(3), 659–672. https://doi.org/10.1111/bcp.12987 (accessed on 23rd June 2025).
16. Wang, F., Li, P., Chu, H. C., & Lo, P. K. (2022). Nucleic acids and their analogues for biomedical applications. *Biosensors (Basel), 12*(2), 93. https://doi.org/10.3390/bios12020093 (accessed on 23rd June 2025).
17. Julian, D., Vanegas, T., Cruz, J. C., & Reyes, L. H. (2021). Delivery systems for nucleic acids and proteins: Barriers, cell capture pathways and nanocarriers. *Pharmaceutics, 13*(3), 428. https://doi.org/10.3390/pharmaceutics13030428 (accessed on 23rd June 2025).
18. Jote, T., Bulcha, Y., Wang, H., Ma, H., Tai, P. W. L., & Gao, G. (2021). Viral vector platforms within the gene therapy landscape. *Signal Transduction and Targeted*

Therapy, 6, 53. https://doi.org/10.1038/s41392-021-00487-6 (accessed on 23rd June 2025).

19. van den Berg, A. I. S., Yun, C. O., Schiffelers, R. M., & Hennink, W. E. (2021). Polymeric delivery systems for nucleic acid therapeutics: Approaching the clinic. *Journal of Controlled Release, 331*, 121–141. https://doi.org/10.1016/j.jconrel.2021.01.014 (accessed on 23rd June 2025).
20. Scott, L. J. (2015). Alipogene tiparvovec: A review of its use in adults with familial lipoprotein lipase deficiency. *Drugs, 75*(2), 175–182. https://doi.org/10.1007/s40265-014-0339-9 (accessed on 23rd June 2025).
21. Morris, G., O'Brien, D., & Henshall, D. C. (2021). Opportunities and challenges for microRNA-targeting therapeutics for epilepsy. *Trends in Pharmacological Sciences, 42*(7), 605–616. https://doi.org/10.1016/j.tips.2021.04.007 (accessed on 23rd June 2025).
22. Dhuri, K., Clara, B., Quijano, E., Pham, H., Gupta, A., Vikram, A., & Bahal, R. (2020). Antisense oligonucleotides: An emerging area in drug discovery and development. *Journal of Clinical Medicine, 9*(6), 1–24. https://doi.org/10.3390/jcm9062004 (accessed on 23rd June 2025).
23. Melo, A. R. da S., de Macêdo, L. S., Invenção, M. da C. V., de Moura, I. A., da Gama, M. A. T. M., de Melo, C. M. L., Silva, A. J. D., Batista, M. V. de A., & de Freitas, A. C. (2022). Third-generation vaccines: Features of nucleic acid vaccines and strategies to improve their efficiency. *Genes, 13*(12), 2287–2301. https://doi.org/10.3390/genes13122287 (accessed on 23rd June 2025).
24. Han, X., Mitchell, M. J., & Nie, G. (2020). Nanomaterials for therapeutic RNA delivery. *Matter, 3*, 1948–1975.
25. Schoenmaker, L., Witzigmann, D., Kulkarni, J., Verbeke, R., Kersten, G., Jiskoot, W., & Crommelin, D. (2021). mRNA-lipid nanoparticle COVID-19 vaccines: Structure and stability. *International Journal of Pharmaceutics, 601*, 120586.
26. Ingle, R. G., & Fang, W. J. (2023). An overview of the stability and delivery challenges of commercial nucleic acid therapeutics. *Pharmaceutics, 15*(4), 1158. https://doi.org/10.3390/pharmaceutics15041158 (accessed on 23rd June 2025).
27. Ols, S., Yang, L., Thompson, E. A., Pushparaj, P., Tran, K., Liang, F., Lin, A., Eriksson, B., Hedestam, G. B. K., Wyatt, R. T., & Loré, K. (2020). Route of vaccine administration alters antigen trafficking but not innate or adaptive immunity. *Cell Reports, 30*(12), 3964–3971. https://doi.org/10.1016/j.celrep.2020.02.111 (accessed on 23rd June 2025).
28. Xue, L., Yan, Y. F., Kos, P., Chen, X., & Siegwart, D. J. (2021). PEI fluorination reduces toxicity and promotes liver-targeted siRNA delivery. *Drug Delivery and Translational Research, 11*(1), 255–260.
29. Merkel, O. M., Beyerle, A., Librizzi, D., Pfestroff, A., Behr, T. M., Sproat, B., Barth, P. J., & Kissel, T. (2009). Nonviral siRNA delivery to the lung: Investigation of PEG-PEI polyplexes and their *in vivo* performance. *Molecular Pharmaceutics, 6*(4), 1246–1260. https://doi.org/10.1021/mp900107v (accessed on 23rd June 2025).
30. Deng, Z. C., Kalin, G. T., Shi, D. L., & Kalinichenko, V. V. (2021). Nanoparticle delivery systems with cell-specific targeting for pulmonary diseases. *American Journal of Respiratory Cell and Molecular Biology, 64*(3), 292–307. https://doi.org/10.1165/rcmb.2020-0306TR (accessed on 23rd June 2025).

31. Zoulikha, M., Xiao, Q. Q., Boafo, G. F., Marwa, A., Chen, S. Z., & He, W. (2022). Pulmonary delivery of siRNA against acute lung injury/acute respiratory distress syndrome. *Acta Pharmaceutica Sinica B, 12*(2), 600–620. https://doi.org/10.1016/j.apsb.2021.08.009 (accessed on 23rd June 2025).
32. Del, S. L., Costamagna, A., Muraca, G., Rotondo, G., Civiletti, F., Vizio, B., Bosco, O., Conte, E. L. M., Frati, G., Delsedime, L., Lupia, E., Fanelli, V., & Ranieri, V. M. (2016). Intratracheal administration of small interfering RNA targeting FAS reduces lung ischemia reperfusion injury. *Critical Care Medicine, 44*(8), e604–e613. https://doi.org/10.1097/CCM.0000000000001601 (accessed on 23rd June 2025).
33. Laube, B. L. (2015). Aerosolized medications for gene and peptide therapy. *Respiratory Care, 60*(6), 806–824. https://doi.org/10.4187/respcare.03554 (accessed on 23rd June 2025).
34. Farkas, A., Tomisa, G., Szénasi, G., Furi, P., Kugler, S., Nagy, A., Varga, J., & Horváth, A. (2023). The effect of lung emptying before the inhalation of aerosol drugs on drug deposition in the respiratory system. *International Journal of Pharmaceutics: X, 6*, 100192. https://doi.org/10.1016/j.ijpx.2023.100192 (accessed on 23rd June 2025).
35. Qin, Y., Ou, L., Zha, L., & Zeng, Y., & Li, L. (2023). Delivery of nucleic acids using nanomaterials. *Molecular Biomedicine, 4*, 48. https://doi.org/10.1186/s43556-023-00160-0 (accessed on 23rd June 2025).
36. Balian, A., & Hernandez, F. J. (2021). Nucleases as molecular targets for cancer diagnosis. *Biomarker Research, 9*(1), 86–102. https://doi.org/10.1186/s40364-021-00342-4 (accessed on 23rd June 2025).
37. Xu, L., & Anchordoquy, T. (2011). Drug delivery trends in clinical trials and translational medicine: Challenges and opportunities in the delivery of nucleic acid-based therapeutics. *Journal of Pharmaceutical Sciences, 100*(1), 38–52. https://doi.org/10.1002/jps.22243 (accessed on 23rd June 2025).
38. Mahmoudi, M., Landry, M. P., Moore, A., & Coreas, R. (2023). The protein corona from nanomedicine to environmental science. *Nature Reviews Materials, 8*(7), 422–438. https://doi.org/10.1038/s41578-023-00552-2 (accessed on 23rd June 2025).
39. He, X. Y., Wang, J., Tang, Y. Q., Chiang, S. T., Han, T., Chen, Q., Qian, C., Shen, X., Li, R., & Ai, X. (2023). Recent advances of emerging spleen-targeting nano vaccines for immunotherapy. *Advanced Healthcare Materials, 12*(23), 18. https://doi.org/10.1002/adhm.202300351C (accessed on 23rd June 2025).
40. Zhang, M. M., Gao, S., Yang, D. J., Fang, Y., Lin, X., Jin, X., Liu, Y., Liu, X., Su, K., & Shi, K. (2021). Influencing factors and strategies of enhancing nanoparticles into tumors *in vivo*. *Acta Pharmaceutica Sinica B, 11*(8), 2265–2285. https://doi.org/10.1016/j.apsb.2021.03.033 (accessed on 23rd June 2025).
41. Pangeni, R., Meng, T., Poudel, S., Sharma, D., Hutsell, H., Ma, J., Rubin, B. K., Longest, W., Hindle, M., & Xu, Q. (2023). Airway mucus in pulmonary diseases: Muco-adhesive and muco-penetrating particles to overcome the airway mucus barriers. *International Journal of Pharmaceutics, 634*, 17. https://doi.org/10.1016/j.ijpharm.2023.122661 (accessed on 23rd June 2025).
42. Ernst, M., John, T., Guenther, M., Wagner, C., Schaefer, U. F., & Lehr, C. M. (2017). A model for the transient sub diffusive behavior of particles in mucus. *Biophysical Journal, 112*(1), 172–179. https://doi.org/10.1016/j.bpj.2016.11.900 (accessed on 23rd June 2025).

43. d'Angelo, I., Costabile, G., Durantie, E., Brocca, P., Rondelli, V., Russo, A., Russo, G., Miro, A., Quaglia, F., Petri-Fink, A., Rutishauser, B. R., & Ungaro, F. (2018). Hybrid lipid/polymer nanoparticles for pulmonary delivery of siRNA: Development and fate upon *in vitro* deposition on the human epithelial airway barrier. *Journal of Aerosol Medicine and Pulmonary Drug Delivery, 31*(3), 170–181. https://doi.org/10.1089/jamp.2017.1364 (accessed on 23rd June 2025).
44. Hu, M., Li, X., You, Z., Cai, R., & Chen, C. (2023). Physiological barriers and strategies of lipid-based nanoparticles for nucleic acid drug delivery. *Advanced Materials*. https://doi.org/10.1002/adma.202303266 (accessed on 23rd June 2025).
45. Kubota, K., Onishi, K., Sawaki, K., Li, T., Mitsuoka, K., Sato, T., & Takeoka, S. (2017). Effect of the nano formulation of siRNA-lipid assemblies on their cellular uptake and immune stimulation. *International Journal of Nanomedicine, 12*, 5121–5133. https://doi.org/10.2147/IJN.S136426 (accessed on 23rd June 2025).
46. Suberi, A., Grun, M. K., Mao, T., Israelow, B., Reschke, M., Grundler, J., Akhtar, L., Lee, T., Shin, K., Piotrowski-Daspit, A. S., Homer, R. J., Iwasaki, A., Suh, H. W., & Saltzman, W. M. (2023). Polymer nanoparticles deliver mRNA to the lung for mucosal vaccination. *Science Translational Medicine, 15*(709), eabq0603. https://doi.org/10.1126/scitranslmed.abq0603 (accessed on 23rd June 2025).
47. Hatakeyama, H., Akita, H., Ito, E., Hayashi, Y., Oishi, M., Nagasaki, Y., Danev, R., Nagayama, K., Kaji, N., Kikuchi, H., Baba, Y., & Harashima, H. (2011). Systemic delivery of siRNA to tumors using a lipid nanoparticle containing a tumor-specific cleavable PEG-lipid. *Biomaterials, 32*(18), 4306–4316. https://doi.org/10.1016/j.biomaterials.2011.02.045 (accessed on 23rd June 2025).
48. Zeng, J., Shirihai, O. S., & Grinstaff, M. W. (2020). Modulating lysosomal pH: A molecular and nanoscale materials design perspective. *Journal of Life Sciences (Westlake Village, Calif), 2*(4), 25–37. https://doi.org/10.36069/jols/20201204 (accessed on 23rd June 2025).
49. Zuhorn, I. S., Bakowsky, U., Polushkin, E., Visser, W. H., Stuart, M. C. A., Engberts, J. B. F. N., & Hoekstra, D. (2005). Nonbilayer phase of lipoplex-membrane mixture determines endosomal escape of genetic cargo and transfection efficiency. *Molecular Therapy, 11*(5), 801–810. https://doi.org/10.1016/j.ymthe.2004.12.018 (accessed on 23rd June 2025).
50. Shui, M., Chen, Z., Chen, Y., Yuan, Q., Li, H., Vong, C. T., Farag, M. A., & Wang, S. (2023). Engineering polyphenol-based carriers for nucleic acid delivery. *Theragnostic, 13*(10), 3204–3223. https://doi.org/10.7150/thno.81604 (accessed on 23rd June 2025).
51. Farshbaf, M., Davaran, S., Zarebkohan, A., Annabi, N., Akbarzadeh, A., & Salehi, R. (2018). Significant role of cationic polymers in drug delivery systems. *Artificial Cells, Nanomedicine, and Biotechnology, 46*(8), 1872–1891. https://doi.org/10.1080/21691401.2017.1395344 (accessed on 23rd June 2025).
52. Farber, F. E., Melnick, J. L., & Butel, J. S. (1975). Optimal conditions for uptake of exogenous DNA by Chinese hamster lung cells deficient in hypoxanthine-guanine phosphoribosyl transferase. *Biochemical et Biophysical Acta–Nucleic Acids and Protein Synthesis, 390*, 298–311. https://doi.org/10.1016/0005-2787(75)90350-0 (accessed on 23rd June 2025).

53. Ramsay, E., Hadgraft, J., Birchall, J., & Gumbleton, M. (2000). Examination of the biophysical interaction between plasmid DNA and the polycations, polylysine and polyornithine, as a basis for their differential gene transfection *in-vitro*. *International Journal of Pharmaceutics, 210*, 97–107. https://doi.org/10.1016/S0378-5173(00)00571-8 (accessed on 23rd June 2025).
54. Wu, G. Y., & Wu, C. H. (1987). Receptor-mediated *in vitro* gene transformation by a soluble DNA carrier system. *Journal of Biological Chemistry, 262*(10), 4429–4432.
55. Schreiber, S., Kämpgen, E., Wagner, E., Pirkhammer, D., Trcka, J., Korschan, H., Lindemann, A., Dorffner, R., Kittler, H., Kasteliz, F., Küpcü, Z., Sinski, A., Zatloukal, K., Buschle, M., Schmidt, W., Birnstiel, M., Kempe, R. E., Voigt, T., Weber, H. A., & Stingl, G. (1999). Immunotherapy of metastatic malignant melanoma by a vaccine consisting of autologous interleukin 2-transfected cancer cells: Outcome of a phase I study. *Human Gene Therapy, 10*(6), 983–993. https://doi.org/10.1089/10430349950018382 (accessed on 23rd June 2025).
56. Luthman, H., & Magnusson, G. (1983). High efficiency polyoma DNA transfection of chloroquine treated cells. *Nucleic Acids Research, 11*(5), 1295–1308. https://doi.org/10.1093/nar/11.5.1295 (accessed on 23rd June 2025).
57. Cotten, M., Langle-Rouault, F., Kirlappos, H., Wagner, E., Mechtler, K., Zenke, M., Beug, H., & Birnstiel, M. L. (1990). Transferrin-polycation-mediated introduction of DNA into human leukemic cells: Stimulation by agents that affect the survival of transfected DNA or modulate transferrin receptor levels. *Proceedings of the National Academy of Sciences of the United States of America, 87*, 4033–4037. https://doi.org/10.1073/pnas.87.11.4033 (accessed on 23rd June 2025).
58. Erbacher, P., Roche, A. C., Monsigny, M., & Midoux, P. (1996). Putative role of chloroquine in gene transfer into a human hepatoma cell line by DNA/lactosylated polylysine complexes. *Experimental Cell Research, 225*, 186–194. https://doi.org/10.1006/excr.1996.0169 (accessed on 23rd June 2025).
59. Cheng, J., Zeidan, R., Mishra, S., Liu, A., Pun, S. H., Kulkarni, R. P., Jensen, G. S., Bellocq, N. C., & Davis, M. E. (2006). Structure-function correlation of chloroquine and analogues as transgene expression enhancers in nonviral gene delivery. *Journal of Medicinal Chemistry, 49*, 6522–6531. https://doi.org/10.1021/jm060736s (accessed on 23rd June 2025).
60. Zhang, P., & Wagner, E. (2017). History of polymeric gene delivery systems. *Topics in Current Chemistry (Cham), 375*(2), 26. https://doi.org/10.1007/s41061-017-0112-0 (accessed on 23rd June 2025).
61. Katayose, S., & Kataoka, K. (1998). Remarkable increase in nuclease resistance of plasmid DNA through supramolecular assembly with poly (ethylene glycol)-poly(L-lysine) block copolymer. *Journal of Pharmaceutical Sciences, 87*(2), 160–163. https://doi.org/10.1021/js970304s (accessed on 23rd June 2025).
62. Palmer, K., Moore, J., Everard, M., Harris, J. D., Rodgers, S., Rees, R. C., Murray, A. K., Mascari, R., Kirkwood, J., Riches, P. G., Fisher, C., Thomas, J. M., Harries, M., Johnston, S. R., Collins, M. K., & Gore, M. E. (1999). Gene therapy with autologous, interleukin 2-secreting tumor cells in patients with malignant melanoma. *Human Gene Therapy, 10*(8), 1261–1268. https://doi.org/10.1089/10430349950017941 (accessed on 23rd June 2025).

63. Mann, A., Khan, M. A., Shukla, V., & Ganguli, M. (2007). Atomic force microscopy reveals the assembly of potential DNA "nanocarriers" by poly-L-ornithine. *Biophysical Chemistry, 129*(2, 3), 126–136. https://doi.org/10.1016/j.bpc.2007.05.012 (accessed on 23rd June 2025).
64. Kim, P. H., Kim, T. I., Yockman, J. W., Kim, S. W., & Yun, C. O. (2010). The effect of surface modification of adenovirus with an arginine-grafted bio reducible polymer on transduction efficiency and immunogenicity in cancer gene therapy. *Biomaterials, 31*(7), 1865–1874. https://doi.org/10.1016/j.biomaterials.2009.11.043 (accessed on 23rd June 2025).
65. Wyman, T. B., Nicol, F., Zelphati, O., Scaria, P. V., Plank, C., & Szoka, F. C. Jr. (1997). Design, synthesis, and characterization of a cationic peptide that binds to nucleic acids and permeabilizes bilayers. *Biochemistry, 36*(10), 3008–3017. https://doi.org/10.1021/bi9618474 (accessed on 23rd June 2025).
66. Li, W., Nicol, F., & Szoka, F. C. Jr. (2004). GALA: A designed synthetic pH-responsive amphipathic peptide with applications in drug and gene delivery. *Advanced Drug Delivery Reviews, 56*(7), 967–985. https://doi.org/10.1016/j.addr.2003.10.041 (accessed on 23rd June 2025).
67. Palmerston Mendes, L., Pan, J., & Torchilin, V. P. (2017). Dendrimers as nanocarriers for nucleic acid and drug delivery in cancer therapy. *Molecules, 22*(9), 1401. https://doi.org/10.3390/molecules22091401 (accessed on 23rd June 2025).
68. Mintzer, M. A., Merkel, O. M., Kissel, T., & Simanek, E. E. (2009). Polycationic triazine-based dendrimers: Effect of peripheral groups on transfection efficiency. *New Journal of Chemistry, 33*, 1918–1925. https://doi.org/10.1039/b908735d (accessed on 23rd June 2025).
69. Behr, J. (1997). The proton sponge: A trick to enter cells the viruses did not exploit. *Chimia (Aarau), 51*, 34–36.
70. Fischer, D., Li, Y., Ahlemeyer, B., Krieglstein, J., & Kissel, T. (2003). *In vitro* cytotoxicity testing of polycations: Influence of polymer structure on cell viability and hemolysis. *Biomaterials, 24*(7), 1121–1131. https://doi.org/10.1016/s0142-9612(02)00445-3 (accessed on 23rd June 2025).
71. Gjetting, T., Arildsen, N. S., Christensen, C. L., Poulsen, T. T., Roth, J. A., Handlos, V. N., & Poulsen, H. S. (2010). *In vitro* and *in vivo* effects of polyethylene glycol (PEG)-modified lipid in DOTAP/cholesterol-mediated gene transfection. *International Journal of Nanomedicine, 5*, 371–383. https://doi.org/10.2147/ijn.s10462 (accessed on 23rd June 2025).
72. Woo, J., & Lee, J. S. (2021). Effects of lyoprotectants on long-term stability and transfection efficacy of lyophilized poly(lactide-co-glycoside)-graft-polyethyleneimine/plasmid DNA polyplexes. *Nanomedicine (London), 16*(15), 1269–1280. https://doi.org/10.2217/nnm-2021-0065 (accessed on 23rd June 2025).
73. Itaka, K., Harada, A., Yamasaki, Y., Nakamura, K., Kawaguchi, H., & Kataoka, K. (2004). *In situ* single cell observation by fluorescence resonance energy transfer reveals fast intra-cytoplasmic delivery and easy release of plasmid DNA complexed with linear polyethyleneimine. *Journal of Gene Medicine, 6*(1), 76–84. https://doi.org/10.1002/jgm.470 (accessed on 23rd June 2025).
74. Ludtke, J. J., Zhang, G., Sebestyén, M. G., & Wolff, J. A. (1999). A nuclear localization signal can enhance both the nuclear transport and expression of 1 kb DNA. *Journal*

of Cell Science, 112(Pt 12), 2033–2041. https://doi.org/10.1242/jcs.112.12.2033 (accessed on 23rd June 2025).
75. Plank, C., Mechtler, K., Szoka, F. C. Jr., & Wagner, E. (1996). Activation of the complement system by synthetic DNA complexes: A potential barrier for intravenous gene delivery. *Human Gene Therapy, 7*(12), 1437–1446. https://doi.org/10.1089/hum.1996.7.12-1437 (accessed on 23rd June 2025).
76. Tracey, S. R., Smyth, P., Barelle, C. J., & Scott, C. J. (2021). Development of next generation nanomedicine-based approaches for the treatment of cancer: We've barely scratched the surface. *Biochemical Society Transactions, 49*(5), 2253–2269. https://doi.org/10.1042/BST20210343 (accessed on 23rd June 2025).
77. Freeman, E. C., Weiland, L. M., & Meng, W. S. (2013). Modeling the proton sponge hypothesis: Examining proton sponge effectiveness for enhancing intracellular gene delivery through multiscale modeling. *Journal of Biomaterials Science, Polymer Edition, 24*(4), 398–416. https://doi.org/10.1080/09205063.2012.690282 (accessed on 23rd June 2025).
78. Sonawane, N. D., Szoka, F. C. Jr., & Verkman, A. S. (2003). Chloride accumulation and swelling in endosomes enhances DNA transfer by polyamine-DNA polyplexes. *Journal of Biological Chemistry, 278*(45), 44826–44831. https://doi.org/10.1074/jbc.M308643200 (accessed on 23rd June 2025).
79. Mendes, B. B., Conniot, J., Avital, A., Yao, D., Jiang, X., Zhou, X., Sharf-Pauker, N., Xiao, Y., Adir, O., Liang, H., Shi, J., Schroeder, A., & Conde, J. (2022). Nano delivery of nucleic acids. *Nature Reviews Methods Primers, 2*, 24. https://doi.org/10.1038/s43586-022-00104-y (accessed on 23rd June 2025).
80. Mishra, A., & Yadav, S. K. (2016). Development of sustained release metoprolol succinate matrix tablets using kappa carrageenan as monolithic polymer. *Research Journal of Pharmacy and Technology, 9*(9), 1311–1316.
81. Dewangan, H. K., Sharma, A., Mishra, A., & Singour, P. (2021). Mucoadhesive microspheres of atorvastatin calcium: Rational design, evaluation and enhancement of bioavailability. *Indian Journal of Pharmaceutical Education and Research, 55*(3s), S733–S741.
82. Tiwari, P., Shivhare, V., Ahuja, R., Khan, N., Shukla, D. N., Mishra, A. K., Basu, A., & Dutt Konar, A. (2023). A homochiral diphenylalanine analog based mechanoresponsive hydrogel: An insight towards its wound healing efficacy. *Chemistry & Biodiversity, 20*(10), e202300622. https://doi.org/10.1002/cbdv.202300622 (accessed on 23rd June 2025).
83. Tiwari, P., Gupta, A., Shukla, D. N., Mishra, A. K., Basu, A., & Dutt Konar, A. (2021). Chiral orchestration: A tool for fishing out tripeptide-based mechanoresponsive supergelators possessing anti-inflammatory and antimicrobial properties. *ACS Applied Bio Materials, 4*(5), 4119–4130. https://doi.org/10.1021/acsabm.0c01513 (accessed on 23rd June 2025).
84. Ahn, C. H., Chae, S. Y., Bae, Y. H., & Kim, S. W. (2002). Biodegradable poly(ethylenimine) for plasmid DNA delivery. *Journal of Controlled Release, 80*(1–3), 273–282. https://doi.org/10.1016/s0168-3659(01)00547-8 (accessed on 23rd June 2025).
85. Wen, Y., Pan, S., Luo, X., Zhang, X., Zhang, W., & Feng, M. (2009). A biodegradable low molecular weight polyethyleneimine derivative as low toxicity and efficient gene

vector. *Bioconjugate Chemistry, 20*(2), 322–332. https://doi.org/10.1021/bc800428y (accessed on 23rd June 2025).

86. Dang, J. M., & Leong, K. W. (2006). Natural polymers for gene delivery and tissue engineering. *Advanced Drug Delivery Reviews, 58*(4), 487–499. https://doi.org/10.1016/j.addr.2006.03.001 (accessed on 23rd June 2025).
87. Ni, R., Feng, R., & Chau, Y. (2019). Synthetic approaches for nucleic acid delivery: Choosing the right carriers. *Life, 9*(3), 59. https://doi.org/10.3390/life9030059 (accessed on 23rd June 2025).
88. Guo, X., Yuan, Z., Xu, Y., Zhao, X., Fang, Z., & Yuan, W. E. (2019). A low-molecular-weight polyethyleneimine/pDNA-VEGF polyplex system constructed in a one-pot manner for hindlimb ischemia therapy. *Pharmaceutics, 11*(4), 171. https://doi.org/10.3390/pharmaceutics11040171 (accessed on 23rd June 2025).
89. Li, B., Niu, H., Zhao, X., Huang, X., Ding, Y., Dang, K., Yang, T., Chen, Y., Ma, J., Liu, X., Zhang, K., Xie, H., & Ding, P. (2024). Targeted anti-cancer therapy: Co-delivery of VEGF siRNA and phenethyl isothiocyanate (PEITC) via cRGD-modified lipid nanoparticles for enhanced anti-angiogenic efficacy. *Asian Journal of Pharmaceutical Sciences, 19*(2), 100891. https://doi.org/10.1016/j.ajps.2024.100891 (accessed on 23rd June 2025).
90. Haley, R. M., Gottardi, R., Langer, R., & Mitchell, M. J. (2020). Cyclodextrins in drug delivery: Applications in gene and combination therapy. *Drug Delivery and Translational Research, 10*(3), 661–677. https://doi.org/10.1007/s13346-020-00724-5 (accessed on 23rd June 2025).
91. Ramezani, M., Ebrahimian, M., & Hashemi, M. (2017). Current strategies in the modification of PLGA-based gene delivery system. *Current Medicinal Chemistry, 24*(7), 728–739. https://doi.org/10.2174/0929867324666161205130416 (accessed on 23rd June 2025).
92. Zeng, M., Xu, Q., Zhou, D., A, S., Alshehri, F., Lara-Sáez, I., Zheng, Y., Li, M., & Wang, W. (2021). Highly branched poly (β-amino ester) s for gene delivery in hereditary skin diseases. *Advanced Drug Delivery Reviews, 176*, 113842. https://doi.org/10.1016/j.addr.2021.113842 (accessed on 23rd June 2025).
93. Lv, Z., Zhu, Y., & Li, F. (2021). DNA functional nanomaterials for controlled delivery of nucleic acid-based drugs. *Frontiers in Bioengineering and Biotechnology, 9*, 720291. https://doi.org/10.3389/fbioe.2021.720291 (accessed on 23rd June 2025).
94. Okamoto, A., Asai, T., Hirai, Y., Shimizu, K., Koide, H., Minamino, T., & Oku, N. (2018). Systemic administration of siRNA with anti-HB-EGF antibody-modified lipid nanoparticles for the treatment of triple-negative breast cancer. *Molecular Pharmaceutics, 15*(4), 1495–1504. https://doi.org/10.1021/acs.molpharmaceut.7b01055 (accessed on 23rd June 2025).
95. Wooddell, C. I., Rozema, D. B., Hossbach, M., John, M., Hamilton, H. L., Chu, Q., Hegge, J. O., Klein, J. J., Wakefield, D. H., Oropeza, C. E., Deckert, J., Roehl, I., Jahn-Hofmann, K., Hadwiger, P., Vornlocher, H. P., McLachlan, A., & Lewis, D. L. (2013). Hepatocyte-targeted RNAi therapeutics for the treatment of chronic hepatitis B virus infection. *Molecular Therapy, 21*(5), 973–985. https://doi.org/10.1038/mt.2013.31 (accessed on 23rd June 2025).

96. Zhu, L., & Mahato, R. I. (2010). Lipid and polymeric carrier-mediated nucleic acid delivery. *Expert Opinion on Drug Delivery, 7*(10), 1209–1226. https://doi.org/10.1517/17425247.2010.513969 (accessed on 23rd June 2025).
97. Bolhassani, A. (2023). Lipid-based delivery systems in development of genetic and subunit vaccines. *Molecular Biotechnology, 65*(5), 669–698. https://doi.org/10.1007/s12033-022-00624-8 (accessed on 23rd June 2025).
98. Khalil, I. A., Younis, M. A., Kimura, S., & Harashima, H. (2020). Lipid nanoparticles for cell-specific *in vivo* targeted delivery of nucleic acids. *Biological and Pharmaceutical Bulletin, 43*(4), 584–595. https://doi.org/10.1248/bpb.b19-00743 (accessed on 23rd June 2025).
99. Hou, X., Zaks, T., Langer, R., & Dong, Y. (2021). Lipid nanoparticles for mRNA delivery. *Nature Reviews Materials, 6*(12), 1078–1094. https://doi.org/10.1038/s41578-021-00358-0 (accessed on 23rd June 2025).
100. Kim, M. W., Kwon, S. H., Choi, J. H., & Lee, A. (2018). A promising biocompatible platform: Lipid-based and bio-inspired smart drug delivery systems for cancer therapy. *International Journal of Molecular Sciences, 19*(12), 3859. https://doi.org/10.3390/ijms19123859 (accessed on 23rd June 2025).
101. Hafez, I. M., Maurer, N., & Cullis, P. R. (2001). On the mechanism whereby cationic lipids promote intracellular delivery of polynucleic acids. *Gene Therapy, 8*(15), 1188–1196. https://doi.org/10.1038/sj.gt.3301506 (accessed on 23rd June 2025).
102. Zuhorn, I. S., Engberts, J. B., & Hoekstra, D. (2007). Gene delivery by cationic lipid vectors: Overcoming cellular barriers. *European Biophysics Journal, 36*(4, 5), 349–362. https://doi.org/10.1007/s00249-006-0092-4 (accessed on 23rd June 2025).
103. Kojima, C., Sawada, M., Nakase, I., & Matsumoto, A. (2023). Gene delivery into T-cells using ternary complexes of DNA, Lipofectamine, and carboxy-terminal phenylalanine-modified dendrimers. *Macromolecular Bioscience, 23*(11), e2300139. https://doi.org/.1002/mabi.202300139 (accessed on 23rd June 2025).
104. Cardarelli, F., Digiacomo, L., Marchini, C., Amici, A., Salomone, F., Fiume, G., Rossetta, A., Gratton, E., Pozzi, D., & Caracciolo, G. (2016). The intracellular trafficking mechanism of Lipofectamine-based transfection reagents and its implication for gene delivery. *Scientific Reports, 6*, 25879. https://doi.org/10.1038/srep25879 (accessed on 23rd June 2025).
105. Zhang, Y. Q., Guo, R. R., Chen, Y. H., Li, T. C., Du, W. Z., Xiang, R. W., Guan, J. B., Li, Y. P., Huang, Y. Y., Yu, Z. Q., Cai, Y., Zhang, P., & Ling, G. X. (2023). Ionizable drug delivery systems for efficient and selective gene therapy. *Military Medical Research, 10*(1), 9. https://doi.org/10.1186/s40779-023-00445-z (accessed on 23rd June 2025).
106. Lee, J. B., Zhang, K., Tam, Y. Y., Tam, Y. K., Belliveau, N. M., Sung, V. Y., Lin, P. J., LeBlanc, E., Ciufolini, M. A., Rennie, P. S., & Cullis, P. R. (2012). Lipid nanoparticle siRNA systems for silencing the androgen receptor in human prostate cancer *in vivo*. *International Journal of Cancer, 131*(5), E781–E790. https://doi.org/10.1002/ijc.27361 (accessed on 23rd June 2025).
107. Liu, S., Cheng, Q., Wei, T., Yu, X., Johnson, L. T., Farbiak, L., & Siegwart, D. J. (2021). Membrane-destabilizing ionizable phospholipids for organ-selective mRNA delivery and CRISPR-Cas gene editing. *Nature Materials, 20*(5), 701–710. https://doi.org/10.1038/s41563-020-00886-0 (accessed on 23rd June 2025).

108. Fenton, O. S., Kauffman, K. J., McClellan, R. L., Appel, E. A., Dorkin, J. R., Tibbitt, M. W., Heartlein, M. W., DeRosa, F., Langer, R., & Anderson, D. G. (2016). Bioinspired alkenyl amino alcohol ionizable lipid materials for highly potent *in vivo* mRNA delivery. *Advanced Materials, 28*(15), 2939–2943. https://doi.org/10.1002/adma.201505822 (accessed on 23rd June 2025).
109. Zhang, Y., Sun, C., Wang, C., Jankovic, K. E., & Dong, Y. (2021). Lipids and lipid derivatives for RNA delivery. *Chemical Reviews, 121*(20), 12181–12277. https://doi.org/10.1021/acs.chemrev.1c00244 (accessed on 23rd June 2025).
110. Han, X., Zhang, H., Butowska, K., Swingle, K. L., Alameh, M. G., Weissman, D., & Mitchell, M. J. (2021). An ionizable lipid toolbox for RNA delivery. *Nature Communications, 12*(1), 7233. https://doi.org/10.1038/s41467-021-27493-0 (accessed on 23rd June 2025).
111. Deng, H., Zhao, X., He, D., Guo, W., Yang, K., Dong, A., & Liang, X. J. (2016). One-step gene delivery into the cytoplasm in a fusion-dependent manner based on a new membrane Fuso genic lipid. *Chemical Communications (Cambridge), 52*(46), 7406–7408. https://doi.org/10.1039/c6cc01996j (accessed on 23rd June 2025).
112. Mochizuki, S., Kanegae, N., Nishina, K., Kamikawa, Y., Koiwai, K., Masunaga, H., & Sakurai, K. (2013). The role of the helper lipid dioleoyl phosphatidylethanolamine (DOPE) for DNA transfection cooperating with a cationic lipid bearing ethylenediamine. *Biochemical et Biophysical Acta, 1828*(2), 412–418. https://doi.org/10.1016/j.bbamem.2012.10.017 (accessed on 23rd June 2025).
113. Pozzi, D., & Caracciolo, G. (2023). Looking back, moving forward: Lipid nanoparticles as a promising frontier in gene delivery. *ACS Pharmacology & Translational Science, 6*(11), 1561–1573. https://doi.org/10.1021/acsptsci.3c00185 (accessed on 23rd June 2025).
114. Paez-Perez, M., Russell, I. A., Cicuta, P., & Di Michele, L. (2022). Modulating membrane fusion through the design of Fuso genic DNA circuits and bilayer composition. *Soft Matter, 18*(37), 7035–7044. https://doi.org/10.1039/d2sm00863g (accessed on 23rd June 2025).
115. Ripoll, M., Bernard, M. C., Vaure, C., Bazin, E., Commandeur, S., Perkov, V., Lemdani, K., Nicolaï, M. C., Bonifassi, P., Kichler, A., Frisch, B., & Haensler, J. (2022). An imidazole modified lipid confers enhanced mRNA-LNP stability and strong immunization properties in mice and non-human primates. *Biomaterials, 286*, 121570. https://doi.org/10.1016/j.biomaterials.2022.121570 (accessed on 23rd June 2025).
116. Huang, R., Gyanani, V., Zhao, S., Lu, Y., & Guo, X. (2022). Imidazole-based pH-sensitive convertible liposomes for anticancer drug delivery. *Pharmaceuticals (Basel), 15*(3), 306. https://doi.org/10.3390/ph15030306 (accessed on 23rd June 2025).
117. Zhao, X., Chen, J., Qiu, M., Li, Y., Glass, Z., & Xu, Q. (2020). Imidazole-based synthetic lipidoses for *in vivo* mRNA delivery into primary T lymphocytes. *Angewandte Chemise International Edition, 59*(45), 20083–20089. https://doi.org/10.1002/anie.202008082 (accessed on 23rd June 2025).
118. Solodin, I., Brown, C. S., Bruno, M. S., Chow, C. Y., Jang, E. H., Debs, R. J., & Heath, T. D. (1995). A novel series of amphiphilic imidazolinium compounds for

in vitro and *in vivo* gene delivery. *Biochemistry, 34*(41), 13537–13544. https://doi.org/10.1021/bi00041a033 (accessed on 23rd June 2025).
119. Dobbs, W., Heinrich, B., Bourgogne, C., Donnio, B., Terazzi, E., Bonnet, M. E., Stock, F., Erbacher, P., Bolcato-Bellemin, A. L., & Douce, L. (2009). Mesomorphic imidazolium salts: New vectors for efficient siRNA transfection. *Journal of the American Chemical Society, 131*(37), 13338–13346. https://doi.org/10.1021/ja903028f (accessed on 23rd June 2025).
120. Huang, Q. D., Chen, H., Zhou, L. H., Huang, J., Wu, J., & Yu, X. Q. (2008). A novel macrocyclic polyamine cationic lipid containing an imidazolium salt group: Synthesis, characterization and its transfection activity as a gene delivery vector. *Chemistry & Biodiversity Drug Design, 71*(3), 224–229. https://doi.org/10.1111/j.1747-0285.2008.00631.x (accessed on 23rd June 2025).
121. Mukherjee, A., Waters, A. K., Kalyan, P., Achrol, A. S., Kesari, S., & Yenugonda, V. M. (2019). Lipid-polymer hybrid nanoparticles as a next-generation drug delivery platform: State of the art, emerging technologies, and perspectives. *International Journal of Nanomedicine, 14*, 1937–1952. https://doi.org/10.2147/IJN.S198353 (accessed on 23rd June 2025).
122. Gajbhiye, K. R., Salve, R., Narwade, M., Sheikh, A., Kesharwani, P., & Gajbhiye, V. (2023). Lipid polymer hybrid nanoparticles: A custom-tailored next-generation approach for cancer therapeutics. *Molecular Cancer, 22*(1), 160. https://doi.org/10.1186/s12943-023-01849-0 (accessed on 23rd June 2025).
123. Sivadasan, D., Sultan, M. H., Madkhali, O., Almoshari, Y., & Thangavel, N. (2021). Polymeric lipid hybrid nanoparticles (PLNs) as emerging drug delivery platform—A comprehensive review of their properties, preparation methods, and therapeutic applications. *Pharmaceutics, 13*(8), 1291. https://doi.org/10.3390/pharmaceutics13081291 (accessed on 23rd June 2025).
124. Liu, G. W., Guzman, E. B., Menon, N., & Langer, R. S. (2023). Lipid nanoparticles for nucleic acid delivery to endothelial cells. *Pharmaceutical Research, 40*(1), 3–25. https://doi.org/10.1007/s11095-023-03471-7 (accessed on 23rd June 2025).
125. Golubovic, A., Tsai, S., & Li, B. (2023). Bioinspired lipid nanocarriers for RNA delivery. *ACS Bio & Medicinal Chemistry Au, 3*(2), 114–136. https://doi.org/10.1021/acsbiomedchemau.2c00073 (accessed on 23rd June 2025).
126. Barba, A. A., Bochicchio, S., Dalmoro, A., & Lamberti, G. (2019). Lipid delivery systems for nucleic-acid-based drugs: From production to clinical applications. *Pharmaceutics, 11*(8), 360. https://doi.org/10.3390/pharmaceutics11080360 (accessed on 23rd June 2025).
127. Cheng, X., & Lee, R. J. (2016). The role of helper lipids in lipid nanoparticles (LNPs) designed for oligonucleotide delivery. *Advanced Drug Delivery Reviews, 99*(Pt A), 129–137. https://doi.org/10.1016/j.addr.2016.01.022 (accessed on 23rd June 2025).
128. Li, S., & Huang, L. (2000). Nonviral gene therapy: Promises and challenges. *Gene Therapy, 7*(1), 31–34. https://doi.org/10.1038/sj.gt.3301110 (accessed on 23rd June 2025).
129. Pardi, N., Hogan, M. J., Porter, F. W., & Weissman, D. (2018). mRNA vaccines–A new era in vaccinology. *Nature Reviews Drug Discovery, 17*(4), 261–279. https://doi.org/10.1038/nrd.2017.243 (accessed on 23rd June 2025).

130. Baden, L. R., El Sahly, H. M., Essink, B., Kotloff, K., Frey, S., Novak, R., Diemert, D., Spector, S. A., Rouphael, N., Creech, C. B., McGettigan, J., Khetan, S., Segall, N., Solis, J., Brosz, A., Fierro, C., Schwartz, H., Neuzil, K., Corey, L., & COVE Study Group. (2021). Efficacy and safety of the mRNA-1273 SARS-CoV-2 vaccine. *The New England Journal of Medicine, 384*(5), 403–416. https://doi.org/10.1056/NEJMoa2035389 (accessed on 23rd June 2025).
131. Nabel, G. J., Nabel, E. G., Yang, Z. Y., Fox, B. A., Plautz, G. E., Gao, X., Huang, L., Shu, S., Gordon, D., & Chang, A. E. (1993). Direct gene transfer with DNA-liposome complexes in melanoma: Expression, biologic activity, and lack of toxicity in humans. *Proceedings of the National Academy of Sciences of the United States of America, 90*(23), 11307–11311. https://doi.org/10.1073/pnas.90.23.11307 (accessed on 23rd June 2025).
132. Caplen, N. J., Alton, E. W., Middleton, P. G., Dorin, J. R., Stevenson, B. J., Gao, X., Durham, S. R., Jeffery, P. K., Hodson, M. E., Coutelle, C., et al. (1995). Liposome-mediated CFTR gene transfer to the nasal epithelium of patients with cystic fibrosis. *Nature Medicine, 1*(1), 39–46. https://doi.org/10.1038/nm0195-39 (accessed on 23rd June 2025). Erratum in: *Nature Medicine, 1*(3), 272.
133. Kowalski, P. S., Rudra, A., Miao, L., & Anderson, D. G. (2019). Delivering the messenger: Advances in technologies for therapeutic mRNA delivery. *Molecular Therapy, 27*(4), 710–728. https://doi.org/10.1016/j.ymthe.2019.02.012 (accessed on 23rd June 2025).
134. Davis, M. E. (2009). The first targeted delivery of siRNA in humans via a self-assembling, cyclodextrin polymer-based nanoparticle: From concept to clinic. *Molecular Pharmaceutics, 6*(3), 659–668. https://doi.org/10.1021/mp900015y (accessed on 23rd June 2025).

CHAPTER 5

Regulatory Aspects Related to Nanomedicine and Gene Therapy Applications

ASTHA, MAHENDRA SINGH ASHAWAT, AJAY KUMAR, and PRAVIN KUMAR*

Laureate Institute of Pharmacy, Kathog, Himachal Pradesh, India

*Corresponding author

ABSTRACT

Nanomedicine and gene therapy are revolutionary approaches in the field of modern medicine, offering unparalleled opportunities for personalized and targeted treatments. However, the successful integration of these innovative methods into clinical practice necessitates a strong regulatory framework that prioritizes patient safety, effectiveness, and ethical standards. This summary provides an overview of the key regulatory aspects that govern the applications of nanomedicines and gene therapy, highlighting the evolving landscape shaped by advancements in these fields. The regulatory process begins with a clear classification and definition, recognizing the unique characteristics of nanomedicines and gene therapies. Regulatory agencies such as the FDA in the United States and the EMA in the European Union play crucial roles in evaluating and approving these groundbreaking therapies. These tests aim to establish the therapeutic effectiveness of these treatments in human subjects. The risk-benefit assessment is a critical step in this process, weighing the potential advantages against the possible risks, taking into account factors such as disease severity and alternative treatments. Ensuring quality control and

Nanotechnology for Nucleic Acid Delivery: Pankaj Sharma, Saloni Jain, and Vinay Jain (Eds.)

DOI: 10.1201/9781998511853-5

adherence to manufacturing standards is essential to guarantee the consistency and reliability of nanomedicines and gene therapies. Ethical considerations, particularly in gene therapy involving germline editing, require careful examination, addressing issues such as informed consent, privacy, and potential unintended consequences. Post-marketing surveillance becomes crucial for continuous monitoring, identifying any long-term or rare adverse effects that may arise after market approval. This abstract highlight the need for interdisciplinary collaboration among researchers, regulatory bodies, and gene therapy applications. It is crucial to regularly update and revise regulatory frameworks to adapt to the ever-changing nature of these medical technologies.

5.1 INTRODUCTION

The usage and application of materials in the nanometer range is the basis of the broad definition of nanotechnology. This minuscule range offers numerous advantages in an extensive array of applications, encompassing electronics, sunscreens, cosmetics, energy storage, and medication administration. When these particles are in their nanoscale form, their size frequently bestows desirable and unique traits, such as chemical, physical, and biological qualities that may be advantageous over their bigger counterparts. Given that numerous biologically relevant molecules, including water, antibodies, proteins, glucose, enzymes, hemoglobin, and receptors, all fall within this range, nanoscale medications have the potential to be extremely beneficial [1]. It was anticipated that the use of nanotechnology in medicine would completely transform the delivery of healthcare. Though most in the industry attribute this to the fact that nanomedicine is still in its infancy and lack of clarity regarding regulation for clinical use is severely impeding their translation, expectations have not lived up to the early excitement.

There are a number of clear advantages to these technologies, despite the fact that our understanding of the pharmacokinetics, pharmacodynamics, and toxicity of many nanomaterials in humans is extremely limited. There is still a lot of excitement surrounding the field of nanomedicine and how it will affect the pharmaceutical industry, but regulatory guidance in this area is desperately needed in order to give manufacturers, legislators, healthcare providers, and the general public legal certainty [2]. Due to their many qualities, nanomaterials can be used in a wide range of clinical settings. One of the main advantages of nanoparticles is their tiny size (10–200 nm), which enables them to bypass the renal and complement systems and traverse the body without obstructing blood flow. It was initially believed that one of the ways that nanoparticles might effectively infiltrate tumor tissues was through their enhanced permeability and retention impact; the size of clinically employed nanomaterials is also significant in cancer treatments [3]. This idea, however, has been hotly debated in the scientific community as compelling evidence has emerged to demonstrate that tumor formation is caused by active transport processes that dominate nanoparticle trafficking.

Although there is still disagreement on this among many in the community, it is becoming increasingly obvious that localized pressure within the tumor site would not be advantageous for passive targeting through Enhanced Permeability and Retention and may be the primary limiting factor to this phenomenon as more attention is paid to the tumor microenvironment.

These characteristics stem from the surface Plasmon resonance theory, which describes the oscillation of free electrons within metal nanoparticles [4]. A few metal oxide nanoparticles are also magnetic, which makes them useful for a variety of tasks like medication administration, cell targeting and separation, and imaging. On a small scale, it is typically easy and inexpensive to produce, but scaling up and maintaining stability throughout large-scale manufacturing has proven to be challenging. The majority of nanomaterials are syringe filtered below the molecular cut off for biological impurities (Table 5.1) like bacteria, making them quite easy to sterilize after manufacturing and uage in healthcare [5].

TABLE 5.1 Schematic Illustration Depicting the Size of Nanomaterial in Relation to Various Biological Molecules

Particles	**Size**
Atoms	10–1nm
Bacterial Cell	103 nm
Antibody	10 nm
Liposomes	102 nm
Red Blood Cell	104 nm
Fibroblast	105 nm
Pencil Tip	106 nm
Metal Nanoparticles	10 nm
NanoCrystals	102 nm

5.1.1 NANOMEDICINE

Nanomedicine integrates nanotechnology principles with medicines to create new strategies for disease diagnosis, treatment, and prevention. Materials at the nanoscale possess distinct properties that can be utilized to design cutting-edge medical tools and devices [6]. The incorporation of nanotechnology in healthcare has paved the way for the advancement of nanomedicine, presenting fresh possibilities for overcoming health obstacles [7]. It includes:

5.1.1.1 DIAGNOSTIC NANO PROBES

Nano scales materials like nanoparticles can be designed to act as contrast agents for imaging techniques such as magnetic resonance imaging, computed tomography or fluorescence imaging [8]. These tiny probes allow for improved detection of diseases in their initial stages with greater sensitivity and accuracy which includes:

1. **Drug Delivery System:** Nanoparticles have the ability to be designed in a way that allow them to encapsulated drugs, safeguarding them from degradation and enabling them to be delivered specifically to certain cells or tissues [9]. This enhances the effectiveness of the treatment while minimizing any negative effects on healthy tissues.
2. **Therapeutic Nanomaterial:** Nanomaterial's have the capability to directly interact with biological systems in order to achieve therapeutic effects. This includes the use of Nano scale material for treatment such as hyperthermia, photodynamic therapy and gene therapy. These approaches take advantages of the unique properties of nanomaterial to selectively target and treat diseases cells [10].
3. **Diagnostic Nano Sensors:** The field of nanotechnology has greatly contributed to the development of highly sensitive and specific diagnostic tools. Nano sensors have the ability to detect biomolecule, pathogen or specific cellular changes providing rapid and accurate diagnostic information. This is particularly valuable for early detection and monitoring of diseases [11].

4. **Regenerative Medicine:** Nanotechnology plays a significant role in tissue engineering and regenerative medicine by providing scaffolds at the Nano scale that support the growth of cells and promote tissue regeneration. These nano-materials are designed to mimic the natural extracellular matrix and aid in the repair of damaged tissues.
5. **Theranostics:** The integration of diagnostics and therapeutics is a fundamental concept in the field of Nano medicine known as Theranostics [12]. Nanoparticles can be engineered to simultaneously diagnose and treat diseases, offering a personalized and targeted approach to healthcare.

5.2 NEED OF NANOMEDICINE REGULATION

The rapidly developing subject of nanomedicine is a source of great excitement; however, as of right now, there is a dearth of direction in this area. Numerous nanomedicines function by either directly interacting with genetic materials or by interacting with biomolecules necessary for cell division and normal genome function, all of which have the potential to be mutagenic and genotoxic. The inflammatory response of neutrophils and macrophages, which results in the formation of reactive oxygen and nitrogen species that induce oxidative and nitrosamine stress, mediates this toxicity to nanomedicines. Such free radicals can accumulate and do serious harm to the organism [13].

This damage can happen in a number of ways, such as by inducing oxidative DNA damage that results in strand breakage, cancer-causing protein denaturation and lipid peroxidation, damaging mitochondrial membranes that result in cell death and necrosis, and transcription of genes linked to fibrosis and carcinogenesis. The accumulation of these particles in the liver upon intravenous administration, as well as their translocation to several organ systems, including the cardiovascular, neurological, and renal systems [14].

There are just too many unknowns in the case of particles that are unable to be traced after administration, which might potentially jeopardize public safety. Because many nanomedicines' specific interactions with biological systems are still poorly known, it can be challenging to comprehend, detect, or draw inferences regarding the physicochemical and toxicological characteristics of these medications [15]. Still, not much is expected to change in this sector in the absence of standardized regulatory advice. It must also be acknowledged that there is no "one-size-fits-all" approach to this process, as the distinct properties seen at the nanoscale depend heavily on the type of nanoparticle, its surface characteristics, how it is administered, and most importantly, its morphology, which can vary (Figure 5.1) [16]. This is something that is undoubtedly slowing down the regulatory process.

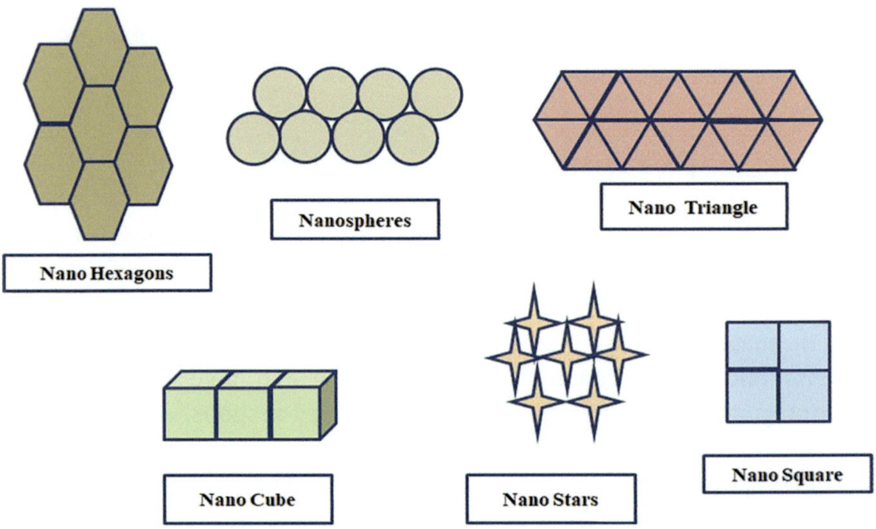

FIGURE 5.1 Diagram illustrating the various shapes of nanomaterial used in clinical applications.

The regulatory bodies are justified in their caution since, after receiving market permission for nanoparticles employed in medical imaging, those approvals were later revoked due to the appearance of unexpected patient problems following administration. Concerns revealed in clinical trials led the European Medicines Agency (EMA) to withdraw Sincere, an ultra-small super paramagnetic iron oxide (USPIO) contrast agent for magnetic resonance imaging, from the market in 2008 after declining a recommendation for marketing authorization. These included serious adverse responses that included lower back pain and, more concerning, allergic reactions that were fatal in one case [17]. Therefore, market authorization for this specific nanomolecule was rejected since it was determined that the hazards greatly outweighed any potential advantages. Nonetheless, it seems that an excessively cautious approach is leading to a great deal of inertia in the sector; frequently, the benchmark checks needed for approval remain opaque and are in line with the regulations for tiny medicinal molecules, which do not fully capture the promise of nanomaterials [18].

The public, manufacturers, healthcare providers, and legislators lack clarity and legal certainty in the absence of guidance, which is why it is so important. The Environmental Protection Agency (EPA) has taken action to address the dangers associated with nanoparticles [19].

5.2.1 REGULATORY FRAMEWORK FOR NANO MEDICINE

The fact that regulatory agencies like the FDA rely on safety data from bulk materials, which don't exhibit the same pharmacodynamics and pharmacokinetic activity as nanomedicines, may be the largest obstacle to the regulation of nanomedicines (Figure 5.2) [20]. This means that once a nanomedicine has received marketing permission, statistics on safety and efficacy will not accurately reflect what might happen when it is utilized in clinical settings.

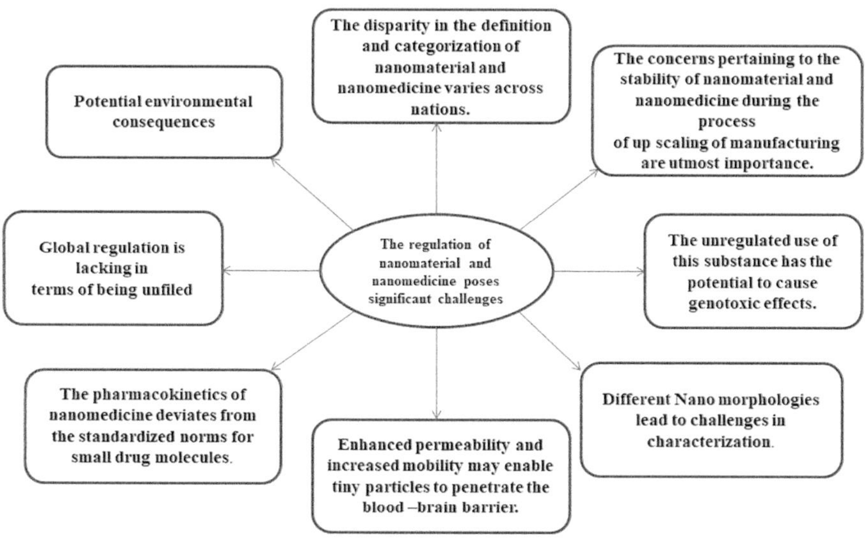

FIGURE 5.2 Highlighting the major challenges faced in the regulation of nanomaterial.

Before being approved for clinical usage, the mechanism and action of drug delivery in nanomedicine development require extensive preclinical safety data, including information on side effects. Furthermore, because the particles are smaller than their larger counterparts, they could be dangerous to patients. This enables them to get through the blood-brain barrier, which may eventually impair brain function or at the very least result in edema [21].

One of the biggest obstacles to the regulation of nanomedicines is defining their pharmacokinetics. This is because they diverge from the anticipated and typical path that tiny medicinal molecules take. Because of their prolonged bioavailability, there could be a serious health risk to the general public if nanomedicine products were ever sold over-the-counter. Regulatory agencies are required to determine if a particular nanomedicine should be sold as an over-the-counter drug or placed on the market under close monitoring. However, the dearth of data and information on toxicity that is currently accessible makes it exceedingly difficult to reach a definitive conclusion in this area [22]. Over the past 10 years, nanomedicines and its offspring, nanosimilars, have been brought to market. The difficulties encountered in the research and production of pharmaceuticals applies not only to nanomedicines but also to their derivative products. However, as people's awareness has grown, regulatory agencies have been forced to review their current rules. In the EU, the EMA may accept follow-on goods as shortened applications falling within the generic or hybrid categories. Here are some key factors to consider in the regulatory framework for nanomedicine.

Nanomedicines frequently involve nanoparticles, which may have safety profiles distinct from traditional pharmaceuticals. Regulatory bodies emphasize thorough risk assessments to identify potential hazards and ensure patient safety, which includes [23]:

1. **Characterization and Standardization:** Accurate characterization of nanoparticles is essential, and standardized methods for their production and characterization are crucial. Regulatory authorities may request detailed information on the physiochemical properties of nanomedicine.

2. **Quality Control and Manufacturing Practices:** Strict quality control measures and adherence to good manufacturing practices are vital. The manufacturing processes for nanomedicine should be well documented and capable of producing consistent results [24].

3. **Toxicology Studies:** Comprehensive toxicological studies are typically necessary to evaluate the potential adverse effects of nanomedicine. This includes research on biodistribution, metabolism, and long-term impacts.
4. **Regulatory Agencies:** Various countries and regions may have different regulatory bodies' responsibilities for approving and monitoring nanomedicine [25]. For instance, the Food and Drug Administration plays a significant role in the United States, while the European Medicines Agency oversees regulation in the European Union.
5. **Guidance Documents:** Regulatory agencies frequently issue specific guidance documents for the development and approval of nanomedicines. These documents provide valuable insights into regulatory expectations and requirements [26].
6. **International Cooperation:** Given the worldwide reach of the pharmaceutical sector, international cooperation and the alignment of standards play a vital role. Entities like the International Council for Harmonization of Technical Requirements for Pharmaceuticals for Human Use strive to achieve global harmonization of regulatory demands.
7. **Ethical Reflections:** Ethical dimensions, particularly in relation to the utilization of nanotechnology in medical research and therapy, are also taken into account [27]. This encompasses informed consent, privacy, and the broader societal implications.

5.2.2 NANO-MEDICINE APPROVED FOR CLINICAL USES

Amphotericin B is an antifungal medication that cannot be administered on its own because of its limited tolerance, poor solubility in water, and patient adverse effects. Initially, amphotericin B was prepared as mixed micelle dispersion (Fungizone) in deoxycholate. Research into Fungizone's toxicity to human cells has shown that this specific nanoparticle system might not be appropriate for application [28]. Since then, other investigations into amphotericin B formulations driven by nanotechnology have successfully entered clinical trials. These consist of Amphotec, AmBisome, and Abelcet. AmBisome, which encapsulates amphotericin B in a liposome and has been incredibly successful, was the first nanomedicine licensed in Europe. Another type of nanomedicine that was approved in 2004 was approved for the treatment of persistent pain, composed of multivesicular liposomes encasing morphine sulfate, allowing for a longer-lasting medication release. To avoid abuse, addiction, and overdose, the goal was to move patients who needed opioid therapies down to single dosage formulations [29].

Additional nanotechnology formulations consist of polypeptides, aptamers like Micera and Cimzia, and polyethylene glycosylated proteins. 2008 saw the approval of Cimzia, a polyethylene glycosylated antibody suggested for Crohn's disease, and Mircera, an anemia linked with chronic renal failure in adults. Nanocrystals have also been licensed for clinical usage as nanomedicines. Because of its extended, consistent release of the medication, metal-based nano formulations like Feraheme have also been licensed. This enables patients with anemia in chronic renal disease to take their medication less frequently [30].

5.2.3 GLOBAL STRATEGIES TO NANOMEDICINE REGULATION

1. **United States of America:** Until now, the FDA has regulated nanotechnology products, including nanomedicines, using its existing regulatory authority and statutory authority, in addition to product-specific requirements. The FDA has published guidelines on nanomaterials in food, cosmetics, and animal feed over the years. There aren't any published guidelines specifically for nanomedicine, though. The FDA released draft guidance in 2017 regarding drug items that contain nanomaterials, including biological products. Furthermore, the FDA assesses each nanotechnology individually rather than trying to classify them as safe or dangerous. It is noteworthy that the FDA recognized a number of characteristics related to their regulatory strategy [31].

2. **United Kingdom:** The Medicines and Healthcare Products Regulatory Authority (MHRA) is responsible for regulating medicines in the United Kingdom. Similar to the FDA, there is a lack of explicit guidelines regarding nanomedicine approval, and cases are handled according to need. It is recommended that researchers

working on nanomedicines communicate with the MHRA Innovation Office for support and direction during the procedure. Similar to the US, other institutions, like the European Nanomedicine Characterization Laboratory (EU-NCL), with locations around the UK and EU, offer and continuously improve preclinical characterization assay knowledge [32].

3. **European Union:** The EU has made headway in defining the official meaning of the term "nanomaterial" by forming task forces and consortiums. These groups have produced a number of reports and recommendations that address food, the environment, and human health. The EU-NCL and REFINE project, among other previously mentioned initiatives, have received funding from government awards to further progress this sector. The European Medicines Union (EMU), the EU's regulatory agency, has released a number of detailed draft rules for various nanomedicine production criteria, in contrast to the UK [33].
4. **Canada:** "Considers any manufactured product, material, substance, ingredient, device, system, or structure to be nanomaterial if it is at or within the Nano scale (1–100 nm) in at least one spatial dimension, or is smaller or larger than the Nano scale in all spatial dimensions and exhibits one or more Nano scale phenomena," according to Health Canada's Working Definition of Nanomaterials. Canada depends on current regulatory systems for the approval of items involving nanotechnology. Health Canada recommends that in order to identify and evaluate the risks and qualities of a product, manufacturers should confer with the relevant regulatory body early in the development process [34].
5. **Japan:** The Pharmaceuticals and Medical Devices Agency (PMDA) and the Ministry of Health, Labor and Welfare (MHLW) oversee medicine regulations in Japan. The regulatory organizations in Japan are still working on developing a definition and regulations unique to nanomedicines. Guidelines for the creation of liposome-based pharmaceutical products were released in 2016. It should be mentioned that data on nanomedicine is being gathered and examined by regulators and reviewers. Additionally, the MHLW/PMDA and the EMA have worked together to publish reflection articles [35].

5.3 GENE THERAPY

Gene therapy is a medical technique that involves manipulating genetic material within individual cells to address or prevent diseases [36]. Through the insertion of a functional, non-mutated gene into the patient's genome, gene therapy aims to treat genetic disorders. The patient would not be able to make a functioning protein if the non-mutated gene wasn't present.

Sometimes the functional gene is introduced using viral vectors like adenoviruses, in which case the desired gene replaces the deleted portion of the viral genome. More sophisticated gene therapy techniques, such as those used to treat severe combined immunodeficiency (SCID), aim to fix the mutation at the original location in the genome. The goal of gene therapy is to replace a damaged gene with a healthy, normal one. Rare diseases like sickle cell anemia, which is brought on by a single mutation, and fatal illnesses like severe combined immunodeficiency can both be treated using gene therapy (SCID). Recombinant therapeutic biochemicals, such as insulin, somatotropin, somatostatin, interferon, human blood clotting factor VIII, and so forth, are produced using gene therapy. Numerous protocols have been devised for the production and introduction of genes in humans; however, substantial evidence regarding the clinical efficiency is still pending.

The creation of more effective gene transfer vectors for the long-term, sustained expression of foreign genes and an improved comprehension of the gene physiology underlying human disease are prerequisites for the success of gene therapy. One day, medical biotechnologists may be able to treat human gene problems thanks to advancements in gene editing techniques and a better understanding of how genes function in the body. Gene therapy is the process of treating a hereditary condition by gene manipulation. Contrary to various media assertions, gene therapy has not yet proved to provide patients with any meaningful relief.

Through the application of recombinant DNA technology, a genetic condition caused by a single defective allele may theoretically be corrected by substituting or augmenting the defective allele with a normal, functional allele. The transplanted allele may be duplicated and continuously expressed if the new allele was introduced into the bone marrow cells, which continue to increase throughout the patient's life. All blood and immune system cells originate from bone marrow stem cells. Then, the immune system might fight against illness.

Gene therapy is being researched for a variety of hereditary diseases, including sickle cell anemia and SCID. The ADA gene is faulty in the SCID patient. He or she lacks functioning T-lymphocytes and is unable to combat the infections that are attacking them. After removing lymphocytes from the patient's bone marrow, a functional copy of the human gene encoding for ADA is transferred into the lymphocytes by retrovirus. The patient's bone marrow is replenished with the treated cells. Many genetic disorders, such as sickle cell anemia and SCID, are being studied for potential treatments via gene therapy. The SCID patient has a defective ADA gene. He or she is unable to fight off the illnesses that are targeting them since they do not have functional T-lymphocytes. A functional copy of the human gene code for ADA is introduced into the lymphocytes by retrovirus after the patient's bone marrow lymphocytes have been extracted. The treated cells are added back into the patient's bone marrow.

5.3.1 METHODS FOR GENE THERAPY

Many strategies have been attempted to successfully transfer genes to the right target place. These methods can be roughly divided into four groups:

1. **Gene Modification:**
   a. Replacement therapy;
   b. Corrective gene therapy.
2. **Gene Transfer:**
   a. Physical (Microinjection, Gene gun, Electroporation, etc.);
   b. chemical (Liposomes, Oligonucleotides, Cationic liposomes, etc.);
   c. Biological (Viral vectors, mammalian artificial chromosomes, etc.).
3. **Gene Transfer in Specific Cell Lines:**
   a. Somatic cell therapy;
   b. Germ line gene therapy.
   4. Eugenic Approach (Gene Insertion).

5.3.1.1 GENE MODIFICATION

A faulty gene is implanted anywhere in the genome during replacement treatment so that its product can take the place of the defective gene.

Recessive disorders, which are characterized by an enzyme or other protein shortage, might benefit from this strategy. This method may not be effective in treating dominant disease, which is linked to the creation of an aberrant gene product that interferes with the normal gene's product, even though genes function in the genome by providing the proper regulatory sequence.

Corrective gene therapy, on the other hand, calls for substituting a normal sequence for a mutant gene or a portion of a mutant gene. The application of recombinant technologies can do this. Corrective therapy also includes the introduction of transfer RNA into the cell to repress a specific mutation.

5.3.1.2 GENE TRANSFER

A particular disease may be improved through gene transfer. To boost height, for instance, a growth hormone gene could be introduced. It is possible to transfer genes into cells physically, chemically, or biologically.

5.3.1.3 GENE TRANSFER TO SPECIFIC CELL LINES

Somatic gene therapy is a novel strategy to treating many genetic and acquired diseases by inserting a gene into a particular type of somatic cell. If all goes according to plan, it works throughout a person's lifetime to treat a hereditary illness. Even though it sounds good, there are several real-world issues. However, germ line therapy, as opposed to somatic cell therapy, involves injecting or inserting a gene into a germ cell, or a fertilized egg. In this case, the added gene would also be passed on to subsequent generations.

5.3.1.4 EUGENIC APPROACH (GENE INSERTION)

The eugenics method involves introducing genes into a person to change or enhance complicated features. Take intelligence, for instance. It is, however, much beyond the realm of existing technological capability.

5.3.2 NEW DEVELOPMENTS IN GENE THERAPY

Reaching the goal of effective gene therapies for human diseases has been a difficult one. Some of the problems that remain to be solved include: How to avoid an immune response in the patient, which can interfere with gene therapy in two ways:

- The vector causes irritation.
- The vector elicits antibodies that destroy the vector when it is administered again.

5.3.2.1 ADENO-ASSOCIATED VIRUS (AAV)

The term "Adeno-associated virus" refers to the fact that AAV is frequently detected in cells that are also infected with adenovirus, yet it appears to be benign on its own, such as:

- Does not cause the host to become inflamed;
- Can reach cells that are not dividing;
- Successfully integrates into a single location on human chromosome 19, the host's genome. AAV vectors can only be used once because they do, however, cause a robust immune response. The issue of achieving optimal transgene expression could potentially be resolved by utilizing two AAV vectors at the same time: one that introduces the desired gene (e.g., erythropoietin in this instance, adenosine deaminase, or factor VIII) into the host cells, and the other carries genes for the transcription factor components required to activate that particular gene.

5.3.2.2 REGULATED PRODUCTION OF ERYTHROPOIETIN (EPO)

1. **Vector 1:** Among other things, this DNA fragment included the AAV DNA. A gene that codes for a protein with two domains: a section of the molecule called p65 is required to trigger the transcription of genes, but it is unable to bind to DNA. Part of it (FRB) binds the medication rapamycin. A gene that codes for a second,

dual-domain protein: a section of the molecule (ZFHD1) that binds selectively to the DNA in the erythropoietin gene promoter but is unable to initiate gene transcription on its own; a section that binds to rapamycin as well (FKBP12). The two genes' continuous expression (transcription and translation) is made possible by a promoter (not depicted). However, take note that the two gene products are inactive on their own.

2. **Vector 2:** Among other things, this DNA fragment included the AAV DNA. There are 12 erythropoietin gene promoters that are identical (green boxes). The EPO gene directly.

   The main objective of gene therapy is to rectify or compensate for genetic abnormalities that contribute to illnesses. There are multiple approaches to gene therapy which includes:

1. **Gene Replacement Therapy:** This method entails substituting a defective or absent gene with a functional one it is commonly employed for genetic disorders caused by a single gene mutation [37].
2. **Gene Editing:** Advanced technologies such as CRISPR-Cas9 allow precise modification to specific genes with in an organism DNA. This can be utilized to correct genetic mutation or introduce therapeutic genes [38].
3. **Gene Addition Therapy:** In situations where a specific gene is missing or functioning improperly, additional copies of the functional gene can be introduced into the cells to restore normal function [39].
4. **Gene Silencing:** This technique involves suppressing the expression of a particular gene. It can be beneficial in condition where overactive gene contributes to diseases.

Gene therapy shows immense potential in treating various genetic and acquired disorders, including specific types of cancer, genetic disorders like cystic fibrosis, and certain forms of inherited blindness [38]. However, it also presents challenges and ethical considerations, such as concerns regarding long-term safety, potential unintended consequences, and the necessity for rigorous clinical trials [40]. This encompasses informed consent, privacy, and the broader societal implications.

5.3.3 REGULATORY LANDSCAPE FOR GENE THERAPY

The regulatory environment for gene therapy is constantly changing and dynamic. It is important to note that there may have been developments since the information provided and dynamic [41]. There may have been development since the information provided and it is advisable to consult the latest source of information, which includes:

1. **United States (FDA):** The U.S. Food and Drug Administration (FDA) has actively participated in regulating gene therapy products. To oversee gene therapy, cell therapy, and regenerative medicine products, the FDA has established the Office of Tissues and Advanced Therapies (OTAT) [42]. Several gene therapy products have received FDA approval, and the regulatory approach has been adaptable, taking into account the unique challenges and characteristics of gene therapies.
2. **European Union (EMA):** The European Medicines Agency (EMA) plays a crucial role in authorizing and supervising gene therapies in the European Union. The Committee for Advanced Therapies (CAT) is responsible for evaluating advanced therapy medicinal products (ATMPs), which include gene therapies [43]. To address the specific challenges associated with gene therapy products, the EU has implemented the advanced.
3. **Therapy Medicinal Products (ATMP) Regulation China (NMPA):** China's National Medical Products Administration has actively participated in the regulation of gene therapies. The regulatory framework for gene therapy in China has evolved to accommodate advancements in the fields [44].
4. **International Harmonization:** Efforts have been made to harmonize regulations globally. Organizations like the International Council for Harmonization of Technical Requirements for Pharmaceuticals for Human Use are working towards standardizing regulatory requirements for pharmaceutical products, including gene therapies.
5. **Regulatory Pathways:** Various regulatory routes could be accessible for gene therapies, such as expedited approval initiatives and orphan drug designations, contingent upon the characteristics of the therapy and the specific diseases being targeted.

6. **Challenges and Consideration:** The regulatory environment surrounding gene therapy presents distinct obstacles stemming from the intricate nature of the technology, lingering safety apprehensions, and ethical dilemmas that may arise [45]. Authorities are striving to find a middle ground between fostering progress in innovation and upholding the well-being of patients.

5.3.4 EMERGING TRENDS IN REGULATORY SCIENCE

Several emerging trends have been influencing the field of regulatory science. It is important to note that the regulatory landscape is constantly evolving, and new trends may have emerged since then. Here are some key emerging trends in regulatory sciences [46]:

1. **Advanced Therapies and Personalized Medicine:** The emergence of advanced therapies, such as gene therapies, cell therapies, and personalized medicine, has led regulatory agencies to adapt and establish specific guidelines for these innovative treatments.
2. **Real-World Evidence:** There is a growing focus on integrating real-world evidence, which includes data from routine clinical practice and patient experiences, into the regulatory decision-making process. This can offer additional insights into the safety and efficacy of treatments [47].
3. **Patient –Centric Approaches:** Regulatory bodies are increasingly prioritizing patient engagement and integrating patient viewpoints into the drug development and approval processes. This involves collecting patient-reported outcomes and considering patient preferences.
4. **Digital Health and Wearables:** The adoption of digital health tools, such as wearable devices and mobile applications, is becoming more widespread [48]. Regulatory agencies are working on establishing frameworks for evaluating and regulating digital health products.
5. **Regulatory Harmonization:** Efforts towards global regulatory harmonization persist, with organizations like the International Council for Harmonization of Technical Requirements for

Pharmaceuticals for Human Use focusing on standardizing regulatory requirements across different regions [49].

6. **Block Chain Technology:** As the biosimilars market expands, regulatory agencies are enhancing guidelines for approving and switching between biosimilars products, especially in the realm of complex biology. Establishing a suitable framework for assessing the safety and effectiveness of products in these fields is a top priority. The utilization of blockchain technology for ensuring data integrity, traceability, and security in regulatory procedures is gaining recognition. This technology holds the potential to improve transparency and streamline regulatory processes. There is a growing emphasis on evaluating the environmental impact of pharmaceutical products. Regulatory agencies are taking into account the environmental sustainability of drug manufacturing processes and product life cycle [50].

5.4 CONCLUSION

In spite of the absence of precise regulatory guidelines, more than 50 nanomedicines have been released onto the market, and this figure is increasing gradually. These are primarily related to cancer therapy because of the difficult tumor landscape that prevents efficient pharmacological treatment and the toxic substances that are necessary. The most well-known of them are the liposomal preparations Doxil and AmBisome, which have more recently shown promise when combined with albumin-drug nanoparticles like Abraxane and polymeric micelles like Eligard, to mention a few. A global problem is the absence of official regulation of the manufacturing of nanomaterials and nanomedicines for use in health-related applications. Certain nanomedicines are classified as medical devices and others as medications due to discrepancies amongst government bodies. The nanomedicine community needs urgent coherence across the governance sector to enable development to proceed as expected. While small molecules are frequently not licensed globally for this reason, what is deemed fit for purpose in one jurisdiction does not translate to another. Since nanomaterials are not new, the creation of working groups and clusters has not resulted in any action thus far, and the current regulatory framework is unable to meet the necessity or urgency of treating certain diseases.

Although there have been some initiatives to establish National Characterization Laboratories by government agencies and academic groups, more clear and strict guidelines from the major regulatory authorities, such as the FDA and MHRA, are required. A worldwide consortium for the regulation of nanomaterials should be formed in order to advance these objectives and provide official guidelines to the research communities, as many diseases do not discriminate based on factors such as race or geography.

ACKNOWLEDGMENT

None

CONFLICT OF INTEREST

The author declared no conflict of interest

FUNDING

None

KEYWORDS

- **antibodies**
- **enzymes**
- **gene therapy**
- **glucose**
- **hemoglobin**
- **nano medicines**
- **proteins**
- **receptors**
- **regulatory aspects**
- **risk benefits assessment.**
- **therapeutic effectiveness**

REFERENCES

1. Yadav, R., Bhawale, R., Srivastava, V., Pardhi, E., Bhalerao, H. A., Sonti, R., & Mehra, N. K. (2024). Innovative nanoparticulate strategies in colon cancer treatment: A paradigm shift. *AAPS Pharm SciTech, 25*(3), 52. https://doi.org/10.1208/s12249-024-02759-0 (accessed on 23rd June 2025).
2. Ting, S. G., Lea-Banks, H., & Hynynen, K. (2023). Physical characterization to improve scalability and potential of anesthetic-loaded nanodroplets. *Pharmaceutics, 15*(8), 2077. https://doi.org/10.3390/pharmaceutics15082077 (accessed on 23rd June 2025).
3. Vander Zee, M., de Vries, C., Masa, M., Morales, M., Rayo, M., & Hegger, I. (2023). Regulatory aspects of a nanomaterial for imaging therapeutic cells. *Drug Delivery and Translational Research, 13*(11), 2693–2703. https://doi.org/10.1007/s13346-023-01359-y (accessed on 23rd June 2025).
4. Hanigan, D., Truong, L., Schoepf, J., Nosaka, T., Mulchandani, A., Tanguay, R. L., & Westerhoff, P. (2018). Trade-offs in ecosystem impacts from nanomaterial versus organic chemical ultraviolet filters in sunscreens. *Water Research, 139*, 281–290. https://doi.org/10.1016/j.watres.2018.03.062 (accessed on 23rd June 2025).
5. Pomerantseva, E., Bonaccorso, F., Feng, X., Cui, Y., & Gogotsi, Y. (2019). Energy storage: The future enabled by nanomaterial. *Science, 366*(6468), eaan8285. https://doi.org/10.1126/science.aan8285 (accessed on 23rd June 2025).
6. Min, Y., Caster, J. M., Eblan, M. J., & Wang, A. Z. (2015). Clinical translation of nanomedicine. *Chemical Reviews, 115*(19), 11147–11190. https://doi.org/10.1021/acs.chemrev.5b00116 (accessed on 23rd June 2025).
7. Seigneuric, R., Markey, L., Nuyten, D. S., Dubernet, C., Evelo, C. T., Finot, E., & Garrido, C. (2010). From nanotechnology to nanomedicine: Applications to cancer research. *Current Molecular Medicine, 10*(7), 640–652. https://doi.org/10.2174/156652410792630634 (accessed on 23rd June 2025).
8. He, H., Liu, L., Morin, E. E., Liu, M., & Schwendeman, A. (2019). Survey of clinical translation of cancer nanomedicines—Lessons learned from successes and failures. *Accounts of Chemical Research, 52*(9), 2445–2461. https://doi.org/10.1021/acs.accounts.9b00228N (accessed on 23rd June 2025).
9. Golombek, S. K., May, J. N., Theek, B., Appold, L., Drude, N., Kiessling, F., & Lammers, T. (2018). Tumor targeting via EPR: Strategies to enhance patient responses. *Advanced Drug Delivery Reviews, 130*, 17–38. https://doi.org/10.1016/j.addr.2018.07.007 (accessed on 23rd June 2025).
10. Sindhwani, S., Syed, A. M., Ngai, J., Kingston, B. R., Maiorino, L., Rothschild, J., MacMillan, P., Zhang, Y., Rajesh, N. U., Hoang, T., Wu, J. L. Y., Wilhelm, S., Zilman, A., Gadde, S., Sulaiman, A., Ouyang, B., Lin, Z., Wang, L., Egeblad, M., & Chan, W. C. W. (2020). The entry of nanoparticles into solid tumors. *Nature Materials, 19*(5), 566–575. https://doi.org/10.1038/s41563-019-0566-2 (accessed on 23rd June 2025).
11. Paliwal, R., Babu, R. J., & Palakurthi, S. (2014). Nanomedicine scale-up technologies: Feasibilities and challenges. *AAPS Pharm SciTech, 15*(6), 1527–1534. https://doi.org/10.1208/s12249-014-0177-9 (accessed on 23rd June 2025).

12. Zhang, X. Q., Xu, X., Bertrand, N., Pridgen, E., Swami, A., & Farokhzad, O. C. (2012). Interactions of nanomaterial and biological systems: Implications to personalized nanomedicine. *Advanced Drug Delivery Reviews, 64*(13), 1363–1384. https://doi.org/10.1016/j.addr.2012.08.005 (accessed on 23rd June 2025).
13. Liu, L., & Kong, L. (2021). Research progress on the carcinogenicity of metal nanomaterial. *Journal of Applied Toxicology, 41*(9), 1334–1344. https://doi.org/10.1002/jat.4145 (accessed on 23rd June 2025).
14. Singh, N., Manshian, B., Jenkins, G. J., Griffiths, S. M., Williams, P. M., Maffeis, T. G., Wright, C. J., & Doak, S. H. (2009). Nano genotoxicology: The DNA damaging potential of engineered nanomaterial. *Biomaterials, 30*(23, 24), 3891–3914. https://doi.org/10.1016/j.biomaterials.2009.04.009 (accessed on 23rd June 2025).
15. Smolkova, B., Dusinska, M., & Gabelova, A. (2017). Nanomedicine and epigenome: Possible health risks. *Food and Chemical Toxicology, 109*(Pt. 1), 780–796. https://doi.org/10.1016/j.fct.2017.07.020 (accessed on 23rd June 2025).
16. Manke, A., Wang, L., & Rojanasakul, Y. (2013). Mechanisms of nanoparticle-induced oxidative stress and toxicity. *BioMed Research International, 2013*, 942916. https://doi.org/10.1155/2013/942916 (accessed on 23rd June 2025).
17. Kermanizadeh, A., Balharry, D., Wallin, H., Loft, S., & Møller, P. (2015). Nanomaterial translocation—The bio kinetics, tissue accumulation, toxicity and fate of materials in secondary organs—A review. *Critical Reviews in Toxicology, 45*(10), 837–872. https://doi.org/10.3109/10408444.2015.1058747 (accessed on 23rd June 2025).
18. Farinha, P., Coelho, J. M. P., Reis, C. P., & Gaspar, M. M. (2021). A comprehensive updated review on magnetic nanoparticles in diagnostics. *Nanomaterials, 11*(12), 3432. https://doi.org/10.3390/nano11123432 (accessed on 23rd June 2025).
19. Rankin-Turner, S., Vader, P., O'Driscoll, L., Giebel, B., Heaney, L. M., & Davies, O. G. (2021). A call for the standardized reporting of factors affecting the exogenous loading of extracellular vesicles with therapeutic cargos. *Advanced Drug Delivery Reviews, 173*, 479–491. https://doi.org/10.1016/j.addr.2021.04.012 (accessed on 23rd June 2025).
20. Cuccione, E., Chhour, P., Si-Mohamed, S., Dumot, C., Kim, J., Hubert, V., Da Silva, C. C., Vandamme, M., Chereul, E., Balegamire, J., Chevalier, Y., Berthezène, Y., Boussel, L., Douek, P., Cormode, D. P., & Wiart, M. (2020). Multicolor spectral photon counting CT monitors and quantifies therapeutic cells and their encapsulating scaffold in a model of brain damage. *Nano Theragnostic, 4*(3), 129–141. https://doi.org/10.7150/ntno.45354 (accessed on 23rd June 2025).
21. Tawakoni, C., Cuccione, E., Dumot, C., Balegamire, J., Si-Mohamed, S. A., Kim, J., Crola-da-Silva, C., Chevalier, Y., Boussel, L., Douek, P., Cormode, D., Elleaume, H., Brun, E., & Wiart, M. (2023). High-resolution synchrotron K-edge subtraction CT allows tracking and quantifying therapeutic cells and their scaffold in a rat model of focal cerebral injury and can serve as a reference for spectral photon counting CT. *Nano Theragnostic, 7*(2), 176–186. https://doi.org/10.7150/ntno.79575 (accessed on 23rd June 2025).
22. Said, M., Tawakoni, C., Dumot, C., Toupet, K., Dong, Y. C., Collomb, N., Auxenfans, C., Moissan, A., Favier, B., Chovelon, B., Barbier, E. L., Jorgensen, C., Cormode, D. P., Noël, D., Brun, E., Elleaume, H., Wiart, M., Detante, O., Rome, C., & Auzély-Velty, R. (2023). A novel injectable radiopaque hydrogel with potent properties for

multicolor CT imaging in the context of brain and cartilage regenerative therapy. *bioRxiv*. https://doi.org/10.1101/2023.04.20.537520 (accessed on 23rd June 2025).

23. Ahmad, E., Athar, A., Nimisha, Zia, Q., Sharma, A. K., Sajid, M., Bharadwaj, M., Ansari, M. A., & Saluja, S. S. (2024). Harnessing nature's potential: *Alpinia galanga* methanolic extract mediated green synthesis of silver nanoparticle, characterization and evaluation of anti-neoplastic activity. *Bioprocess and Biosystems Engineering*. https://doi.org/10.1007/s00449-024-02993-7 (accessed on 23rd June 2025).
24. Vagena, I. A., Gatou, M. A., Theocharous, G., Pantelis, P., Gazouli, M., Pippa, N., Gorgoulis, V. G., Pavlatou, E. A., & Lagopati, N. (2024). Functionalized ZnO-based nanocomposites for diverse biological applications: Current trends and future perspectives. *Nanomaterials, 14*(5), 397. https://doi.org/10.3390/nano14050397 (accessed on 23rd June 2025).
25. Krishna, S. B. N., Jakmunee, J., Mishra, Y. K., & Prakash, J. (2024). ZnO based 0–3D diverse nano-architectures, films and coatings for biomedical applications. *Journal of Materials Chemistry B, 12*(12), 2950–2984. https://doi.org/10.1039/d4tb00184 (accessed on 23rd June 2025).
26. Gupta, J., Hassan, P. A., & Barick, K. C. (2023). Multifunctional ZnO nanostructures: A next generation nanomedicine for cancer therapy, targeted drug delivery, bio imaging, and tissue regeneration. *Nanotechnology, 34*(28), 10.1088/1361-6528/accc35. https://doi.org/10.1088/1361-6528/accc35 (accessed on 23rd June 2025).
27. Oh, J. Y., Kim, H. S., Palanikumar, L., Go, E. M., Jana, B., Park, S. A., Kim, H. Y., Kim, K., Seo, J. K., Kwak, S. K., Kim, C., Kang, S., & Ryu, J. H. (2018). Cloaking nanoparticles with protein corona shield for targeted drug delivery. *Nature Communications, 9*(1), 4548. https://doi.org/10.1038/s41467-018-06979-4 (accessed on 23rd June 2025).
28. Brouwer, H., Porbahaie, M., Boeren, S., Busch, M., & Bouwmeester, H. (2024). The *in vitro* gastrointestinal digestion-associated protein corona of polystyrene nano- and microplastics increases their uptake by human THP-1-derived macrophages. *Particle and Fiber Toxicology, 21*(1), 4. https://doi.org/10.1186/s12989-024-00563 (accessed on 23rd June 2025).
29. Burns, J., Buck, A. C., D'Souza, S., Dube, A., & Bardien, S. (2023). Nano phytomedicines as therapeutic agents for Parkinson's disease. *ACS Omega, 8*(45), 42045–42061. https://doi.org/10.1021/acsomega.3c04862 (accessed on 23rd June 2025).
30. Lozano, D., Larraga, V., Vallet-Regí, M., & Manzano, M. (2023). An overview of the use of nanoparticles in vaccine development. *Nanomaterials, 13*(12), 1828. https://doi.org/10.3390/nano13121828 (accessed on 23rd June 2025).
31. Sainz, V., Conniot, J., Matos, A. I., Peres, C., Zupanoio, E., Moura, L., Silva, L. C., Florindo, H. F., & Gaspar, R. S. (2015). Regulatory aspects on nanomedicines. *Biochemical and Biophysical Research Communications, 468*(3), 504–510. https://doi.org/10.1016/j.bbrc.2015.08.023 (accessed on 23rd June 2025).
32. Edmondson, R., Broglie, J. J., Adcock, A. F., & Yang, L. (2014). Three-dimensional cell culture systems and their applications in drug discovery and cell-based biosensors. *Assay and Drug Development Technologies, 12*(4), 207–218. https://doi.org/10.1089/adt.2014.573 (accessed on 23rd June 2025).

33. Shyam, R., Reddy, L. V. K., & Palaniappan, A. (2023). Fabrication and characterization techniques of *in vitro* 3D tissue models. *International Journal of Molecular Sciences, 24*(3), 1912. https://doi.org/10.3390/ijms24031912 (accessed on 23rd June 2025).
34. Zhao, J., Zhou, C., Xiao, Y., Zhang, K., Zhang, Q., Xia, L., Jiang, B., Jiang, C., Ming, W., Zhang, H., Long, H., & Liang, W. (2024). Oxygen generating biomaterials at the forefront of regenerative medicine: Advances in bone regeneration. *Frontiers in Bioengineering and Biotechnology, 12*, 1292171. https://doi.org/10.3389/fbioe.2024.1292171 (accessed on 23rd June 2025).
35. Mamidi, N., Ijadi, F., & Norahan, M. H. (2023). Leveraging the recent advancements in GelMA scaffolds for bone tissue engineering: An assessment of challenges and opportunities. *Biomacromolecules*. https://doi.org/10.1021/acs.biomac.3c00279 (accessed on 23rd June 2025).
36. Ten Ham, R. M. T., Hövels, A. M., Hoekman, J., Frederix, G. W. J., Leufkens, H. G. M., Klungel, O. H., Jedema, I., Veld, S. A. J., Nikolic, T., Van Pel, M., Zwaginga, J. J., Lin, F., de Goede, A. L., Schreibelt, G., Budde, S., de Vries, I. J. M., Wilkie, G. M., Dolstra, H., Ovelgönne, H., Meij, P., & Hoefnagel, M. H. N. (2020). What does cell therapy manufacturing cost? A framework and methodology to facilitate academic and other small-scale cell therapy manufacturing costings. *Cytotherapy, 22*(7), 388–397. https://doi.org/10.1016/j.jcyt.2020.03.432 (accessed on 23rd June 2025).
37. Mussolino, C., & Cathomen, T. (2012). TALE nucleases: Tailored genome engineering made easy. *Current Opinion in Biotechnology, 23*(5), 644–650. https://doi.org/10.1016/j.copbio.2012.01.013 (accessed on 23rd June 2025).
38. Ylä-Herttuala, S. (2012). Endgame: Glybera finally recommended for approval as the first gene therapy drug in the European Union. *Molecular Therapy, 20*(10), 1831–1832. https://doi.org/10.1038/mt.2012.194 (accessed on 23rd June 2025).
39. Salmon, F., Grosios, K., & Petry, H. (2014). Safety profile of recombinant adeno-associated viral vectors: Focus on alipogene tiparvovec (Glybera®). *Expert Review of Clinical Pharmacology, 7*(1), 53–65. https://doi.org/10.1586/17512433.2014.852065 (accessed on 23rd June 2025).
40. Modi, N. (2023). The future of perinatal research. *European Journal of Pediatrics, 182*(5), 1935–1939. https://doi.org/10.1007/s00431-022-04671 (accessed on 23rd June 2025).
41. Zarogouldis, P., Karamanos, N. K., Porpodis, K., Domvri, K., Huang, H., Hohenforst-Schimdt, W., Goldberg, E. P., & Zarogoulidis, K. (2012). Vectors for inhaled gene therapy in lung cancer: Application for nano oncology and safety of bio nanotechnology. *International Journal of Molecular Sciences, 13*(9), 10828–10862. https://doi.org/10.3390/ijms130910828 (accessed on 23rd June 2025).
42. Xie, L., Xie, D., Du, Z., Xue, S., Wang, K., Yu, X., Liu, X., Peng, Q., & Fang, C. (2024). A novel therapeutic outlook: Classification, applications and challenges of inhalable micron/nanoparticle drug delivery systems in lung cancer (Review). *International Journal of Oncology, 64*(4), 38. https://doi.org/10.3892/ijo.2024.5626 (accessed on 23rd June 2025).
43. Wang, H., Qin, L., Zhang, X., Guan, J., & Mao, S. (2022). Mechanisms and challenges of nanocarriers as non-viral vectors of therapeutic genes for enhanced pulmonary

delivery. *Journal of Controlled Release, 352*, 970–993. https://doi.org/10.1016/j.jconrel.2022.10.061 (accessed on 23rd June 2025).

44. Yuan, M., Han, Z., Liang, Y., Sun, Y., He, B., Chen, W., & Li, F. (2023). mRNA nano delivery systems: Targeting strategies and administration routes. *Biomaterials Research, 27*(1), 90. https://doi.org/10.1186/s40824-023-00425-3 (accessed on 23rd June 2025).
45. Gemayel, J., Chebly, A., Kourie, H., Hanna, C., Mheidly, K., Mhanna, M., Karam, F., Ghoussaini, D., Najjar, P. E., & Khalil, C. (2024). Genome engineering as a therapeutic approach in cancer therapy: A comprehensive review. *Advanced Genetics, 5*(1), 2300201. https://doi.org/10.1002/ggn2.202300201 (accessed on 23rd June 2025).
46. Rossi, M., Steklov, M., Huberty, F., Nguyen, T., Marijsse, J., Jacques-Hespel, C., Najm, P., Lonez, C., & Breman, E. (2023). Efficient shRNA-based knockdown of multiple target genes for cell therapy using a chimeric miRNA cluster platform. *Molecular Therapy–Nucleic Acids, 34*, 102038. https://doi.org/10.1016/j.omtn.2023.102038 (accessed on 23rd June 2025).
47. Bukhari, I., Zhang, Y., Thorne, R. F., & Mi, Y. (2023). Editorial: Complexity of tumor microenvironment: A major culprit in cancer development, volume II. *Frontiers in Endocrinology, 13*, 1126778. https://doi.org/10.3389/fendo.2022.1126778 (accessed on 23rd June 2025).
48. Huang, T., Gao, J., Cai, L., Xie, H., Wang, Y., Wang, Y., & Zhou, Q. (2022). Treating pulmonary fibrosis with non-viral gene therapy: From bench to bedside. *Pharmaceutics, 14*(4), 813. https://doi.org/10.3390/pharmaceutics14040813 (accessed on 23rd June 2025).
49. Yan, L., Hou, C., Liu, J., Wang, Y., Zeng, C., Yu, J., Zhou, T., Zhou, Q., Duan, S., & Xiong, W. (2023). Local administration of liposomal-based Plekhf1 gene therapy attenuates pulmonary fibrosis by modulating macrophage polarization. *Science China Life Sciences, 66*(11), 2571–2586. https://doi.org/10.1007/s11427-022-2314-8 (accessed on 23rd June 2025).
50. Wu, W., Wang, Z., Zhang, H., Zhang, X., & Tian, H. (2024). CircGRHPR inhibits aberrant epithelial–mesenchyme transformation progression of lung epithelial cells associated with idiopathic pulmonary fibrosis. *Cell Biology and Toxicology, 40*(1), 7. https://doi.org/10.1007/s10565-024-09839-8 (accessed on 23rd June 2025).

CHAPTER 6

Fundamentals of Artificial Intelligence

ALAM MOHD. ADIL,[1] GURDEEP SINGH,[1,*] and MUKESH KR. SINGH[2]

[1]*Lovely Institute of Technology (Pharmacy), Lovely Professional University, Phagwara, Punjab, India*

[2]*School of Pharmaceutical Sciences, Faculty of Pharmacy, IFTM University, Moradabad, Uttar Pradesh, India*

*Corresponding author

ABSTRACT

Artificial intelligence (AI) is all about creating machines or computer systems that can do work that people can do, like learning, reasoning, problem-solving, Natural Language Processing (NLP), robotics, and computer vision. Basically, it's all about simulating human intelligence in machines. Machine learning and deep learning are both subsets of AI, which are the basic components of it. The ability to analyze and process large amounts of data quickly and accurately is the main advantage of AI. Because of its technology's practical uses in a wide range of technological and research sectors, it has become an extremely important component of industry. The future of AI holds tremendous potential for transformative advancements across various domains like healthcare, finance, manufacturing, autonomous vehicles, education, and human resources. Looking ahead, the future of AI is anticipated to witness advancements in autonomous systems, human-AI collaboration, explainable AI (XAI), and AI ethics. Addressing challenges related to interpretability, transparency, and trust in AI systems will be pivotal for their widespread acceptance and ethical utilization across various domains. This article aims to offer an

Nanotechnology for Nucleic Acid Delivery: Pankaj Sharma, Saloni Jain, and Vinay Jain (Eds.)

DOI: 10.1201/9781998511853-6

overview of the fundamental concepts of AI with their potential application in the development of healthcare.

6.1 INTRODUCTION

Before understanding Artificial Intelligence, first understand what intelligence is. Intelligence is the ability for learning, reasoning, understanding, and mental activity. It covers the capacity to learn, comprehend new situations, reason, and apply knowledge to one's environment [1]. Artificial intelligence (AI) refers to the encouragement of human intelligence in machines, enabling them to achieve tasks like interpreting speech, predicting patterns, and making decisions. It's a group or collection of algorithms that let machines and computers simulate what humans can do, like learning from experience and figuring out solutions to problems. It's different from traditional methods of computing, which rely on people doing logical operations to process data. These methods are used to speed up things that are hard or time-consuming for humans to do, like doing a linear regression on data [2]. AI works by using special hardware and software for writing and machine learning training with algorithms, with famous languages like Python, R, Java, C++, and Julia being used by developers [3].

In a simple way, AI is when computers are trained to mimic human behavior by using large amounts of data from previous examples of similar behaviors. A computer learns when its software can predict and respond to changing conditions based on past results. Machine learning is the procedure of computers learning from and making predictions based on data. Machines can make changes without being specifically programmed. Machine learning is a form of AI that automatically runs the analytical model-making process and allows machines to change to new conditions independently [4]. Deep Learning (DL) is a part of machine learning. It works with algorithms based on the brain's structure and functions, known as "neural networks." This technology has enabled the development of image-based search engines, personalized marketing based on preferences, fraud detection, and cybersecurity incident detection based on people's behavior. Deep Learning enables artificial intelligence applications by understanding complex data and environments [5]. Figure 6.1 shows the elements of artificial intelligence; artificial learning is having only two elements: machine learning and deep learning.

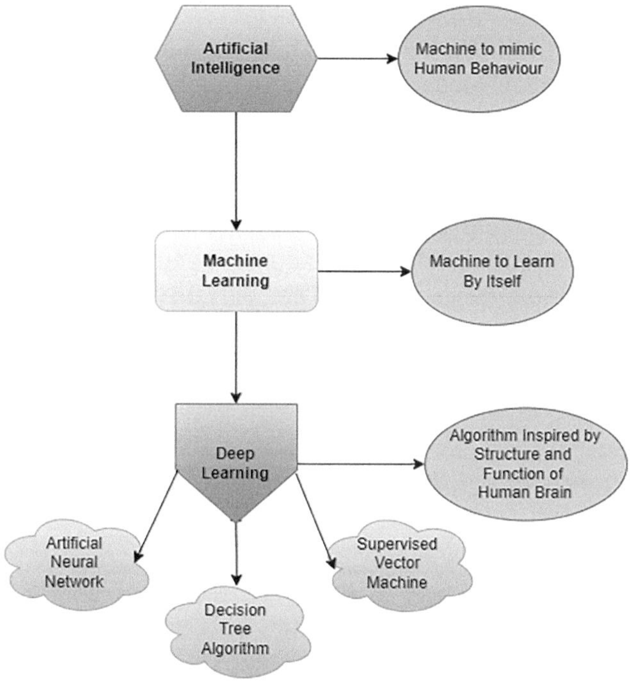

FIGURE 6.1 Elements of artificial intelligence (AI)

6.1.1 ARTIFICIAL INTELLIGENCE (AI) CAN BE DIVIDED INTO TWO MAIN TYPES

- **Narrow or Weak AI:** Narrow or weak AI is designed to present specific tasks, such as speech recognition or image classification.
- **General or Strong AI:** General or Strong AI is designed to have intelligence like a human and the ability to perform a wide range of cognitive tasks..

The capabilities and areas of interest of general and narrow AI are different. While general AI is more adaptable, less dependent on particular data, and devoid of human-like reasoning skills, narrow AI is task-specific and concentrates on labeled data and predefined functions [6, 7]. While general AI can accomplish a greater variety of tasks and is not constrained to predefined functions, narrow AI uses machine learning algorithms to be trained on specific data to identify patterns and make predictions [8].

AI encompasses various approaches that shape how machines behave and interact with their environment. There are perhaps two major perspectives to developing AI methods today: (i) acting like humans; and (ii) acting rationally. AI aims to create computers with thinking, seeing, hearing, walking, talking, and feeling capabilities. The creation of computer abilities typically associated with human intelligence, such as learning, reasoning, and problem-solving, is a key component of AI. The systems of AI aim to revolutionize different industries and change daily life with a variety of functionalities and goals. The goals drive the development of AI technologies that range from problem-solving, decision-making, natural language processing, machine learning, robotics, healthcare advancements, to fostering creativity and innovation [6–8] (Figure 6.1).

6.1.2 THE PRIMARY GOAL OF ARTIFICIAL INTELLIGENCE (AI) INCLUDE

1. **Generating Expert Systems:** Developing intelligent systems capable of learning, reasoning, and advising users efficiently, AI systems can capture and utilize expert knowledge in specific departments, creating expert systems that can give solutions to problems, provide recommendations, and make conclusions based on established rules and logical reasoning.
2. **Reasoning:** Implementing different forms of reasoning to interpret ideas and transitions between sets of facts.
3. **Robotic Machines:** Enabling machines to understand, think, behave, solve problems, and mimic human-like cognitive abilities, AI is essential to robotics because it allows robots to see their surroundings, decide for themselves, and carry out tasks on their own. Applications for robotics include assembly lines, industrial automation, autonomous drones, self-driving cars, and robotic assistants in a variety of circumstances.
4. **Enhancing Efficiency and Automation:** Improving efficiency by automating tasks and decision-making processes.
5. **Decision-Making and Predictive Analytics:** Developing a system that can examine data, identify patterns, and make data-driven decisions, AI systems can analyze large datasets and

identify patterns within them, enabling tasks such as predictive modeling, anomaly detection, classification, and clustering.

6. **Personalization and User Experience:** Enhancing user experience through personalized interactions, the systems of AI examine user behavior and preferences to offer tailored experiences, content, and recommendations. Digital marketing, social media, streaming services, and e-commerce platforms all make extensive use of this.
7. **Natural Language Processing (NLP) and Understanding:** Allowing machines to know and communicate in natural language, NLP allows AI systems to understand, interpret, and produce human language. This capability allows tasks like language translation, sentiment analysis, text summarization, and chatbots, making interactions between humans and machines more natural and intuitive.
8. **Creativity and Innovation:** AI systems are becoming more and more capable of producing artistic, musical, literary, and design content. Text generation, making music, product design, and realistic image creation are all possible with generative models such as GANs (Generative Adversarial Networks) and transformers.
9. **Healthcare Advancements:** Improving diagnostics, treatment planning, and patient care in the healthcare sector.
10. **Ethical and Fair AI:** Ensuring AI systems are developed ethically without biases to benefit all individuals regardless of background. With the growing impact of AI on society, there's a rising focus on ensuring that AI systems are developed and utilized responsibly, considering factors like fairness, transparency, privacy, accountability, and bias mitigation.

6.1.3 HISTORICAL DEVELOPMENT

AI has its origins in the early philosophical discussions concerning the behavior of intelligence and the possibility of AI resembling that of humans. In the 16th and 17th centuries, philosophers like Descartes, Hobbes, and Leibniz debated the viability of creating artificial entities that possessed intelligence akin to that of humans.

In the year 1818, the publication of Mary Shelley's "Frankenstein" drew attention to the concept of artificial beings during the 18th century. This book examined the ethical ramifications of producing artificial life and its effects [9].

John McCarthy first proposed that "every aspect of learning or any other feature of intelligence can in principle be so precisely described that a machine can be made to simulate it" at the 1956 Dartmouth Conference, which is when he first used the term "artificial intelligence." The current era of AI research and development began with this conference [10].

Symbolic artificial intelligence, which participated in representing knowledge as symbols and using rules to manipulate and reason with these symbols, was the focus of AI research in the 1960s and 1970s. Expert systems were created as a result of this strategy, and they were intended to replicate how human experts in particular fields made decisions [11]. The focus of AI research in the 1980s and 1990s shifted to connectionism, which makes use of neural networks to identify patterns in data. Deep learning algorithms were created as a result of this strategy, and they have been crucial to recent developments in AI, including speech and picture recognition.

In the 1990s and 2000s, advances in machine learning, particularly neural networks and statistical methods, revitalized the field of AI. Techniques such as deep learning have led to steps forward in areas like computer vision, natural language processing, and robotics. AI has been impacting many different aspects of society in recent years, from virtual assistants and self-driving cars to recommendation engines on websites. Concerns about ethics and the effects of AI on society have also gained traction.

6.1.4 BENEFITS OF ARTIFICIAL INTELLIGENCE (AI)

AI has numerous advantages that have revolutionized the way humans live and work in day-to-day life. Some of the key advantages of AI are as follows [12–14]:

1. **Increased Efficiency:** AI can perform tasks much quickly and more precise than humans, reducing the time and more work required for repetitive or complex tasks.

2. **Enhancement of Decision-Making:** AI can analyze large amounts of data, detect patterns and make predictions, helping humans make informed decisions.
3. **Personalization:** AI can analyze customer performance and preferences to create customized recommendations and experiences.
4. **Cost Savings:** The task which can are performed by human, AI can automate that work by reducing labor costs and improving efficiency.
5. **Enhanced Safety:** In dangerous or hazardous environments where human safety is at risk, such as in mining or construction in such place, AI in can be replaced by human.
6. **Continuous Learning:** AI systems can learn and improve over time, becoming more accurate and efficient as they process more data.
7. **24/7 Availability:** AI can work or available 24/7 at that place where task is going continuously without breaks.
8. **Improved Quality:** AI can detect errors or defects in products, enhancing quality of the product and reducing waste.
9. **Increased Innovation:** AI can be used to explore new ideas and develop innovative products and solutions.
10. **Improved Customer Service:** Chatbots and virtual assistants can provide 24/7 customer support, improving customer satisfaction and reducing response times, with the help of AI.

6.1.5 LIMITATIONS OF ARTIFICIAL INTELLIGENCE (AI)

While AI has numerous benefits, there are also some disadvantages associated with its use. Some of the main disadvantages of AI include [12–14]:

1. **Job Loss:** One of the most significant concerns about AI is that it could runs many jobs automatically that are currently done by humans, which leads to job displacement and unemployment.
2. **Lack of Emotional Intelligence:** AI lacks the emotional intelligence of humans, which can be crucial in certain industries, such as healthcare and customer service.

3. **Bias:** Discriminatory outcomes arrives on system when, AI algorithms can be biased if they are trained on biased data.
4. **Cost:** Developing and implementing AI systems can be costly, especially for small businesses.
5. **Dependence:** As human are becoming more reliant on AI, there is a risk that we will lose our ability to perform certain tasks without it, leading to dependence.
6. **Security Risks:** Sometimes AI systems is becoming weak, which makes easy for hacking and cyber-attacks, which can compromise sensitive data.
7. **Ethical Concerns:** There are ethical concerns comes around the by the use of AI, particularly in areas such as surveillance, autonomous weapons, and privacy.

6.2 PROBLEM SOLVING AND SEARCH

The predominant AI framework for problem-solving, which includes planning, learning, scientific discovery, and mathematical theorem proof, is state-space search. This method shows that these actions can be viewed as search problems in an abstract sense. As the large amount of research in AI focuses on the methodical decomposition of complicated problems into search problems and the development of efficient strategies for solving them, some real-time examples are shown in Table 6.1 [15].

TABLE 6.1 Artificial Intelligence (AI) has the Wide Range of Real-Life Applications Across Various Industries and Sectors

Real Life application of Artificial Intelligence (AI)			
Sl. No.	**Areas of Application**	**Examples**	**Real Life Application**
1.	*Neural Networks*	Face recognition, Character recognition, handwriting recognition, pattern prediction	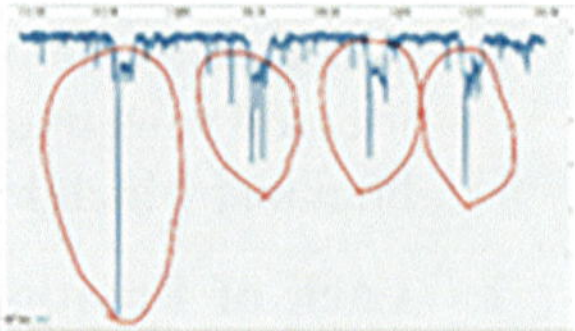

TABLE 6.1 *(Continued)*

Real Life application of Artificial Intelligence (AI)			
Sl. No.	**Areas of Application**	**Examples**	**Real Life Application**
2.	*Natural Language Processing*	Google Voice, Speech Recognition	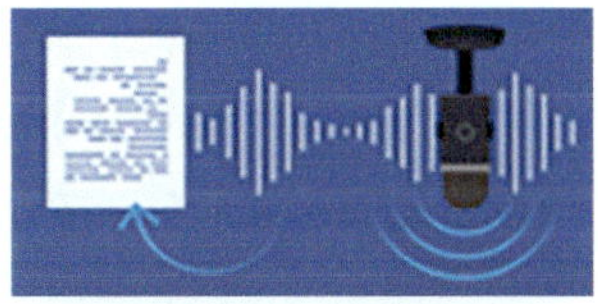
3.	*Robotics*	In industry for spraying, moving, checking, cleaning, carving, coating, automobiles	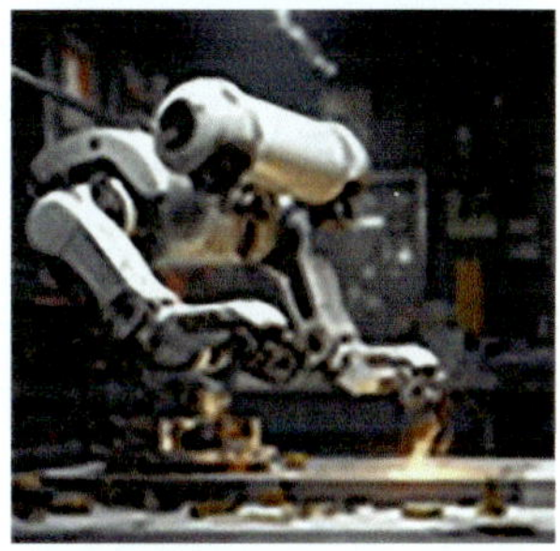
4.	*Expert System*	Clinical Systems, Flight Tracking Systems	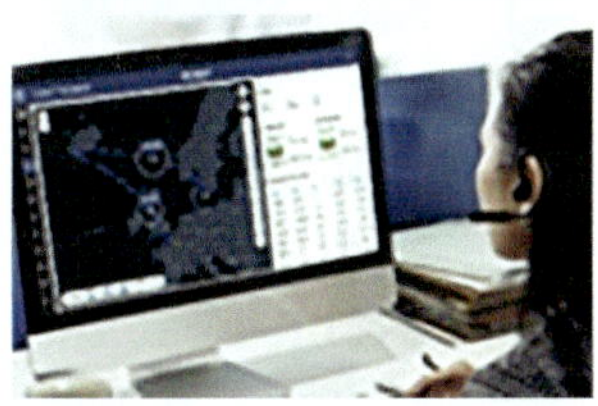
5.	*Computer Vision*	Medical image processing, action recognition, transportation	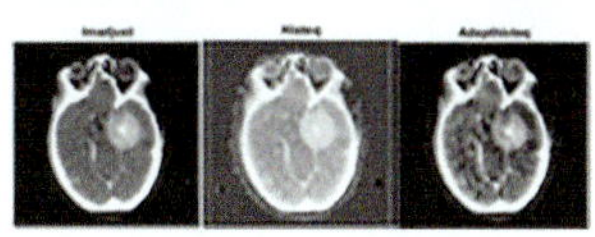

6.2.1 PROBLEM-SOLVING TECHNIQUES IN ARTIFICIAL INTELLIGENCE (AI)

Problem-solving is a fundamental aspect of AI, involving various techniques to find solutions efficiently. Here is an overview of key search algorithms and problem-solving methods:

1. Search Algorithms:

   a. **Depth-First Search:** This algorithm explores possible outcomes along each branch before backtracking. It searches far down the search tree, possibly getting to the goal more quickly, but it might not always find the best answer [16; 17].

b. **Breadth-First Search:** In contrast, breadth-first search explores all neighbor branching at the present depth before moving on to the next level. It ensures the shortest path to the goal but requires more memory due to storing all nodes at each level.

c. **A* Search:** A* search combines the advantages of both depth-first and breadth-first searches by using a heuristic to advise the search towards the crucial paths. It moderates the nodes based on a combination of actual price and estimated cost to reach the goal, ensuring an optimal solution if certain conditions are met [18].

6.2.2 PROBLEM-SOLVING METHODS

1. **State Space Problems:** These problems involve defining states, operators, initial state, goal state, and path costs. By navigating through states and operators, AI systems can find solutions efficiently by searching through a problem space [19].

2. **Problem Reduction:** This method involves breaking down complex problems into simpler subproblems until reaching a solution. It is commonly used in planning, expert systems, and theorem proving to tackle intricate challenges step by step.

These problem-solving techniques play a crucial role in AI applications, enabling systems to navigate complex scenarios, make decisions, and find optimal solutions efficiently. By leveraging search algorithms and problem-solving methods effectively, AI systems can address a wide range of challenges across various domains. Here, Figure 6.2 shows the work flowchart of problem-solving methods in AI.

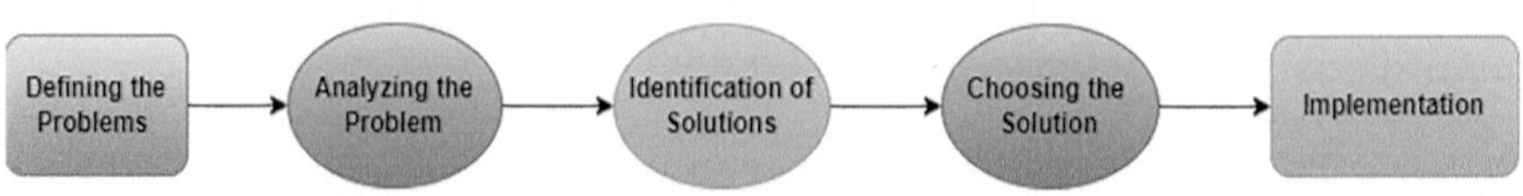

FIGURE 6.2 Problem-solving method in artificial intelligence (AI).

6.3 KNOWLEDGE REPRESENTATION AND REASONING

Reasoning, decision-making, and problem-solving in AI systems depend on the representation and manipulation of knowledge. Different techniques have been developed to represent text in a machine-readable format. Some common methods used for representing and manipulating knowledge in AI systems are discussed in the subsections.

6.3.1 LOGICAL REPRESENTATIONS

Logical representations express knowledge using formal logic, which consists of symbols, predicates, and rules. The most common logical representation used in AI is predicate logic, which includes propositions, variables, quantifiers, and logical operators. Propositional logic represents facts using simple true/false statements. It is suitable for representing knowledge about the state of the world or the relationship between different objects.

First-order logic, also known as predicate logic, extends propositional logic by defining variables, quantifiers, and predicates [20]. It allows for more complex statements about objects, properties, and relationships. Rules in this representation define relationships and infer new knowledge based on existing facts. For example, "if X is a parent of Y and Y is a parent of Z, then X is a grandparent of Z." It enables formal reasoning and inference, allowing AI systems to derive new knowledge from existing knowledge bases.

6.3.2 SEMANTIC NETWORKS

Semantic networks represent knowledge using a network structure composed of nodes (concepts) and edges (relationships) between them. Each node specifies a concept or object, and each edge represents a relationship between the two concepts. They are intuitive and easy to understand, making them suitable for capturing conceptual knowledge and hierarchical relationships. Nodes in semantic networks can have attributes or properties associated with them, providing additional information about concepts. Semantic networks support various operations such as inheritance (propagating properties from parent nodes to child nodes), similarity assessment, and semantic querying. Examples of semantic networks include ConceptNet, WordNet, and the Cyc knowledge base [21].

6.3.3 ONTOLOGIES

Ontologies specify concepts, attributes, and relationships within a particular domain by defining a standardized vocabulary. They improve the comprehension of AI systems by offering a standard framework for knowledge inference and representation [22]. With every method having its own benefits in terms of efficiently capturing, organizing, and applying information for tasks like reasoning, decision-making, and problem-solving, these approaches provide a variety of ways to represent and manipulate knowledge in AI systems. AI systems can effectively process information and make defensible decisions based on structured knowledge representations by utilizing these techniques.

Automated reasoning is the process of using computational techniques to derive new knowledge from existing knowledge bases or sets of rules. These are the systems that leverage various forms of reasoning to automate logical inference processes, enabling machines to make decisions, solve problems, and draw conclusions efficiently. Each type of reasoning plays a distinct role in AI applications, including the system's ability to analyze data, learn patterns, predict, and make decisions based on available information [23]. Different forms of automated reasoning can be employed, including deductive, inductive, and abductive reasoning. Each type of reasoning has its own features and function. Here's an overview of these techniques [24, 25, 26]:

1. **Deductive Reasoning:** This type of reasoning includes specific conclusions that are drawn from general principles or premises. It is a fundamental form of reasoning used in mathematics and logic to derive logical conclusions from given information.

2. **Inductive Reasoning:** This reasoning contributes to making generalizations based on particular observations. This type of reasoning is used to predict future outcomes or patterns based on previous data, allowing AI systems to learn from examples and make probabilistic predictions.

3. **Abductive Reasoning:** Abductive reasoning involves inferring the best explanation for observed phenomena. It is used to generate hypotheses or explanations that best fit the available evidence, aiding in problem-solving and decision-making processes.

6.4 MACHINE LEARNING (ML)

ML is a subpart of AI that focuses on the growth of algorithms and models that enable computers to learn patterns and make decisions from data without being explicitly programmed [27]. ML algorithms enable systems to enhance their performance over time through experience, making them increasingly capable of performing tasks and making predictions accurately.

6.4.1 SUBFIELDS OF MACHINE LEARNING (ML) [28]

1. **Supervised Learning:** It involves training a model on a labeled dataset, in which each example contains input features and target labels. The aim of supervised learning is to train a mapping from input features to output labels that allows the model to make predictions on unseen data. Examples of supervised learning tasks include classification, where the model predicts discrete labels (e.g., spam detection, image recognition), and regression, where the model forecasts continuous values (e.g., house price prediction, stock price forecasting). Common algorithms in supervised learning include decision trees, support vector machines (SVM), k-nearest neighbors (k-NN), logistic regression, and deep neural networks.
2. **Unsupervised Learning:** It conducts training a system on a dataset that is not labeled, where the aim is to find hidden patterns, structures, or relationships within the data. Unlike supervised learning, unsupervised learning does not require explicit target labels, and the model must find its own internal representations of the data. Examples of unsupervised learning tasks involve clustering, where the aim is to form groups of similar data points together (e.g., customer segmentation, document clustering), and dimensionality reduction, where the goal is to reduce the number of features while preserving the important information in the data (e.g., principal component analysis, t-distributed stochastic neighbor embedding). Common algorithms in unsupervised learning include k-means clustering, hierarchical clustering, Gaussian mixture models (GMM), and autoencoders.

3. **Reinforcement Learning:** It conducts training of a model to arrange decisions in sequence within an environment to yield a large cumulative proceed signal. The model interacts with the environment by taking actions, receiving feedback in the form of rewards or penalties, and learning to improve its decision-making policy over time. Reinforcement learning is characterized by psychology and is often likened to how humans and animals learn through training and mistakes. Examples of RL applications include playing games (e.g., AlphaGo), robotics, autopilot driving, recommendation systems, and resource management. Common algorithms in reinforcement learning include Q-learning, policy gradients, deep Q-networks (DQN), and actor-critic methods. These are subfields of machine learning that encompass a wide range of algorithms, techniques, and applications, enabling AI systems to learn from data, generalize patterns, and make accurate decisions in many domains. Supervised learning is used for tasks with labeled data, unsupervised learning is applied to discover hidden structures in unlabeled data, and reinforcement learning is employed for sequential decision-making in dynamic environments.

6.5 NEURAL NETWORKS (NNS)

Artificial neural networks (ANNs) or NNs are a part of machine learning algorithms which are characterized by the structure and function of biological neural networks present in living beings, which are found in the brains of animals, including humans. An ANN is made up of layers of connected nodes, like neurons or units. An input layer, one or more hidden layers, and an output layer are the most common types of these layers [29, 30].

The Key Components and Concepts of Anns, Along with Their Biological Inspiration Are as Follows:

1. **Neurons:** Biological inspiration: The fundamental units of the neural networks in the brain are neurons. Via dendrites, they receive signals from other neurons, process them in the cell body, and then send signals via an axon to other neurons.

   - **Artificial Representation:** In ANNs, Neurons are designed as nodes that process information, generate an output, and receive input. Every neuron modifies its input before sending the outcome to the layer below.

2. **Layers:** Biological inspiration: Neural networks in the brain include of many layers which are interconnected to neurons, including input, output, and intermediate hidden layers.
   - **Artificial Representation:** ANNs also are made of layers present in neurons. One or more hidden layers process the information between the input and output after the input layer receives data and the output layer generates the network's output.
3. **Connections:** Biological inspiration: Neurons in biological networks are connected to each other via synapses, which allow them to transmit signals electrochemically.
   - **Artificial Representation:** In ANNs, connections between neurons are characterized by weights. These weights define the power of link between the neurons and which are made during the learning process to optimize how the network's performed.
4. **Activation Function:** Biological inspiration: Neurons in the brain exhibit complex activation patterns in response to input signals.
   - **Artificial Representation:** In ANNs, an activation function is applied by each neuron to the weighted sum of its inputs. By doing this, the network gains non-linearity, which enables it to recognize intricate patterns and connections in the data.
5. **Learning Algorithms:** Biological inspiration: The brain learns through a process of synaptic plasticity, where the strength of attachments between neurons is adjusted which is based on experience.
   - **Artificial Representation:** ANNs learn from data using various learning algorithms, such as backpropagation. In order to minimize the discrepancy between its predicted and true outputs in the training data, the network modifies its weights during the learning process.

ANNs mimic the basic principles of biological neural networks to regulate tasks like classification, regression, pattern prediction, and more

[31]. While they simplify and abstract many aspects of neural function, ANNs have proven to be powerful tools to give solution for a wide range of machine learning problems.

6.7 DEEP LEARNING

Artificial neural networks are used in deep learning, a subfield of machine learning and AI, to learn from and make predictions or judgments about data. In addition, unlike traditional machine learning techniques, which include manual extraction of features from raw data, deep learning algorithms learn hierarchical representations (HDRs) directly from raw data. This ability to learn features automatically makes deep learning especially useful for image prediction, Natural language processing (NLP), and speech recognition [32, 33]. Deep learning architectures are neural network models composed of many layers, allowing them to gain complex representations of data [34]. Here's an explanation of three prominent architectures [35, 36].

6.7.1 FEEDFORWARD NEURAL NETWORKS

The most basic type of neural network is called a feedforward neural network, in which information only moves in one direction from input to output. They are made up of an output layer, an input layer, and one or more hidden layers. Several neurons, sometimes known as nodes or units, make up each layer. A fully connected network is formed when all of the neurons in one layer are connected to all of the neurons in the layer below it. In order to produce an output, each neuron in a layer takes in inputs, weights them, adds them together, and then runs the mixture through an activation function. Sigmoid, hyperbolic tangent (tanh), and rectified linear unit (ReLU) are examples of common activation functions. Feedforward networks are appropriate for function approximation, regression, and classification.

6.7.2 CONVOLUTIONAL NEURAL NETWORKS (CNNS)

Special neural networks are made to process structured, grid-like data, such as images. They make use of fully connected, pooling, and convolutional layers. Convolutional layers apply convolution operations to the input by extracting features from local input regions using learnable filters or kernels. Convolutional layers create feature maps, which are then down sampled by pooling layers to reduce spatial dimensions while maintaining significant features. CNNs have the capacity to train hierarchical representations of visual data, capturing spatial hierarchies of features like edges, textures, and object parts. This is remarkably achieved in image characterization, model identification, image classification, and various other computer vision tasks. Popular CNN architectures include LeNet, AlexNet, VGGNet, GoogLeNet, and ResNet.

6.7.3 RECURRENT NEURAL NETWORKS (RNNS)

RNNs are used to process arrangements of data where the order of elements matters, such as time-series data, text, and speech. They have feedback loops, which enable the persistence of information over time. An RNN's hidden states, which serve as a kind of memory to store details about prior inputs, are linked to each neuron. RNNs are useful for tasks like language modeling, machine translation, speech recognition, and time-series prediction because they can display temporal dynamics and dependencies. However, the vanishing gradient problem impedes the ability of standard RNNs to capture long-term dependencies. Popular RNN variations like long short-term memory (LSTM) and Gated Recurrent Unit (GRU) are made to better capture long-range dependencies and solve the vanishing gradient issue. These architectures are the cornerstone of deep learning and have made major strides possible in a number of domains, including speech recognition, computer vision, and natural language processing.

6.8 NATURAL LANGUAGE PROCESSING (NLP)

NLP is a subfield of AI that concerns the interaction between computers and human languages. It makes it possible for computers to produce meaningful, intelligible, and practical human language through understanding, interpreting, and generation. Text classification, sentiment analysis, machine translation, named entity recognition, language modeling, and many other tasks and applications are all included in the broad field of NLP [37]. Some applications of NLP are included in the subsections [38, 39, 40].

6.8.1 SENTIMENT ANALYSIS

Sentiment analysis, sometimes referred to as opinion mining, is the process of examining textual data to ascertain the sentiment expressed, be it neutral, positive, or negative. It is employed in many different contexts, such as market research, product reviews, social media monitoring, and customer feedback analysis. Machine learning models are trained to classify the general sentiment of a document or sentence, and NLP techniques are used to extract sentiment-bearing words or phrases from text.

6.8.2 TEXT CLASSIFICATION

Text classification consists of categorizing text documents into different classes. It is mostly applicable for spam identification, topic classification, sentiment analysis, and language identification. Natural Language Processing techniques are employed to separate relevant characteristics from text models, such as words, phrases, or n-grams, and then training is given to machine learning models to classify documents into different categories based on these features.

6.8.3 MACHINE TRANSLATION

Machine translation is the performance of translating text or speech automatically from one language to another language. It plays a crucial role in bridging diverse language barriers and makes communication easy across many different cultures and languages. NLP techniques, particularly statistical and neural machine translation models, are used to analyze and translate text at the word, phrase, or sentence level. Modern machine translation systems often leverage large-scale parallel corpora and deep learning architectures such as arrangement models with attention mechanisms to achieve futuristic or modern performance.

6.9 COMPUTER VISION

Computer vision is a part of AI focused on allowing computers to interpret and understand visual information from the world [41]. It involves various tasks, each serving different purposes in processing and analyzing visual data. Some of the key tasks in computer vision include [42, 43]:

6.9.1 IMAGE CLASSIFICATION

It is performed by categorizing a full image into different categories. This task is often used for tasks like identifying objects in images or scenes, such as classifying whether an image contains a cat or a dog.

6.9.2 OBJECT DETECTION

Object detection involves not only categorizing objects within an image but also locating and delineating their positions with bounding boxes. It is used for scenarios where multiple objects need to be identified within an image, such as detecting pedestrians, vehicles, or various items in a retail setting.

6.9.3 IMAGE SEGMENTATION

Image segmentation consists of dividing an image into many layers or regions, where every layer represents a distinct object or area of interest. While object detection uses bounding boxes to identify and localize objects, image segmentation assigns a label to each pixel in the image, providing pixel-level accuracy. It is utilized in many different applications, including autonomous driving, semantic scene understanding, and medical image analysis.

6.9.4 INSTANCE SEGMENTATION

Instance segmentation is an enlargement of object detection and gives accurate information, where the goal is to not only classify and segment objects but also to differentiate between individual instances of the same class. It's used when distinguishing between separate objects of the same category is important, such as in counting objects or tracking them in video streams.

6.9.5 OBJECT TRACKING

Object tracking involves following the trajectory of a particular object across a sequence of frames in a video. It is essential for tasks such as surveillance, action recognition, and autonomous navigation.

These tasks are fundamental to many computer vision applications, ranging from industrial automation and robotics to healthcare, automotive, retail, and entertainment. Advances in computer vision techniques continue to drive innovation in various domains, enabling machines to perceive and interact with the visual world more intelligently.

6.10 ROBOTICS AND AUTONOMOUS SYSTEMS

The study of designing, building, using, and operating robots is known as robotics. A robot is a kind of machine that can perform tasks fully or partially on its own. Robots are frequently programmable and have the ability to interact with their surroundings [44]. AI and robotics are transforming many different industries and facets of daily life. The study of robotics focuses on the design, construction, and management of autonomous or semi-autonomous robots [45]. On the other hand, AI is concerned with developing intelligent systems that replicate cognitive processes that humans do, like learning and making decisions. Robots are now better equipped to adapt, learn, and interact with their surroundings thanks to the amazing advances made possible by the combination of robotics and artificial intelligence [46].

6.10.1 ARTIFICIAL INTELLIGENCE (AI) IN ROBOTICS HAS DIVERSE APPLICATIONS ACROSS INDUSTRIES

1. **Customer Service:** AI-powered chatbots are increasingly used in customer service for handling simple requests without human involvement, learning from interactions to improve service quality.
2. **Assembly:** AI enhances robotic assembly processes, especially in complex manufacturing industries like aerospace, by enabling

real-time course correction and optimizing paths for efficient assembly.

3. **Packaging:** AI improves efficiency and accuracy in the packaging industry by refining motions made by robotic systems, making equipment installation and movement easier.
4. **Imaging:** AI enhances visual acuity and image recognition in robots across industries like assembly and logistics, ensuring greater accuracy in tasks requiring detailed visual analysis.
5. **Machine Learning:** Robots utilize machine learning to explore their surroundings, learn about their environment, navigate obstacles, and solve problems efficiently. This technology is applied in various domains from home robots to manufacturing robots in factories.

6.11 EXPERT SYSTEMS

Expert systems are also a type of AI technology that designs and mimics human experts' decision-making processes in a particular field. These are computer programs that use logic and knowledge to solve issues, offer suggestions, or reach judgments. Knowledge bases and inference engines are two essential parts of expert systems that combine to provide intelligent problem-solving [47–49]. They have two components.

6.11.1 KNOWLEDGE BASE

This component stores facts, rules, and heuristic knowledge relevant to a specific domain. It represents the critical information required for the system to function effectively. It is a central component of an expert system that stores relevant information and expertise about a particular domain. The knowledge base organizes this knowledge in a structured format that the expert system can access and utilize during problem-solving. There are two main types of knowledge:

1. **Factual Knowledge:** This includes information, data, rules, and heuristics acquired from human experts, textbooks, manuals, or other sources.

2. **Procedural Knowledge:** This refers to the problem-solving methods, strategies, and algorithms used by experts to analyze and solve problems within the domain.

6.11.2 INFERENCE ENGINE

The inference engine processes information from the knowledge base, combines it with specific case facts, and generates recommendations or solutions. It applies rules to known facts to deduce new information, guiding the system's decision-making process. It is responsible for reasoning and drawing conclusions based on the data stored in the knowledge base. It applies various inference techniques, including deduction, induction, abduction, and reasoning by analogy, to derive new knowledge from existing facts and rules.

The inference engine uses algorithms and rules of inference to process input data, apply relevant knowledge, and generate output in the form of recommendations, solutions, or decisions. It controls a strategy to choose and execute appropriate inference rules, considering factors such as the certainty of the information, the relevance of rules, and the goals of problem-solving.

6.12 ETHICAL AND SOCIETAL IMPLICATIONS

The responsible development and implementation of artificial intelligence systems are significantly influenced by ethical considerations in AI, such as bias, fairness, transparency, and accountability. These moral precepts are crucial for guaranteeing that AI systems uphold accountability, advance justice, safeguard privacy, and respect human rights throughout their entire lifecycle [50]. There are some key ethical considerations in AI [51]:

Ethical considerations in AI are increasingly important as AI technologies become more pervasive in various aspects of our lives. Here's a discussion of some key ethical considerations in AI.

6.12.1 BIAS

Bias in AI refers to the unfair or discriminatory treatment of individuals or groups based on characteristics such as race, gender, ethnicity, or socioeconomic status. Bias can appear in AI systems due to biased training data, flawed algorithms, or biased decision-making processes. Addressing bias in AI requires proper attention to data collection and curation, algorithm design, and model evaluation to ensure fairness and equity.

6.12.2 FAIRNESS

Fairness in AI involves ensuring that AI systems treat all individuals and groups fairly and without discrimination. Fairness considerations include mitigating biases, avoiding unfair outcomes or disparities, and promoting equal opportunities and access to AI technologies. Fairness metrics and techniques, such as fairness-aware algorithms and fairness constraints, can help evaluate and promote fairness in AI systems.

6.12.3 TRANSPARENCY

Transparency in AI refers to the ability to understand and explain the decisions and behavior of AI systems. Transparent AI systems provide explanations for their decisions, disclose their underlying algorithms and data sources, and enable external scrutiny and accountability. Transparency enhances trust, accountability, and user acceptance of AI technologies, particularly in high-stakes applications such as healthcare, criminal justice, and finance.

6.12.4 ACCOUNTABILITY

Accountability in AI entails holding individuals, organizations, and AI systems responsible for their actions, decisions, and outcomes. Establishing accountability mechanisms requires a clear delineation of roles and responsibilities, adherence to ethical guidelines and regulations, and mechanisms for oversight, auditing, and redress. Accountability promotes ethical behavior, ensures compliance with legal and regulatory frameworks, and mitigates the risks of harm or misuse associated with AI technologies.

6.12.5 PRIVACY

The gathering, storing, and processing of personal data by AI systems increase privacy concerns because it may violate people's right to privacy.

Implementing privacy-preserving methods like data anonymization, encryption, and differential privacy, as well as abiding by ethical and legal requirements, are necessary to protect privacy in artificial intelligence.

6.12.6 SAFETY AND SECURITY

Ensuring the safety and security of AI systems is crucial to prevent accidents, errors, or malicious attacks that could lead to harm or damage. Safety measures include rigorous testing, validation, and verification of AI systems, as well as designing fail-safe mechanisms and safeguards to mitigate risks and vulnerabilities.

The societal impacts of AI are multifaceted, encompassing job displacement, privacy concerns, and AI-driven discrimination. These issues are central to the ethical considerations surrounding the development and deployment of AI technologies. Here's an exploration of some societal impacts of AI, including job displacement, privacy concerns, healthcare and education, and AI-driven discrimination:

1. **Job Displacement:** AI has the potential to automate tasks traditionally performed by humans, leading to concerns about job displacement. While AI can enhance efficiency and productivity, there is a fear that widespread automation could result in significant job losses, particularly in industries with routine tasks. However, it is also acknowledged that AI can create new job opportunities and lead to increased productivity, necessitating a balance between automation and job creation.

2. **Privacy Concerns:** The collection and analysis of vast amounts of data by AI systems raise significant privacy concerns. Ensuring that personal data is collected and used ethically and with consent is crucial. AI systems used for surveillance purposes can infringe on privacy rights, and unauthorized access to personal data can result in identity theft or financial loss. Addressing privacy concerns requires robust regulations and guidelines to govern the development and use of AI technologies.

3. **Impact on Healthcare and Education:** AI technologies have the potential to improve healthcare outcomes through personalized medicine, disease diagnosis, drug discovery, and patient care

optimization. However, concerns exist regarding the ethical use of AI in healthcare, including issues related to patient privacy, medical ethics, and the potential for AI to exacerbate healthcare disparities. In education, AI-driven personalized learning systems can adapt to individual student needs, enhance student engagement, and improve learning outcomes. However, concerns about data privacy, algorithmic transparency, and the depersonalization of education remain important considerations.

6.12.7 ETHICAL AND REGULATORY CHALLENGES

The societal impacts of AI raise complex ethical, legal, and regulatory challenges that require careful consideration and action. Ethical guidelines, principles, and frameworks for responsible AI development and deployment are being developed by governments, industry groups, and academic institutions. Regulatory frameworks and standards for AI governance, accountability, and transparency are also being established to address risks and ensure ethical AI practices.

6.12.8 ARTIFICIAL INTELLIGENCE (AI)-DRIVEN DISCRIMINATION

Bias in AI algorithms can perpetuate and exacerbate social inequalities, leading to discriminatory outcomes. For example, facial recognition software has shown lower accuracy rates for individuals with darker skin tones, potentially resulting in unfair treatment. AI systems used in hiring processes may also perpetuate bias against certain groups. Addressing AI-driven discrimination requires awareness of bias in algorithms, diverse and representative datasets, and ongoing efforts to mitigate bias in AI systems.

6.13 FUTURE DIRECTIONS

In this fast-paced life, artificial intelligence is rapidly evolving, with emerging trends for achieving specific goals in the future of AI research and development [52–54]. There are three trends of these:

6.13.1 EXPLAINABLE AI (XAI)

XAI focuses on the progression of AI systems that can provide information for their decisions and actions. This transparency and comprehensibility are crucial, especially in fields where trust and accountability are of the highest significance. XAI aims to address the "black-box" nature of AI models by making their decision-making processes more understandable and interpretable. It enables humans to understand how AI systems arrive at specific conclusions, increasing trust and facilitating better decision-making. XAI has applications in various domains, including finance, healthcare, and autonomous vehicles.

6.13.2 META-LEARNING

Meta-learning is the process of developing AI systems that can learn how to learn. This approach focuses on increasing the learning capabilities of AI models by allowing them to adapt to new tasks and environments more efficiently. Meta-learning holds promise for improving AI performance and versatility.

6.13.3 ARTIFICIAL INTELLIGENCE (AI) SAFETY

The role of AI safety is to ensure the safety, reliability, and robustness of AI systems to prevent unintended consequences, accidents, or harmful behaviors. Research in AI safety covers various dimensions, including robustness to adversarial attacks, ethical considerations, consistency of AI systems with human values, and the prevention of unintended side effects. Techniques for AI safety include designing provably safe and verifiably correct AI systems, developing methods for adversarial robustness and error analysis, and integrating ethical principles into AI development processes.

6.14 CONCLUSIONS

AI refers to the encouragement of human intelligence in machines, enabling them to achieve tasks like interpreting speech, prediction of patterns, and making decisions. Machine learning and deep learning are subsets of AI. Machine learning relies heavily on data quality, quantity, and diversity, directly impacting operational performance. The importance of AI lies in its ability to automate tasks which are impractical for human programming, leading to the development of productivity and performance in areas like pattern recognition, language translation, and speech transcription. In order to ensure AI's peaceful coexistence with society while maintaining moral principles and human welfare, a balanced approach is required due to the ethical considerations and societal advancements brought about by AI. Gaining an understanding of the fundamentals required for successful AI systems is essential to understanding how AI works and develops; the fundamentals include algorithms, data, and computing power. The practical gains of AI adoption across a range of industries are illustrated by the potential increase in efficiency, financial gains, and organizational value that can result from promoting AI use in businesses. People can help ensure that AI advancements are in line with human values and the well-being of society by advocating for ethical AI governance, transparency, and responsible AI development. This will help ensure that AI technologies are integrated into society in an ethical and sustainable manner.

ACKNOWLEDGMENT

None

CONFLICT OF INTEREST

The authors declare no conflict of interest

FUNDING

None

KEYWORDS

- **artificial intelligence**
- **deep learning**
- **explainable AI**
- **healthcare**
- **machine learning**
- **natural language processing**

REFERENCES

1. Breakspear, A. (2013). A new definition of intelligence. *Intelligence and National Security, 28*(5), 678–693. https://doi.org/10.1080/02684527.2012.699285 (accessed on 23rd June 2025).
2. Cavasotto, C. N., & Di Filippo, J. I. (2021). Artificial intelligence in the early stages of drug discovery. *Archives of Biochemistry and Biophysics, 698*, 108730. https://doi.org/10.1016/j.abb.2020.108730 (accessed on 23rd June 2025).
3. Acemoglu, D., & Restrepo, P. (2018). Artificial intelligence, automation, and work. In *The Economics of Artificial Intelligence* (Vol. 10, pp. 197–236).
4. Lele, A. (2019). Artificial intelligence (AI). In *Disruptive Technologies for the Militaries and Security* (Vol. 139, p. 54).
5. Hinton, G., LeCun, Y., & Bengio, Y. (2015). Deep learning. *Nature, 521*(7553), 436–444. https://doi.org/10.1007/978-1-4842-5028-0_4 (accessed on 23rd June 2025).
6. Corea, F. (2019). AI knowledge map: How to classify AI technologies. In *An Introduction to Data* (pp. 25–29). https://doi.org/10.1007/978-3-030-04468-8_4 (accessed on 23rd June 2025).
7. Goertzel, B. (2018). Artificial general intelligence: Concept, state of the art, and future prospects. *Journal of Artificial General Intelligence, 5*(1), 1–48. https://doi.org/10.2478/jagi-2014-0001 (accessed on 23rd June 2025).
8. Bundy, A. (2017). Preparing for the future of artificial intelligence. *AI & Society, 32*, 285–287. https://doi.org/10.1007/s00146-016-0685-0 (accessed on 23rd June 2025).
9. Reynoso, R. (2020). A complete history of artificial intelligence. *Learning Hub*. Retrieved from: https://learninghub.com (accessed on 23rd June 2025).
10. Ertel, W. (2018). *Introduction to Artificial Intelligence*. Springer.
11. Kaul, V., Enslin, S., & Gross, S. A. (2020). History of artificial intelligence in medicine. *Gastrointestinal Endoscopy, 92*(4), 807–812. https://doi.org/10.1016/j.gie.2020.06.040 (accessed on 23rd June 2025).

12. Silver, D., Schrittwieser, J., Simonyan, K., Antonoglou, I., Huang, A., & Guez, A. (2017). Mastering the game of Go without human knowledge. *Nature, 550*(7676), 354–359. https://doi.org/10.1038/nature24270 (accessed on 23rd June 2025).
13. Merk, D., Friedrich, L., Grisoni, F., & Schneider, G. (2018). De novo design of bioactive small molecules by artificial intelligence. *Molecular Informatics, 37*(1, 2), 1700153. https://doi.org/10.1002/minf.201700153 (accessed on 23rd June 2025).
14. Jiang, F., Jiang, Y., Zhi, H., Dong, Y., Li, H., & Ma, S. (2017). Artificial intelligence in healthcare: Past, present and future. *Stroke and Vascular Neurology, 2*(4), 230–243. https://doi.org/10.1136/svn-2017-000101 (accessed on 23rd June 2025).
15. Jackson, P. C. (2019). *Introduction to Artificial Intelligence*. Courier Dover Publications.
16. Korf, R. E. (1999). Artificial intelligence search algorithms. *Special Topics and Techniques*. https://dl.acm.org/doi/pdf/10.5555/1882723.1882745 (accessed on 23rd June 2025).
17. Nilsson, N. J. (1969). A mobile automaton: An application of artificial intelligence techniques. *Stanford Research Institute*. https://doi.org/10.21236/ADA459660 (accessed on 23rd June 2025).
18. Pearl, J., & Korf, R. E. (1987). Search techniques. *Annual Review of Computer Science, 2*(1), 451–467.
19. Viharos, Z. J., & Kemény, Z. (2007). AI techniques in modelling, assignment, problem solving and optimization. *Engineering Applications of Artificial Intelligence, 20*(5), 691–698. https://doi.org/10.1016/j.engappai.2006.11.007 (accessed on 23rd June 2025).
20. Li, Z., Liu, X., Wang, X., Liu, P., & Shen, Y. (2023). Transo: A knowledge-driven representation learning method with ontology information constraints. *World Wide Web, 26*(1), 297–319. https://doi.org/10.1007/s11280-022-01016-3 (accessed on 23rd June 2025).
21. Bench-Capon, T. J. (2014). *Knowledge Representation: An Approach to Artificial Intelligence*. Elsevier.
22. Delgrande, J. P., & Mylopoulos, J. (1986). Knowledge representation: Features of knowledge and fundamentals of artificial intelligence. *Lecture Notes in Computer Science, 232*. https://doi.org/10.1007/BFb0022679 (accessed on 23rd June 2025).
23. Ndungi, R., & Uyun, S. (2023). A review of automated reasoning and its applications in the 21st century. *Indonesian Journal of Computer Science, 12*(2), 483–491. https://doi.org/10.33022/ijcs.v12i2.3175 (accessed on 23rd June 2025).
24. Wang, H. (2010). Toward mechanical mathematics. *IBM Journal of Research and Development, 1*, 2–22. https://doi.org/10.1147/rd.41.0002 (accessed on 23rd June 2025).
25. Bradley, A. R., & Manna, Z. (2007). *The Calculus of Computation: Decision Procedures with Applications to Verification* (pp. 1–269).
26. Manna, Z., & Pnueli, A. (1995). *Temporal Verification of Reactive Systems*.
27. Huang, X. L., Ma, X., & Hu, F. (2018). Machine learning and intelligent communications. *Mobile Networks and Applications, 23*, 68–70. https://doi.org/10.1007/s11036-017-0962-2 (accessed on 23rd June 2025).
28. Brownlee, J. (2014). Different types of learning in machine learning. *Machine Learning Mastery*.

29. Raj, R., & Kos, A. (2023). Artificial intelligence: Evolution, developments, applications, and future scope. *Przegląd Elektrotechniczny, 99*(2). https://doi.org/10.15199/48.2023.02.01 (accessed on 23rd June 2025).
30. Nath, M. P., Pandey, P., Somu, K., & Amalraj, P. (2018). Artificial intelligence & machine learning: The emerging milestones in software development. *International Journal of Research and Scientific Innovation, 5*(9), 36–44.
31. Rere, L. R., Fanany, M. I., & Arymurthy, A. M. (2015). Simulated annealing algorithm for deep learning. *Procedia Computer Science, 72*, 137–144.
32. Sharifani, K., & Amini, M. (2023). Machine learning and deep learning: A review of methods and applications. *World Information Technology and Engineering Journal, 10*(07), 3897–3904.
33. Prince, S. J. D. (2023). *Understanding Deep Learning*. MIT Press.
34. Taye, M. M. (2023). Understanding of machine learning with deep learning: Architectures, workflow, applications and future directions. *The Journal of Computers, 12*(5), 1–26. https://doi.org/10.3390/computers12050091 (accessed on 23rd June 2025).
35. Alzubaidi, L., Zhang, J., Humaidi, A. J., Al-Dujaili, A., Duan, Y., & Al-Shamma, O. (2021). Review of deep learning: Concepts, CNN architectures, challenges, applications, future directions. *Journal of Big Data, 8*, 1–74. https://doi.org/10.1186/s40537-021-00444-8 (accessed on 23rd June 2025).
36. Du, W., Rao, N., Liu, D., Jiang, H., Luo, C., Li, Z., Gan, T., & Zeng, B. (2019). Review on the applications of deep learning in the analysis of gastrointestinal endoscopy images. *IEEE Access, 7*, 142053–142069. https://doi.org/10.1109/ACCESS.2019.2944676 (accessed on 23rd June 2025).
37. Khurana, D., Koli, A., Khatter, K., & Singh, S. (2023). Natural language processing: State of the art, current trends and challenges. *Multimedia Tools and Applications, 82*(3), 3713–3744. https://doi.org/10.1007/s11042-022-13428-4 (accessed on 23rd June 2025).
38. Shivahare, B. D., Singh, A. K., Uppal, N., Rizwan, A., Vaathsav, V. S., & Suman, S. (2022). Survey paper: Study of natural language processing and its recent applications. In *Proceedings–2022 2nd International Conference on Innovative Sustainable Computational Technologies*. https://doi.org/10.1109/CISCT55310.2022.10046440 (accessed on 23rd June 2025).
39. Dande, A. A., & Pund, M. A. (2023). A review study on applications of natural language processing. *Indonesian Journal of Electrical Engineering and Computer Science, 3*(25), 122–126.
40. Lhoest, Q., Moral, A. V., Jernite, Y., Thakur, A., von Platen, P., & Patil, S. (2021). Datasets: A community library for natural language processing. *arXiv Preprint arXiv:2109.02846*. https://doi.org/10.48550/arXiv.2109.02846 (accessed on 23rd June 2025).
41. Bajammal, M., Stocco, A., Mazinanian, D., & Mesbah, A. (2020). A survey on the use of computer vision to improve software engineering tasks. *IEEE Transactions on Software Engineering, 48*(5), 1722–1742.
42. Sinha, R. K., Pandey, R., & Pattnaik, R. (2018). Deep learning for computer vision tasks: A review. *Computer Vision and Pattern Recognition*. https://doi.org/10.48550/arXiv.1804.03928 (accessed on 23rd June 2025).

43. Szeliski, R. (2022). *Computer Vision: Algorithms and Applications*. Springer Nature.
44. Vrontis, D., Christofi, M., Pereira, V., Tarba, S., Makrides, A., & Trichina, E. (2022). Artificial intelligence, robotics, advanced technologies and human resource management: A systematic review. *The International Journal of Human Resource Management, 33*(6), 1237–1266. https://doi.org/10.1080/09585192.2020.1871398 (accessed on 23rd June 2025).
45. Bordegoni, M., & Ferrise, F. (2023). Exploring the intersection of metaverse, digital twins, and artificial intelligence in training and maintenance. *Journal of Computer and Information Science in Engineering, 23*(6), 060806. https://doi.org/10.1115/1.4062455 (accessed on 23rd June 2025).
46. Hammer, A., & Karmakar, S. (2021). Automation, AI and the future of work in India. *Employee Relations: The International Journal, 43*(6), 1327–1341. https://doi.org/10.1108/ER-12-2019-0452 (accessed on 23rd June 2025).
47. Turban, E. (1992). *Expert systems and applied artificial intelligence.* In *Expert Systems and Applied Artificial Intelligence* (p. 804).
48. Gupta, I., & Nagpal, G. (2020). *Artificial Intelligence and Expert Systems*. Mercury Learning and Information.
49. Gaba, D. M. (2022). Artificial intelligence and expert systems. In *Control and Automation in Anesthesia* (pp. 22–36). Springer. https://doi.org/10.1007/978-3-642-79573-2_3 (accessed on 23rd June 2025).
50. Mensah, G. B. (2023). *Artificial Intelligence and Ethics: A Comprehensive Review of Bias Mitigation, Transparency, and Accountability in AI Systems*. EGRC Africa Regulation Research.
51. Huriye, A. Z. (2023). The ethics of artificial intelligence: Examining the ethical considerations surrounding the development and use of AI. *American Journal of Technology, 2*(1), 37–44.
52. Madhuri, P. S. (2020). Emerging trends in artificial intelligence. In *Advances in Computational and Bio-Engineering: International Conference on Computational and Bio Engineering* (pp. 357–365). https://doi.org/10.1007/978-3-030-46943-6_40 (accessed on 23rd June 2025).
53. Gursoy, D., & Cai, R. (2024). Artificial intelligence: An overview of research trends and future directions. *International Journal of Contemporary Hospitality Management*. https://doi.org/10.1108/IJCHM-03-2024-0322 (accessed on 23rd June 2025).
54. Chen, M. Y., Chiang, H. S., Lughofer, E., & Egrioglu, E. (2020). Deep learning: Emerging trends, applications and research challenges. *Soft Computing, 24*, 7835–7838. https://doi.org/10.1007/s00500-020-04939-z (accessed on 23rd June 2025).

CHAPTER 7

Role of Artificial Intelligence in Optimizing Nanocarriers for Nucleic Acid Delivery

PRAVIN KUMAR,* MAHENDRA SINGH ASHAWAT, AMARDEEP ANKALGI, and AJAY KUMAR

Laureate Institute of Pharmacy, Kathog, Himachal Pradesh, India

*Corresponding author

ABSTRACT

The present era is in demand for the design and development of nanocarriers with advanced properties, targeting and treatment of numerous diseases or disorders. As compared to conventional drug delivery systems, nanocarriers exhibit better efficiency, less toxicity, and better stability characteristics. The reason might be the nano size range and spatial targeting and drug delivery using the nanocarriers. Several types of nanocarriers, such as liposomes, dendrimers, polymer-drug conjugates, nanoemulsions, nanocapsules, nanospheres, metallic nanoparticles, and carbon nanotubes, and so forth, have been synthesized for drug delivery. Integration of artificial intelligence (AI)/machine learning (ML) and nanotechnology has pronounced prospective in attaining the objective of precise medicine for the advancement of management options for various diseases or disorders such as cancer. The present chapter discusses the convergence of nanotechnology and AI/ML in the investigation and development of nanocarriers. The discussion also includes the advantages, limitations, and future prospects of AI/ML in the scale-up of nanocarriers.

Nanotechnology for Nucleic Acid Delivery: Pankaj Sharma, Saloni Jain, and Vinay Jain (Eds.)

DOI: 10.1201/9781998511853-7

7.1 INTRODUCTION

Pharmaceutical research is in the process of advancement in terms of improved drug bioavailability, stability, and targeting. The development of nanosized and versatile nanocarriers has played a significant role in this progression. These nanocarriers include polymeric nanoparticles, lipid-based nanoparticles such as solid lipid nanocarriers and liposomes, niosomes, inorganic nanocarriers, metallic nanoparticles, nanocomplexes, dendrimers, carbon nanotubes, quantum dots, and many others. These nanocarriers possess numerous advantages in comparison to conventional drug delivery systems owing to the ease in modifying their size, surface properties, and charge, and target directing agents to control uptake, delivery, and removal from the body. The drugs can be delivered by either dispersing into a matrix or encapsulating within layers of nanocarriers. The nanocarriers can be made target-specific by attachment of ligands on the nanocarrier's surface. The nanocarriers can be delivered inside the body via parenteral, topical, oral, and nasal routes [1]. In consideration of the above advantages, the nanocarriers have gained importance in the treatment of several diseases with a broad range of properties. To develop polydisperse nanocarriers with desired therapeutic efficacy and stability, optimization of various parameters of nanocarriers viz. polymer:drug, drug:lipid, temperature, pH, stirring speed, surfactants, size distribution, sterility, surface charge, drug loading, *in vivo* behavior, and the relationship between *in vitro* and *in vivo* results is a difficult task for the manufacturers. It is also a challenging job for the regulatory bodies to grant approval for the nanocarriers. Only 21 nanocarriers got approval from regulatory bodies in the last three decades. The approved nanocarriers are mostly liposomes with oral or intravenous routes of administration [2]. Scaling up nanocarriers from the lab scale to commercial scale is a challenging job due to the lack of standard and *in vivo* relevant guidelines; for example, there are no universally acceptable guidelines for the *in vitro* release study of nanocarriers [3].

In pharmaceutical manufacturing, time, cost, and productivity are important concerns, and it becomes more significant in the case of nano-carrier scale-up and production. Further, drug development and manufacturing are more focused on the trial-and-error approach with increased time, cost, and decreased productivity. The pharmaceutical industry has started to look forward to scientific and technological developments such as computational algorithms and *in silico* models in research and development. The industry and scientists are looking forward to the integration of AI in pharmaceutical manufacturing. Owing to the remarkable development in computer technology for data analysis speed over the past years, a novel field known as "computational pharmaceutics" has emerged into pharmaceutical research with considerable prospective in changing the overall approach of drug delivery development. Computational pharmaceutics is an approach of integrating large data, multi-scale modeling approach, and AI for drug development. In the present era, some focused researches have been carried out or are in process to apply AI strategies in predicting physicochemical properties, stability parameters, drug release, *in vivo* pharmacodynamics and pharmacokinetics characteristics, and *in vitro–in vivo* relationships.

7.2 ARTIFICIAL INTELLIGENCE (AI) AND NANOTECHNOLOGY

The development of an optimal nanocarrier drug delivery system is a challenging task. The integration of AI in the scale-up process has good potential for the development of a lab-scale nanocarrier to commercial scale with desired efficacy, stability, and market potential. The goal of combining AI and automation offers the potential to improve targeted therapeutic nanocarriers for particular patient populations and cell types. The computational algorithms, AI, and machine learning (ML) for the nanocarriers have mostly focused on the formulation of nanocarriers, evaluating their surface properties and interaction with different cells or receptors for drug delivery and therapeutic action [4]. Table 7.1 highlights the important advantages and applications of integrating AI and nanotechnology for the development of nanocarriers.

TABLE 7.1 Advantages and Applications of Artificial Intelligence (AI) in Development of Nanocarriers

Artificial Intelligence (AI) In Nanocarrier's Development
Precise prediction of input parameters to manufacture stable and efficacious nanocarriers
Precise prediction of percent drug loading and entrapment efficiency of nanocarriers
Precise control on particle size and surface charge of nanocarriers
Continuous production and control on nanocarrier's manufacturing process
Precise targeting of nanocarriers for drug delivery and therapeutic efficiency

TABLE 7.1 *(Continued)*

Artificial Intelligence (AI) In Nanocarrier's Development
Precise prediction of nanocarrier's movement in hard to reach cellular locations and targets
Precise prediction of nanocarrier's movement inside the cancerous cells
Precise prediction of nanocarrier's movement for brain drug delivery and targeting across blood brain barrier
Development of a 3D library of nanocarriers and molecular targets
Scale up from laboratory to commercial scale manufacturing
Faster regulatory approval process
Less time and cost for development of a commercial nanocarrier for biomedical application

7.2.1 ARTIFICIAL INTELLIGENCE (AI) AND FORMULATION OF NANOCARRIERS

The continuous and swift advancement of AI has shown newer inspirations in many areas of pharmaceutical research, and microfluidic technology for the development of nanocarriers is one of the beneficiaries. The performance of nanocarriers *in vivo* is directly influenced by their size and quality, which justifies the necessity for production techniques that can consistently produce high-quality nanocarriers that have specific biophysical features [5]. Further, the method of production must be suitable for scale-up from lab scale to pilot scale and to commercial scale. In addition, the variability in excipients (polymers, lipids, inorganic materials, and combinations, etc.) further challenges the commercial manufacturing of a stable and safe nanocarrier. Each requires different manufacturing conditions to achieve the desired quality. A method to formulate the nanocarriers might be showing good results on a lab scale, but the same method might show errors when scaled up for batch volumes for clinical investigations or commercial scale, owing to less precision on control and engineering needed for the set-up.

7.2.1.1 ARTIFICIAL INTELLIGENCE (AI)/MACHINE LEARNING (ML) BASED MICROFLUIDIC TECHNOLOGY

A microfluidic chip is a device for handling fluids that makes use of micron-scale channels. Its compact size allows it to handle fluids at the micron and nanoscale, which significantly lowers sample consumption, lowers bioassay costs, and speeds up reactions (Figure 7.1). Its excellent integration and simplicity of use are further benefits. It has a lot of potential for use in drug development, microbiological research, medical diagnostics, biochemical synthesis, and nanocarrier development. A microchannel reactor is another name for these microreactors. It is further sub-sectioned into microreactors, microexchangers, and micromixers. Precision machining techniques are employed in the manufacturing of these microreactors, which has sizes ranging from 10 to 300 microns. The word "micro" in the microreactor describes that the channels of the fluid in process are at the micron level, rather than referring to the tiny form factor of the microreactor or the less yield of nanocarriers. These reactors can blend components speedily and homogeneously, and they can speed up the reactions by designing hindrances within the channels or by applying an external energy field for efficient mixing of fluids. Due to their small size, microreactors have the benefit of rapid heat transfer, which enhances the heating and reaction rates in the procedures used to prepare nanoparticles requiring specific temperatures to occur [6].

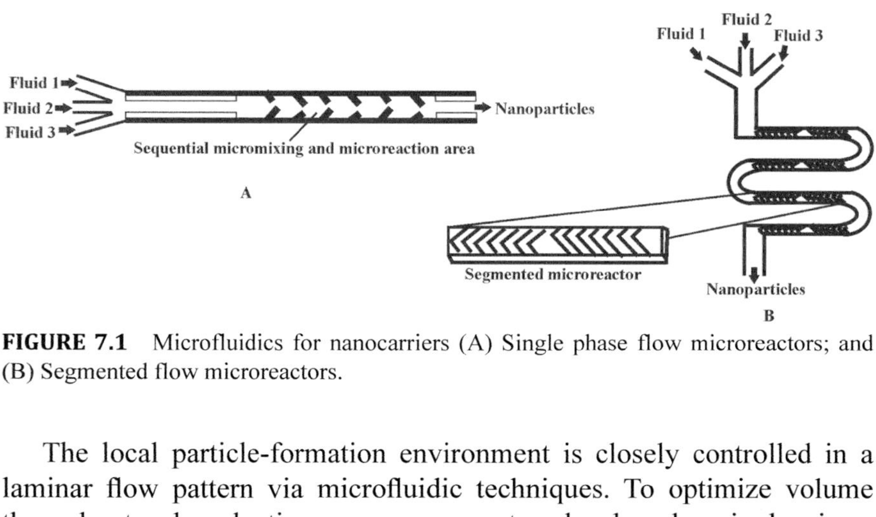

FIGURE 7.1 Microfluidics for nanocarriers (A) Single phase flow microreactors; and (B) Segmented flow microreactors.

The local particle-formation environment is closely controlled in a laminar flow pattern via microfluidic techniques. To optimize volume throughput and production, process parameters developed on single microfluidic mixer devices can be readily transferred to multi-mixer devices with identical channel geometry. Compared to batch-based manufacturing methods, which frequently need sophisticated and time-consuming adjustments in process as the batch size increases, the microfluidic technology offers the continuous manufacturing of nanocarriers with computational adjustments. Integration of AI/ML with microfluidics proposes a pathway for the production of quality nanocarriers, which can be effectively scaled up from the lab to commercial manufacturing.

AI and ML are ideas that are interchangeable, with ML frequently being seen as an application of AI. AI incorporates several computer-based tasks such as reasoning and problem-solving, planning, ML, vision, robotics, natural language processing, and knowledge representation. AI enables software to function like a human brain [7]. ML makes predictions or delivers answers to unknown data by utilizing a vast number of well-known datasets and inputs. The model is developed using a combination of highly advanced non-linear regression analysis and basic linear regressions, which finally enable the model to generate the best predictions [6]. ML uses techniques like decision trees, naïve Bayes, and Markov models to learn on their own. Integration of AI and ML is one of the main areas of future research for microfluidics-based nanocarriers development and evaluation. The data and outcomes of experiments can be utilized to create the predictive data models required for ML algorithms, which may ultimately direct the creation of more superior and efficient drug-loaded nanocarriers [7].

AI/ML integrated microfluidic technology has gained momentum for the development of lipid-based nanocarriers. Lipid-based nanocarriers delivery systems can be classified as liposomes, solid lipid nanoparticles (SLNs), and oligonucleotide-containing lipid nanoparticles (LNPs), based on their morphology [5]. On the other hand, liposomes feature a large aqueous core enveloped by one or more lipid bilayers. Hydrophobic therapeutic agents can be trapped within the phospholipid bilayer of liposomes, whereas hydrophilic therapeutic agents are often encapsulated into the core of liposomes. SLNs often contain hydrophobic molecules within a solid triglyceride core. LNPs consist of numerous nanosize hydrophilic pockets within which nucleotide moieties are entrapped and can be identified by their electron-dense core under electron microscopy. They are used mainly for the delivery of genetic material within cells [8]. Figure 7.2 and Table 7.2 summarize the different nanocarriers such as vesicular nanocarriers, solid lipid nanoparticles, polymeric nanocarriers, inorganic nanocarriers, and metallic nanocarriers investigated using AI/ML integrated technologies for the prediction of different outputs and standardization of different input parameters.

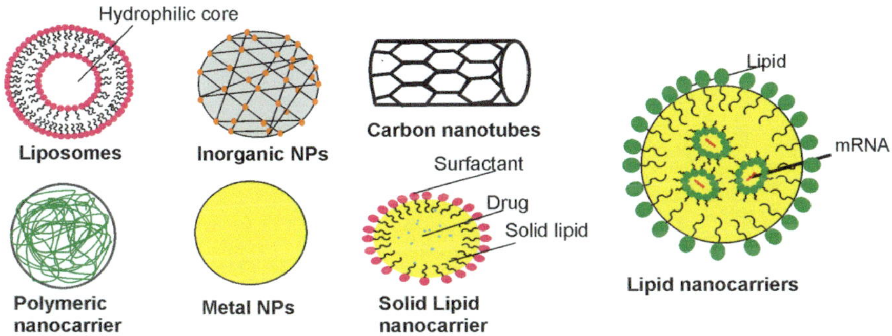

FIGURE 7.2 Important nanocarriers investigated for prediction and optimization using artificial intelligence (AI)/machine learning (ML).

7.2.1.2 ARTIFICIAL INTELLIGENCE (AI)/MACHINE LEARNING (ML), MICROFLUIDICS AND VESICULAR NANOCARRIERS

Liposomes of uniform size distribution were traditionally created using complex methods. However, creating liposomes with microfluidics does not require a complex process [9–13]. Three different proteins—insulin, bovine serum albumin, and ovalbumin—were successfully encapsulated in liposomes using a microfluidics-driven process for encapsulation, purification, evaluation, and control [10]. Another study used a tumor xenograft model to determine the tumor penetration capabilities of nanosized doxorubicin-loaded liposomes manufactured employing microfluidics technology [9]. Similarly, microfluidics technology was used for manufacturing curcumin-loaded liposomes, and anticancer efficacy was established [11]. The microfluidic-based PEGylated DSPC liposomal nanocarrier encapsulating doxorubicin and umbelliprenin was effective against human breast cancer cells [12]. Francesco et al. formulated more than 200 combinations of liposomes by systematically regulating lipid amounts, flow rates, and organic:water mixing volume ratios. On the basis of data collected, feed-forward artificial neural network (ANN) and support-vector machine models were developed to predict the liposome size and PDI [14].

Rebollo et al. formulated liposomal nanocarriers of dioleyl phosphatidylcholine, cholesterol, and 1,2 distearoyl-sn-glycero-3-phosphatidylethanolamine (DSPE)-Polyethylene glycol (PEG) 2000 with various concentrations by application of a microfluidic scheme. An ANN model was developed using the data in order to foresee the particle dimension

TABLE 7.2 Artificial intelligence (AI)/Machine Learning (ML) Technology Investigated for the Development of Nanocarriers

Nanocarrier	AI/ML Technology Investigated	Input Parameters	Output Parameters	Inference
Liposomes of doxorubicin [9]	Microfluidics	Lipid composition	Biodistribution and localization in cancerous cells	• Biodistribution was similar with different sized liposomes (50 nm and 75 nm); Tissue localization and penetration was higher with small size liposomes.
Liposomes of insulin, bovine serum albumin and Ovalbumin [10]	AI integrated microfluidics	Flow rate ratio and total flow rate	Encapsulation efficiency, purification and manufacturing control	• High loading of proteins independent of lipid selection and concentration. • Homogeneous sized liposomes
Liposomes of curcumin [11]	Automated microfluidics	Flow rate ratio and total flow rate	Drug loading, Polydispersibility index (PDI)	• High drug loading compared to conventional methods. • PDI < 0.2 • Synergistic anticancer effect with cisplatin
Liposomes of curcumin [14]	Feed Forward artificial neural network (ANN) integrated microfluidics	Flow rates, lipid concentrations, organic: water mixing volume ratio,	Drug loading, PDI	• PDI<0.2 • High drug loading
Liposomes [15]	ANN integrated microfluidics	Lipid ratio, flow rate and flow rate ratio	PDI	• PDI<0.2
Nanoliposomes of Pilocarpine [16]	ANN	Manufacturing parameters of liposomes	PDI, Entrapment efficiency (EE)	• Homogenous size distribution
Liposomes [17]	Multiple input single output (MISO) and Multiple input multiple output (MIMO)	Hydrocarbon tail length, cholesterol (%), buffer type, solvent temperature and flow rate	Particle size and PDI	• PDI<0.2 • MISO accuracy was more than MIMO

TABLE 7.2 *(Continued)*

Nanocarrier	AI/ML Technology Investigated	Input Parameters	Output Parameters	Inference
Liposomes of curcumin [19]	LSBoost Algorithm	polymer molar ratios, particle size, sonication time and pH	EE (%)	• Accurate prediction of EE (%)
Niosomes [21]	Deep Neural Network (DNN)	Non-ionic surfactant properties and cholesterol concentration	EE (%)	• Hydophilic-lipophilic balance of non-ionic surfactant was most critical parameter for improving EE (%).
Liposomes of insulin [23]	Convolutional neural network algorithm	Therapeutic effect on keratosis	Drug loading, cell activity and anti-inflammatory action on cornea	• Establishment of successful SD rat model for corneal inflammation model.
Liposomes [24]	ML based on differential equations	Liposome size, interstitial fluid pressure (IFP) within tumor cells	Accumulation of liposomes in tumor cells	• Accurately predict the liposome accumulation and IFP in tumor cells.
Solid lipid nanoparticles (SLN) [27]	Gaussian process supervised ML algorithm	Binding energy of drug	Drug loading	• Less percentages bias between the actual and predicted response for binding energies by docking.
SLN [28]	Decision rule and function fitting ML methods	Homogenization time and speed; and concentration of ingredients	Particle size	• Correct prediction of particle size.
SLN of rifabutin [29]	FormRules® and INForm® AI	Lipid components: drug; surfactants, and stirring speed	Surface charge, particle size distribution, and EE (%)	• Accurate predictions of the outcomes variables
Lipid nanoparticles (LNP) for mRNA vaccine [30]	ML technique light GBM	N/P ratio of lipid	Substructures of ionizable lipids	• Significant prediction of N/P ratio and substructures of ionizable lipids.

TABLE 7.2 *(Continued)*

Nanocarrier	AI/ML Technology Investigated	Input Parameters	Output Parameters	Inference
LNP for mRNA vaccine [31]	XGBoost, Bootstrap forest, support vector machines, ANN, k-nearest neighbors, LASSO, ANN-Design of experiment model	Ionizable lipid, an ionizable lipid: cholesterol, total flow rate and flow rate ratio.	Particle size, PDI and EE (%)	• ANN-Design of experiment model outperformed other ML models in prediction.
Chitosan nanoparticles	12 different ML supervised multi-inlet vortex mixer	Flow rate in flash nanoprecipitation technique	Size and PDI	• Random Forest, Decision Tree, Extra Tree, and Bagging algorithm showed better prediction (90%) of outcomes.
Hyaluronic acid and chitosan based polymeric nanoparticles [43]	ANN model of Hydrodenticity	Flow rates and polymer concentrations	Size of nanoparticles for magnetic resonance imaging	• Better prediction of biodistribuiton
Polycaprolactone nanoparticles [44]	Neurofuzzy logic	Mixing conditions, various solvents and stabilizers	Particle size and surface charge	• Most important factor for stable nanoparticles was found to be choice of stabilizers
Poly (lactic-co-glycolic acid)-based nanocarriers [45]	Least Absolute Shrinkage, Selection Operator, Vector regression, Random Forest ML algorithm	Polymer concentration	Particle size, encapsulation efficiency, and drug loading	• Vector regression for particle size and encapsulation efficiency prediction • Random forest for drug loading prediction
Silica nanoparticles [48]	DNN, kernel, and tree based predictive algorithm	Concentration of nanoparticle in cells, serum, cell size, time, surface, and cytotoxic assay type	Cytotoxic and non-cytotoxic silica nanoparticles	• Significant prediction of the outcomes factors for generation of cytotoxic nanoparticles

TABLE 7.2 *(Continued)*

Nanocarrier	AI/ML Technology Investigated	Input Parameters	Output Parameters	Inference
Carbon nanotubes [50]	High speed Raman imaging and Deep learning	-	Identification of carbon nanotubes	• 98% identification accuracy.
Multi-walled carbon nanotubes [51]	Recursive Feature Elimination (RFE) approach	Purity, length, and average zeta potential	Genetoxicity efficiency on exposure	• 80% accuracy in prediction
Metal nanocarriers [52]	Information fusion, perturbation-theory machine learning	Size, shape, and composition vs. biological tests, assay organisms	Antibacterial efficiency	• Accurate prediction of anti-bacterial efficiency
Silver nanoparticles [53]	ML based Decision Tree and Random Forest models	Reducing agent, cell line types, exposure duration, cell viability, particle size, zeta potential, hydrodynamic diameter, concentration, and wavelength.	Cellular toxicity	• Decision tree algorithm showed accurate prediction

and polydispersity index (PDI). Lipid's ratio and process-related parameters viz. flow rate ratio and total flow rate were important variables for the materialization of vesicular nanocarriers with the desired PDI (<0.2) and size (100 nm). The AI, experiment design, and microfluidic method were used to create optimized liposomes manufacturing with good reproducibility [15]. Zhao et al. combined the concept of ANN with response surface methodology to formulate novel ophthalmic flexible nanoliposomes [16].

Sansare et al. investigated an ANN to develop a computational model for the optimization of a continuous liposomes manufacturing process. The input parameters of the ANN were important excipients-related factors such as buffer type, cholesterol percent, and hydrocarbon chain length and important process factors such as flow rate and solvent temperature. Outputs forecasted by ANN included PDI and average particle size of liposomes. Two popular ANN models, multiple-input-multiple-output (MIMO) and multiple-input-single-output (MISO) models, were examined, where MISO showed more accuracy than MIMO. Critical material parameters, process factors, and the ANN model all worked together to significantly reduce the mean relative error during training and testing. Furthermore, an efficient graphic user interface was created so that users could do interactive simulated risk analysis and see model forecasts [17].

The percent entrapment efficiency of drugs within nanocarriers has been predicted and optimized using the ML algorithms [18]. Hoseini et al. investigated the impact of variables—polymer concentration, pH, sonication time, particle size, and PDI—on the percent drug entrapment of nanoliposomes of curcumin by applying the Least-squares boosting (LSBoost) ensemble learning algorithm. The model performance was evaluated using the mean absolute error as the cost function. The results of investigations concluded high capability of the LSBoost algorithm in exactly forecasting and optimizing the entrapment efficiency of the liposomal nanocarriers of curcumin [19]. Mens hawe and colleagues have used feed-forward ANN to develop a terbutaline sulfate-loaded bilosomes for management of asthma by transdermal route [20]. In an investigation for the development of niosomes, ML was used to predict and improve the percent entrapment efficiency. Niosomes are vesicular nanocarriers formed by non-ionic surfactants and cholesterol. To find the most important parameters and its optimal value, data was collected from previous decade articles on niosomes to train a four cost function polynomial regression model, linear regression model, and deep neural network (DNN) model. After that, the sensitivity experiment was used to identify the parameter that had the greatest impact on entrapment efficiency. Ultimately, by holding the other parameters constant and adjusting the most relevant parameter, the most influential parameter's optimal point was found. The best model was found to be DNN, and hydrophilic-lipophilic balance (HLB) was identified as the most influential parameter [21]. A computational algorithm based on the finite element method was developed and investigated for drug concentration and temperature at targeted tumor cells by an intravenously administered doxorubicin-loaded temperature-sensitive liposomes during magnetic hyperthermia. The results of simulation using computational models showed that the killing efficiency was 15% with magnetic hyperthermia, which increased to 50% with combination therapy—magnetic hyperthermia and temperature-sensitive liposomes [22]. A convolutional neural network algorithm-based investigation of insulin-loaded liposomes was performed to optimize drug entrapment, cellular activity, and pharmacodynamics efficiency on corneal inflammation. Convolutional neural network was explored as an AI algorithm to develop a SD rat corneal inflammation model, and the results of investigations concluded the successful establishment of an animal model [23].

Enhanced permeability and retention effect of liposomes-based anticancer agents has inspired the clinical use of nanocarriers in the treatment of tumors. High interstitial fluid pressure (IFP) in tumor cells limits the effect of drug delivery by nanocarriers in the central region. Furthermore, for certain solid tumors, elevated IFP functions as an independent predictive biomarker for the effectiveness of chemotherapy and radiation therapy. Thus, for the best possible treatment planning, precise measurement of the spatial concentration of liposomes and the distribution of IFP within a solid tumor is essential. Investigators developed an ML and partial differential equations-based computation platform to predict accumulation of liposomes within the tumor cells and IFP by pre- and post-administration imaging. The methodology precisely forecasts the accumulation of liposomes at target cells and IFP for a single cancer cell while depending on minimum pre-information [24]. The above-discussed research evidences highlight the potential future of AI/ML in the development of vesicular nanocarriers with optimized particle size and percent drug loading.

7.2.1.3 ARTIFICIAL INTELLIGENCE (AI)/MACHINE LEARNING (ML) AND SOLID LIPID NANOPARTICLES

The evolvement of microfluidics techniques and the integration of AI/ML with microfluidics has changed the paradigm of formulation and optimization of SLNs. SLNs are triglyceride-based solid matrix nanocarriers for hydrophobic drug moieties. The AI/ML integrated microfluidics technology has been investigated for the development of SLNs with homogeneous and stable particle size distribution, and improved entrapment efficiency [5, 25, 26]. Hathout and colleagues optimized a Gaussian process supervised ML-based modeling technique for drug loading of several drugs in SLNs. The results of the investigation concluded that the use of Gaussian Processes showed a lesser amount of bias (%) among the predicted and actual values of binding energies by docking compared to previously adopted ANN approaches. In addition, better mathematical modeling of drug entrapment in relation to binding energy was attained when Molecular Operating Environment® software incorporated with the MMFF94x software suite was investigated [27]. In an investigation, ML-based algorithms were examined for the effect of homogenization time and ingredients on the particle size of SLNs. The results of ML algorithms showed that particle size can be estimated by both decision rule-based ML methods and function fitting ML methods and can be useful for future research [28]. Rauco et al. employed a novel approach to obtain the most optimal, consistent, and stable lipid nanocarrier through a two-step experimental design and the effective modeling of databases through AI approaches. The first approach, which involved a wide choice of numerical levels for the factors, was followed by a second sequence of tests using factor levels within a narrower range. By using hot homogenization, rifabutin-loaded nanoparticles were created, and their surface charge, entrapment efficiency, and particle size distribution were assessed. The use of AI tools has explained the important variables that control the properties of formulations. When the stirring speed and ratio of lipid components:drug:surfactants were altered by INForm® and FormRules®, stable nanocarriers with nano sizes and polydispersions, negative zeta potentials, and good drug loadings were produced [29]. The above discussion highlights the considerable potential for AI application tools on SLN formulation and optimization.

7.2.1.4 ARTIFICIAL INTELLIGENCE (AI)/MACHINE LEARNING (ML) AND LIPID NANOPARTICLES (LNPS)

LNPs are generally used for the transfer of genetic materials inside the cell. LNPs hold their nucleotide cargo within numerous small hydrophilic spaces and can be identified by their electron dense core under electron microscopy [5]. Currently, LNP optimization principally depends on the selection of ionizable lipids by customary experiments, which consume extensive time and cost. Integration of *in silico* models can fast-track the fabrication of mRNA-loaded LNPs. Wang et al. researched a computational technique to speed up the development of LNPs for mRNA vaccines. Initially, data samples from 325 different LNP formulations for the mRNA vaccine with an IgG titer were gathered. A forecast model with respectable reliability and reproducibility (R2 > 0.87) was created using the ML technique lightGBM. Most notably, the system correctly identified the key molecular arrangements of ionizable lipids in LNPs, agreeing closely with previous studies. As predicted by the model, the *in vivo* experiment results demonstrated that LNPs with DLin-MC3-DMA (MC3) as the ionizable lipid with an N/P ratio of 6:1 showed greater efficacy in mice than LNPs with other lipids. The molecular mechanism of the LNPs employed in the experiment was further explored by molecular dynamic modeling. The outcome demonstrated that mRNA molecules twined around the lipid molecules, which assemble together to create LNPs [30]. Maharjan and Colleagues developed a Combinatorial-ANN-Design of experiment model by investigating the effect of ionizable lipid, ionizable lipid:cholesterol, total flow rate, and flow rate ratio on the prediction of outcome parameters for mRNA lipid nanoparticle vaccine. The effect on outcome responses were evaluated using a definitive screening design (DSD) and ML algorithms [31]. ML-based approaches have been investigated to understand the intracellular biology and targeting of mRNA-loaded LNPs. Hunter and Colleagues investigated small molecule profiling and siRNA targeting using cutting-edge imaging techniques and ML. Biological insights were predicted for the mechanism of mRNA delivery using LNPs (MC3-LNP). Advanced Cellular and Endocytic Profiling for Intracellular Delivery (ACE-ID) was the process name for this workflow. To determine comparable impacts on functional mRNA delivery, 178 targets pertinent to trafficking within cells were altered, and an imaging test based on cells was employed. Targets with improved delivery were examined by employing sophisticated image analysis methods to obtain data-rich phenotypic fingerprints from photos. Using ML, important characteristics associated with improved delivery were found, and fluid-phase endocytosis was found to be a successful cellular access pathway. With this new understanding, MC3-LNP was redesigned to specifically target macropinocytosis, leading to a considerable improvement in both *in vivo* and *in vitro* mRNA delivery. The ACE-ID method has the prospective to expedite the establishment of nanocarrier systems for RNA-based treatments and can be widely applied to optimize intracellular delivery systems based on nanomedicine [32].

7.2.1.5 ARTIFICIAL INTELLIGENCE (AI)/MACHINE LEARNING (ML) AND POLYMERIC NANOPARTICLES

Polymeric nanoparticles, fabricated from either natural or synthetic polymers, have been researched extensively and are already in use for clinical purposes. The polymeric nanoparticle's surface can be modified for drug targeting in specific therapeutic treatments. These nanoparticles offer numerous advantages, such as stable particle size and size distribution. Microfluidics technology helps in the development of stable polymeric nanoparticles for various therapeutic purposes, such as PLGA-curcumin nanocarriers for anti-inflammatory action [33, 34], PLGA-paclitaxel nanocarriers for anticancer [35], PLGA-ribavirin nanocarriers for antiviral [36], and PLGA-cyclosporine nanocarriers for mucolytic activity [37]. The ANN is integrated with the development of polymeric nanoparticles. Naggar and Colleagues employed an ANN for the biosynthesis of chitosan nanoparticles using *Olea europaea* leaf extract and *Streptomyces microflavus* [38, 39]. Integration of AI and a quality by design approach was explored for the development of silymarin-loaded lecithin/chitosan nanoparticles [40] and diclofenac sodium-loaded gelatin nanoparticles [41]. ANN integration showed significantly improved prediction ability of critical parameters of developed nanoparticles.

Wu and Colleagues developed and analyzed an ML-directed flash nanoprecipitation technology for unceasing development of chitosan nanocarriers. ML-supervised multi-inlet vortex mixer (MIVM) produced chitosan nanocarriers in a controlled fashion at higher output and having good potential for upscale application. The possible association between the hydrodynamic characteristics of nanoparticles and the independent variables was examined using 12 different ML algorithms. The algorithms identified as Decision Tree, Extra Tree, Random Forest, and Bagging outperformed the others, with an average prediction accuracy of approximately 90% [42]. In pioneered research, Smeraldo and Colleagues studied an ANN model of Hydrodenticity (altering of relaxometric properties of biopolymer matrices) integrated microfluidic technology for the influence of parameters such as polymer concentrations and flow rates on the size of the Gadolinium-DTPA-loaded hyaluronic acid and chitosan-based polymeric nanoparticles for magnetic resonance imaging [43]. Neurofuzzy logic, an AI tool, was investigated by Jara and Colleagues to fabricate uniform-sized polycaprolactone nanoparticles by nanoprecipitation method, having focus on the selection of stabilizers. Relationships between mixing conditions, various solvents and stabilizers, and other factors were determined via the neurofuzzy logic model. Using an AI tool, seven parameters as a function of raw materials and operating conditions were modeled with high prediction. These parameters were tested using dynamic light scattering and laser doppler electrophoresis. The analysis of main component was made possible by the model, which demonstrated that the most important factor in preventing nanoparticle aggregation was the choice of stabilizer [44]. Rezvantalab and Colleagues applied four distinct ML algorithms to develop predictive models based on effective characteristics pertaining to the size, efficiency of encapsulation, and loading of drug in poly (lactic-co-glycolic acid)-based nanocarriers. The most significant features were identified by examining the input parameters using the Least Absolute Shrinkage and Selection Operator. First, tenfold validation techniques were used to train and validate the ML models. Afterward, their reliability and reproducibility were assessed and contrasted in relations of mean absolute error, absolute error, and R2. The comparison end result concluded the suitability of vector regression for the prediction of the size and encapsulation efficiency (%) and random forest for prediction of the percent drug loading of Poly (lactic-co-glycolic acid)-based nanoparticles [45]. The above discussion concludes the future and rising potential of AI/ML-based development of stable polymeric nanoparticles.

7.2.1.6 ARTIFICIAL INTELLIGENCE (AI)/MACHINE LEARNING (ML) AND INORGANIC NANOPARTICLES

Inorganic nanoparticles including silica, carbon nanotubes, quantum dots and graphene have been utilized as efficient drug delivery nanocarriers owing to their remarkable physicochemical characteristics. These nanocarriers have two essential characteristics: surface engineering and controlled synthesis, which provides good flexibility for functional designs and therapeutic targeting [46]. The application of AI/ML in inorganic nanoparticles is mainly researched for the cytotoxic effects for the treatment of diseases or disorders, synthesis of nanoparticles, and diagnosis of diseases.

An impedimetric millifluidic sensor with the ML data processing was investigated as a sensing platform to track the manufacturing of silica nanoparticles in real time. With a global average accuracy of 103.7 ± 1.9%, the ML size descriptor's adaptability was successfully tested on the data collected via independent synthesis using different methods. It is anticipated that the technique will make it possible to monitor more nanomaterials because the sensor offered a universal response concept. This could be beneficial for the advancement of sensor-based devices for commercial purposes and the scaling up of nanocarrier [47]. Martin et al. presented an evidence-based prediction approach using the ML and literature data search to differentiate between cytotoxic and non-cytotoxic silica nanoparticles under specific conditions. Using information from more than 100 publications, researchers created a DNN, tree, and kernel based predictive algorithm based on various aspects of silica nanoparticle's cellular toxicity to date. Internal (4124 samples) and external (905 samples) data sets were used to validate these models. Using the Shapley Additive exPlanation values in the CatBoost model, the model found 13 key features that can explain nanoparticles toxicity that is concentration, cell, serum, time, size, surface, and assay type. The study offers a framework for forecasting and elucidating the toxicity of other manufactured nanocarriers in practical applications [48].

In order to find specifically lethal inorganic nanoparticles, Jyakhwo and Colleagues investigated an *in silico* screening method for large scale targeted discovery. A gradient boosting regression model was created by the researchers to forecast the viability of cell lines targeted with nanoparticles. Additionally, a genetic algorithm based on ML and capable of screening over 14900 candidates per minute was used to choose the most effective selectively cytotoxic nanoparticles. To authenticate the effectiveness of the algorithm, silver nanoparticles with a selective toxicity score of 42% were evaluated on HepG2 cell lines in order to evaluate their suitability for treating liver cancer [49].

7.2.1.7 ARTIFICIAL INTELLIGENCE (AI)/MACHINE LEARNING (ML) AND CARBON NANOTUBES

Carbon nanotubes are cylindrical-shaped carbon structures consisting of benzene rings and have been researched for the delivery of micromolecules or macromolecules via the oral or parenteral route for the treatment of diseases or disorders. Zhang and colleagues proposed a high-throughput methodology to rapidly recognize suspended carbon nanotubes by employing deep learning analysis and high-speed Raman imaging. The developed algorithm achieved 98% identification accuracy for the carbon nanotubes [50]. Many single-walled carbon nanotubes are nested inside one another to generate multi-walled, concentric-cylinder-type carbon nanotubes, which are commonly used in healthcare and industrial applications. However, investigations have shown that exposure to multi-walled carbon nanotubes leads to toxicity due to their physicochemical properties. A validated predictive nanoinformatics model based on machine learning (ML) and statistics was developed for the genotoxicity prediction of different multi-walled carbon nanotubes. Using the recursive feature elimination (RFE) approach, the most important factors were determined. The most effective random forest (RF) model for predicting the genotoxicity of multi-walled carbon nanotubes was found to use just three features, exhibiting high classification probabilities and 80% accuracy on external validation. The model determined that purity, length, and average zeta potential were the most informative features [51].

7.2.1.8 ARTIFICIAL INTELLIGENCE (AI)/MACHINE LEARNING (ML) AND METAL NANOCARRIERS

Metallic nanocarriers have gained interest for the cure and management of diseases such as cancer, diabetes, and skin infections. Metal nanoparticles themselves have shown therapeutic effects through specific cell targeting or by being surface-linked with drugs for selective targeting. Several metal or metal oxide nanocarriers—such as gold, copper, silver, silicon dioxide, zinc oxide, and so forth—have demonstrated antibacterial activity. Due to the various combinations of nanoparticle size, composition, and shape versus assay organisms, biological tests, and several activity variables to be assessed, the examination of antibacterial activity is a challenging and time-consuming process. Tenazaca and Diaz studied the ML based information fusion, perturbation-theory machine learning (IFPTML) approach, fitting it into self-developed SOFT.PTML software for the investigation of antibacterial nanocarriers. The investigated dataset included 15 types of nanocarriers (1–100 nm), with most cases in the size range of 1–50 nm, tested against more than 20 pathogenic bacterial species with different metabolic networks [52]. Desai and colleagues investigated the correlation between the physical characteristics of silver nanoparticles and their cytotoxicity using ML-based Decision Tree (DT) and Random Forest (RF) models. Reducing agent, cell line types, exposure duration, particle size, zeta potential, hydrodynamic diameter, concentration, wavelength, and cell viability were the input variables used for the ML model. These characteristics were taken from the literature, scrutinized, and compiled into a dataset that included information on nanoparticle concentration and cell viability. In predicting toxicity parameters, the DT model outperformed the RF model. Drug delivery and cancer treatments are two potential applications for using algorithms in the design and optimization of silver nanoparticle synthesis [53].

The concept of AI/ML has also been employed for the optimization and scale-up of the synthesis of metallic nanoparticles such as gold nanoparticles. A computational model—central composite design—was compared with ANN modeling for prediction accuracy and fitness to experimental results. Gold nanoparticle biosynthesis values predicted by ANN revealed a more rational relationship with the experimental results compared to the central composite design [54]. In a similar study, response surface methodology and ANN were compared for the optimization of process parameters for the biosynthesis of gold nanoparticles from a plant extract. The input parameters included plant extract volume, auric chloride concentration, reaction duration, pH, and temperature, while absorbance was the output process parameter. Several ANN algorithms were employed, including the Bayesian network, scaled conjugate gradient, and Levenberg–Marquardt algorithms. It was discovered that the Levenberg–Marquardt method provided the best fit results for prediction [55].

7.2.1.9 ARTIFICIAL INTELLIGENCE (AI) AND NANOROBOTS

In the recent past, researchers have focused on the potential of nanorobotics in medicine. For the first time, in 1959, Richard Feynman proposed the application of microrobots in medical science. At that point, the term "nanorobot" came into existence. When it comes to medication delivery, micro/nanorobots may achieve self-directed mobility, which enables the controlled delivery of nanocarriers to locations that are hard to reach. This contrasts with the traditional strategy, which depends on blood flow to reach the target [56]. Drug delivery vehicles should possess several unique features, including controlled navigation, pushing power, cargo transportation and release, as well as penetration within cells and tissues, in order to accurately deliver therapeutic payloads to sites of illness. Although current therapeutic delivery systems are unable to address these issues, nanorobots present a new and exciting class of drug carriers that can fulfill these desired properties. With the ability to move quickly and deliver therapeutic payloads to targeted locations, nanorobots have the potential to enhance treatment efficiency and reduce systemic adverse reactions associated with potentially harmful medications [57]. Although challenges such as design, production scale-up, and toxicity persist in the development of these nanorobots, they have still shown the potential to perform several tasks, such as drug delivery, cancer cell targeting, and microsurgeries (Figure 7.3A–7.3D) [58].

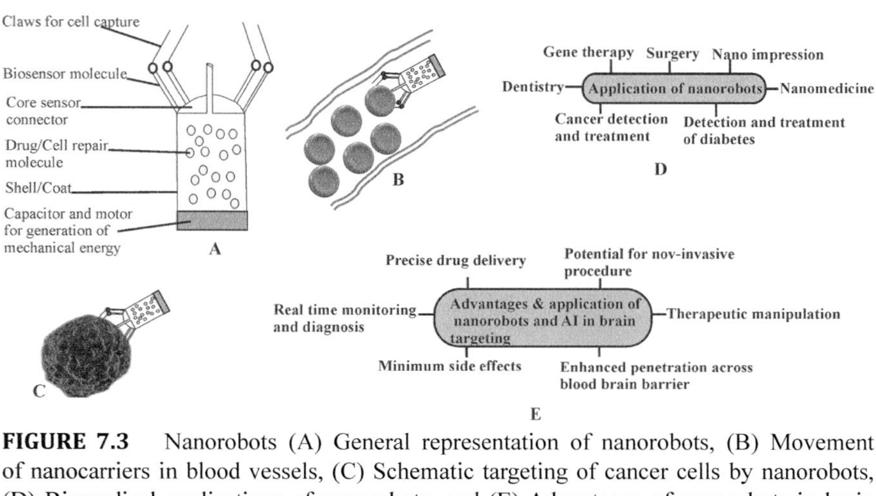

FIGURE 7.3 Nanorobots (A) General representation of nanorobots, (B) Movement of nanocarriers in blood vessels, (C) Schematic targeting of cancer cells by nanorobots, (D) Biomedical applications of nanorobots, and (E) Advantages of nanorobots in brain targeting.

In a study, the self-directed movement of urease-powered nanomotors and their tracking by positron emission tomography (PET), both *in vitro* and *in vivo*, was explored. Nanomotors composed of urease enzyme-containing silica nanoparticles and gold nanoparticles were investigated for radiolabeled *in vivo* imaging. The silica nanoparticles were labeled on urease with ^{18}F, and the gold nanoparticles with ^{125}I. Experiments conducted *in vitro* revealed improved fluid mixing and collective migration of nanomotors, indicating a greater ability to swim along complicated pathways within microfabricated phantoms when compared to static nanomotors. In addition, PET enhanced the tracking of movement behavior and real-time imaging, paving the way for theranostic applications in drug delivery [59]. With ongoing advancements in engineering and biotechnology, pharmaceutical researchers are focusing on the integration of smart sensors, power supplies, and AI in nanorobotics. Researchers are also focusing on AI-based nanorobots for improved drug delivery with effective nanocommunication [60]. ANNs based algorithms are considered to be important in the development of these nanorobots for malignant cell screening and drug delivery. Novel technologies such as DNA nanorobots have also been developed for drug delivery and biosensing [61].

Drug delivery to the brain in neurological disorders is a challenging task for researchers due to the difficulty of crossing the blood–brain barrier (BBB). Computationally powered artificial intelligence/machine learning (AI/ML) tools can be integrated with robotics to forecast and support the development of more advanced nanorobots for drug delivery across the BBB without causing damage, toxicity, or malfunctions (Figure 7.3E). Drug development can proceed more efficiently when research knowledge, BBB physiology, and permeability models are properly combined to generate precise predictions. In this context, computational AI may be classified as application-driven screening for neurodegenerative diseases such as Parkinson's disease, Alzheimer's disease, and multiple sclerosis, as well as CNS infections and neuro-oncology. AI computing may also indirectly support BBB-related neurotechnology by facilitating the design of engineered nanomaterials for BBB imaging and therapeutics, as well as for targeting and control maneuvers within the CNS [62].

7.3 LIMITATIONS/CHALLENGES OF ARTIFICIAL INTELLIGENCE (AI)/MACHINE LEARNING (ML) IN DEVELOPMENT OF NANOCARRIERS

Although the above discussion highlights the advantages of AI/ML in the scale-up and development of stable and efficacious nanocarriers, the integration of AI/ML in the development process has numerous limitations, and overcoming these limitations is a challenging task. The important limitations of AI/ML in the development of nanocarriers are as follows [1, 58, 63–66]:

7.3.1 LIMITATION WITH AVAILABILITY OF UNBIASED DATA

The development of an AI/ML interface depends primarily on the availability of a substantial dataset. One of the biggest challenges in pharmaceutical nanocarriers is the variation in their formulation and development, including differences in raw materials, processing techniques, and evaluation parameter determination. With so many variables and factors, designing AI/ML algorithms for each type of nanocarrier is a difficult task. Furthermore, the complexity and rarity of diseases, as well as population specificity, can result in biased predictions in the development of nanocarriers. The reliability and lack of bias in the available data must be carefully considered when developing AI/ML-based algorithms. Any bias or incompleteness in the data will skew the predictions.

7.3.2 INCAPABILITY TO ADD IN NEW DATA

One the AI model is trained on a data set, the incorporation of new data in the same model is difficult. It is even more difficult in the pharmaceutical nanocarriers in the terms of time-to-time variations and upgradation in raw materials, evaluation parameter and evolution of disease paradigm with availability of new data.

7.3.3 LIMITATION IN ADDRESSING VARIATION IN DRUG RESPONSE

The variation in pharmaceutical dosage forms is not only in terms of raw materials and processing techniques. Sometimes the variation is even present in drug response form patient to patient. One of the reasons for such variation may be the genetic makeup or trait of the patient. This is a challenging task to predict such type of variation by an AI/ML algorithm.

7.3.4 LIMITATION IN INTERPRETATION OF RESULTS

Complex nature of AI algorithms sometimes leads to the output which is difficult to interpret even for the experts. This deficiency of flawless clarifications for forecasts possesses a challenge for the investigators to understand and decoding the research into actionable sights. Better-quality in interpretation and explanation of predicted results fo AI models are essential for effective use.

7.3.5 CHALLENGES OF REGULATORY APPROVAL

AI models are made up of complex algorithms and lacks transparency to explain the predicted outcomes. Therefore, it is difficult to believe on reliability and predictions of AI models and also possess a challenge for the regulatory approval.

7.3.6 UNAVAILABILITY OF REGULATORY GUIDELINES

Due to the complexity of data sets, AI algorithms, unreliability of predictions and problems in updating new data sets, it is challenging to frame the regulatory benchmarks for approval process.

7.4 CONCLUSION AND FUTURE OF AI/ML IN DEVELOPMENT OF NANOCARRIERS

The integration of AI/ML possesses tremendous potential for the development of stable and efficacious nanocarriers. AI technology integration has the ability to significantly accelerate the creation of nanocarriers, enhance patient outcomes, and propel the pharmaceutical industry into the next phase of development. Cost-effective AI/ML-based, theoretically trained computational models will help avoid numerous experiments with various drug and polymer combinations during the development of a specific nanocarrier structure. To provide researchers with the ability to conjugate nanocarriers with different functional groups, it will be necessary in the future to establish a repository of nanocarriers in a three-dimensional (3D) framework. With the use of such a repository, scientists may easily determine which nanocarrier structure is best suited for molecular simulations. It is anticipated that real-time AI/ML monitoring and control capabilities will enhance the efficiency and uniformity of continuous production processes for nanocarriers. AI holds significant promise for regulatory decision-making because it can evaluate vast datasets to accelerate the approval process for medications and improve safety protocols. While AI and computational research will never fully replace laboratory testing, they are essential for expediting and improving target and drug discovery processes, as well as for advancing the development of new and efficient computational tools for nanocarrier simulation. Furthermore, there is a pressing need for more researchers with expertise in data handling and data analysis.

ACKNOWLEDGMENT

None

CONFLICT OF INTEREST

The authors declare no conflict of interest

FUNDING

None

KEYWORDS

- **artificial intelligence**
- **inorganic nanoparticles**
- **lipid nanoparticles**
- **liposomes**
- **machine learning**
- **nanocarriers**
- **nanocarriers**
- **nanorobots**
- **nanotubes**
- **polymeric nanoparticles**

REFERENCES

1. Alshawwa, S. Z., Kassem, A. A., Farid, R. M., Mostafa, S. K., & Labib, G. S. (2022). Nanocarrier drug delivery systems: Characterization, limitations, future perspectives and implementation of artificial intelligence. *Pharmaceutics, 14*(4), 883. https://doi.org/10.3390/pharmaceutics14040883 (accessed on 23rd June 2025).
2. Chariou, P. L., Ortega-Rivera, O. A., & Steinmetz, N. F. (2020). Nanocarriers for the delivery of medical, veterinary, and agricultural active ingredients. *ACS Nano, 14*(3), 2678–2701. https://doi.org/10.1021/acsnano.0c00173 (accessed on 23rd June 2025).
3. Shen, J., & Burgess, D. J. (2013). *In vitro* dissolution testing strategies for nanoparticulate drug delivery systems: Recent developments and challenges. *Drug Delivery and Translational Research, 3*(5), 409–415. https://doi.org/10.1007/s13346-013-0129-z (accessed on 23rd June 2025).
4. Duarte, Y., Márquez-Miranda, V., Miossec, M. J., & González-Nilo, F. (2019). Integration of target discovery, drug discovery and drug delivery: A review on computational strategies. *WIREs Nanomedicine and Nanobiotechnology, 11*(4). https://doi.org/10.1002/wnan.1554 (accessed on 23rd June 2025).
5. Garg, S., Heuck, G., Ip, S., & Ramsay, E. (2016). Microfluidics: A transformational tool for nanomedicine development and production. *Journal of Drug Targeting, 24*(9), 821–835. https://doi.org/10.1080/1061186x.2016.1198354 (accessed on 23rd June 2025).
6. Chen, X., & Lv, H. (2022). Intelligent control of nanoparticle synthesis on microfluidic chips with machine learning. *NPG Asia Materials, 14*(1). https://doi.org/10.1038/s41427-022-00416-1 (accessed on 23rd June 2025).
7. Bhattacharjee, G., Gohil, N., Shukla, M., Sharma, S., Mani, I., Pandya, A., Chu, D., Bui, N. L., Thi, Y. V. N., Khambhati, K., Maurya, R., Ramakrishna, S., & Singh, V. (2023). Exploring the potential of microfluidics for next-generation drug delivery systems. *OpenNano, 12*, 100150. https://doi.org/10.1016/j.onano.2023.100150 (accessed on 23rd June 2025).
8. Leung, A. K. K., Hafez, I., Baoukina, S., Belliveau, N. M., Zhigaltsev, I. V., Afshinmanesh, E., Tieleman, D. P., Hansen, C. L., Hope, M. J., & Cullis, P. R. (2012). Lipid nanoparticles containing siRNA synthesized by microfluidic mixing exhibit an electron-dense nanostructured core. *The Journal of Physical Chemistry C, 116*(34), 18440–18450. https://doi.org/10.1021/jp303267y (accessed on 23rd June 2025).
9. Dong, Y., Tchung, E., Nowell, C. J., Kağa, S., Leong, N., Mehta, D., Kaminskas, L. M., & Boyd, B. J. (2017). Microfluidic preparation of drug-loaded PEGylated liposomes, and the impact of liposome size on tumor retention and penetration. *Journal of Liposome Research, 29*(1), 1–9. https://doi.org/10.1080/08982104.2017.1391285 (accessed on 23rd June 2025).
10. Forbes, N. S., Hussain, M. T., Briuglia, M. L., Edwards, D., Ter Horst, J. H., Szita, N., & Perrie, Y. (2019). Rapid and scale-independent microfluidic manufacture of liposomes entrapping protein incorporating in-line purification and at-line size monitoring. *International Journal of Pharmaceutics, 556*, 68–81. https://doi.org/10.1016/j.ijpharm.2018.11.060 (accessed on 23rd June 2025).

11. Hamano, N., Böttger, R., Lee, S. E., Yang, Y., Kulkarni, J. A., Ip, S., Cullis, P. R., & Li, S. D. (2019). Robust microfluidic technology and new lipid composition for fabrication of curcumin-loaded liposomes: Effect on the anticancer activity and safety of cisplatin. *Molecular Pharmaceutics, 16*(9), 3957–3967. https://doi.org/10.1021/acs.molpharmaceut.9b00583 (accessed on 23rd June 2025).
12. Gkionis, L., Campbell, R. A., Aojula, H., Harris, L. K., & Tirella, A. (2020). Manufacturing drug co-loaded liposomal formulations targeting breast cancer: Influence of preparative method on liposomes characteristics and *in vitro* toxicity. *International Journal of Pharmaceutics, 590*, 119926. https://doi.org/10.1016/j.ijpharm.2020.119926 (accessed on 23rd June 2025).
13. Kastner, E., Kaur, R., Lowry, D., Moghaddam, B., Wilkinson, A., & Perrie, Y. (2014). High-throughput manufacturing of size-tuned liposomes by a new microfluidics method using enhanced statistical tools for characterization. *International Journal of Pharmaceutics, 477*(1, 2), 361–368. https://doi.org/10.1016/j.ijpharm.2014.10.030 (accessed on 23rd June 2025).
14. Di Francesco, V., Boso, D. P., Moore, T. L., Schrefler, B. A., & Decuzzi, P. (2023). Machine learning instructed microfluidic synthesis of curcumin-loaded liposomes. *Biomedical Microdevices, 25*(3). https://doi.org/10.1007/s10544-023-00671-1 (accessed on 23rd June 2025).
15. Rebollo, R., Oyoun, F., Corvis, Y., El-Hammadi, M. M., Saubaméa, B., Andrieux, K., Mignet, N., & Alhareth, K. (2022). Microfluidic manufacturing of liposomes: Development and optimization by design of experiment and machine learning. *ACS Applied Materials & Interfaces, 14*(35), 39736–39745. https://doi.org/10.1021/acsami.2c06627 (accessed on 23rd June 2025).
16. Zhao, F., Lu, J., Jin, X., Wang, Z., Sun, Y., Gao, D., Li, X., & Li, R. (2018). Comparison of response surface methodology and artificial neural network to optimize novel ophthalmic flexible nano-liposomes: Characterization, evaluation, *in vivo* pharmacokinetics and molecular dynamics simulation. *Colloids and Surfaces B: Bio Interfaces, 172*, 288–297. https://doi.org/10.1016/j.colsurfb.2018.08.046 (accessed on 23rd June 2025).
17. Sansare, S., Duran, T., Mohammadiarani, H., Goyal, M., Yenduri, G., Costa, A. P., Xu, X., O'Connor, T., Burgess, D. J., & Chaudhuri, B. (2021). Artificial neural networks in tandem with molecular descriptors as predictive tools for continuous liposome manufacturing. *International Journal of Pharmaceutics, 603*, 120713. https://doi.org/10.1016/j.ijpharm.2021.120713 (accessed on 23rd June 2025).
18. Fahmy, O. M., Eissa, R. A., Mohamed, H. H., Eissa, N. G., & Elsabahy, M. (2023). Machine learning algorithms for prediction of entrapment efficiency in nanomaterials. *Methods, 218*, 133–140. https://doi.org/10.1016/j.ymeth.2023.08.008 (accessed on 23rd June 2025).
19. Hoseini, B., Jaafari, M. R., Golabpour, A., Momtazi-Borojeni, A. A., & Eslami, S. (2023). Optimizing nano liposomal formulations: Assessing factors affecting entrapment efficiency of curcumin-loaded liposomes using machine learning. *International Journal of Pharmaceutics, 646*, 123414. https://doi.org/10.1016/j.ijpharm.2023.123414 (accessed on 23rd June 2025).
20. Menshawe, S. F. E., Aboud, H. M., Elkomy, M. H., Kharshoum, R. M., & Abdeltwab, A. M. (2019). A novel nanogel loaded with chitosan decorated biosomes for

transdermal delivery of terbutaline sulfate: Artificial neural network optimization, *in vitro* characterization and *in vivo* evaluation. *Drug Delivery and Translational Research, 10*(2), 471–485. https://doi.org/10.1007/s13346-019-00688-1 (accessed on 23rd June 2025).
21. Kashani-Asadi-Jafari, F., Aftab, A., & Ghaemmaghami, S. (2022). A machine learning framework for predicting entrapment efficiency in niosomal particles. *International Journal of Pharmaceutics, 627*, 122203. https://doi.org/10.1016/j.ijpharm.2022.122203 (accessed on 23rd June 2025).
22. Tehrani, M. H. H., Soltani, M., Kashkooli, F. M., Mahmoudi, M., & Raahemifar, K. (2021). Computational modeling of combination of magnetic hyperthermia and temperature-sensitive liposome for controlled drug release in solid tumor. *Pharmaceutics, 14*(1), 35. https://doi.org/10.3390/pharmaceutics14010035 (accessed on 23rd June 2025).
23. Liao, Y., Jiang, H., Du, Y., Xiong, X., Zhang, Y., & Du, Z. (2022). Using convolutional neural network as a statistical algorithm to explore the therapeutic effect of insulin liposomes on corneal inflammation. *Computational Intelligence and Neuroscience, 2022*, 1–9. https://doi.org/10.1155/2022/1169438 (accessed on 23rd June 2025).
24. Meaney, C., Stapleton, S., & Kohandel, M. (2023). Predicting intertumoral fluid pressure and liposome accumulation using physics informed deep learning. *Scientific Reports, 13*(1). https://doi.org/10.1038/s41598-023-47988-8 (accessed on 23rd June 2025).
25. Maeki, M., Kimura, N., Sato, Y., Harashima, H., & Tokeshi, M. (2018). Advances in microfluidics for lipid nanoparticles and extracellular vesicles and applications in drug delivery systems. *Advanced Drug Delivery Reviews, 128*, 84–100. https://doi.org/10.1016/j.addr.2018.03.008 (accessed on 23rd June 2025).
26. Capretto, L., Carugo, D., Mazzitelli, S., Nastruzzi, C., & Zhang, X. (2013). Microfluidic and lab-on-a-chip preparation routes for organic nanoparticles and vesicular systems for nanomedicine applications. *Advanced Drug Delivery Reviews, 65*(11, 12), 1496–1532. https://doi.org/10.1016/j.addr.2013.08.002 (accessed on 23rd June 2025).
27. Hathout, R. M., & Metwally, A. A. (2016). Towards better modelling of drug-loading in solid lipid nanoparticles: Molecular dynamics, docking experiments and Gaussian processes machine learning. *European Journal of Pharmaceutics and Biopharmaceutics, 108*, 262–268. https://doi.org/10.1016/j.ejpb.2016.07.019 (accessed on 23rd June 2025).
28. Öztürk, A. A., Gunduz, A. B., & Özışık, O. (2019). Supervised machine learning algorithms for evaluation of solid lipid nanoparticles and particle size. *Combinatorial Chemistry & High Throughput Screening, 21*(9), 693–699. https://doi.org/10.2174/1386207322666181218160704 (accessed on 23rd June 2025).
29. Rouco, H., Díaz-Rodríguez, P., Rama-Molinos, S., & Remuñán-López, C. (2018). Delimiting the knowledge space and the design space of nanostructured lipid carriers through artificial intelligence tools. *International Journal of Pharmaceutics, 553*(1, 2), 522–530. https://doi.org/10.1016/j.ijpharm.2018.10.058 (accessed on 23rd June 2025).
30. Wang, W., Feng, S., Ye, Z., Gao, H., Lin, J., & Ouyang, D. (2022). Prediction of lipid nanoparticles for mRNA vaccines by the machine learning algorithm.

Acta Pharmaceutica Sinica B, 12(6), 2950–2962. https://doi.org/10.1016/j.apsb.2021.11.021 (accessed on 23rd June 2025).

31. Maharjan, R., Hada, S., Lee, J. E., Han, D., Kim, K., Seo, H. J., Foged, C., & Jeong, S. H. (2023). Comparative study of lipid nanoparticle-based mRNA vaccine bioprocess with machine learning and combinatorial artificial neural network-design of experiment approach. *International Journal of Pharmaceutics, 640*, 123012. https://doi.org/10.1016/j.ijpharm.2023.123012 (accessed on 23rd June 2025).
32. Hunter, M. R., Cui, L., Porebski, B. T., Pereira, S., Sonzini, S., Odunze, U., Iyer, P., Engkvist, O., Lloyd, R. L., Peel, S., Sabirsh, A., Ross-Thriepland, D., Jones, A. T., & Desai, A. (2023). Understanding intracellular biology to improve mRNA delivery by lipid nanoparticles. *Small Methods, 7*(9). https://doi.org/10.1002/smtd.202201695 (accessed on 23rd June 2025).
33. Morikawa, Y., Tagami, T., Hoshikawa, A., & Ozeki, T. (2018). The use of an efficient microfluidic mixing system for generating stabilized polymeric nanoparticles for controlled drug release. *Biological & Pharmaceutical Bulletin, 41*(6), 899–907. https://doi.org/10.1248/bpb.b17-01036 (accessed on 23rd June 2025).
34. Leung, M. H. M., & Shen, A. Q. (2018). Microfluidic assisted nanoprecipitation of PLGA nanoparticles for curcumin delivery to leukemia Jurka cells. *Langmuir, 34*(13), 3961–3970. https://doi.org/10.1021/acs.langmuir.7b04335 (accessed on 23rd June 2025).
35. Donno, R., Gennari, A., Lallana, E., De La Rosa, J. M. R., D'Arcy, R., Treacher, K., Hill, K. J., Ashford, M., & Tirelli, N. (2017). Nanomanufacturing through microfluidic-assisted nanoprecipitation: Advanced analytics and structure-activity relationships. *International Journal of Pharmaceutics, 534*(1, 2), 97–107. https://doi.org/10.1016/j.ijpharm.2017.10.006 (accessed on 23rd June 2025).
36. Bramosanti, M., Chronopoulou, L., Grillo, F., Valletta, A., & Palocci, C. (2017). Microfluidic-assisted nanoprecipitation of antiviral-loaded polymeric nanoparticles. *Colloids and Surfaces A: Physicochemical and Engineering Aspects, 532*, 369–376. https://doi.org/10.1016/j.colsurfa.2017.04.062 (accessed on 23rd June 2025).
37. Chiesa, E., Dorati, R., Modena, T., Conti, B., & Genta, I. (2018). Multivariate analysis for the optimization of microfluidics-assisted nanoprecipitation method intended for the loading of small hydrophilic drugs into PLGA nanoparticles. *International Journal of Pharmaceutics, 536*(1), 165–177. https://doi.org/10.1016/j.ijpharm.2017.11.044 (accessed on 23rd June 2025).
38. El-Naggar, N. E., Dalal, S. R., Zweil, A. M., & Eltarahony, M. (2023). Artificial intelligence-based optimization for chitosan nanoparticles biosynthesis, characterization and *in vitro* assessment of its anti-biofilm potentiality. *Scientific Reports, 13*(1). https://doi.org/10.1038/s41598-023-30911-6 (accessed on 23rd June 2025).
39. El-Naggar, N. E., Bashir, S. I., Rabei, N. H., & Saber, W. I. A. (2022). Innovative biosynthesis, artificial intelligence-based optimization, and characterization of chitosan nanoparticles by *Streptomyces microflavus* and their inhibitory potential against *Pectobacterium carotovorum*. *Scientific Reports, 12*(1). https://doi.org/10.1038/s41598-022-25726-w (accessed on 23rd June 2025).
40. Dawoud, M. H. S., Mannaa, I. S., Abdel-Daim, A., & Sweed, N. M. (2023). Integrating artificial intelligence with quality by design in the formulation of lecithin/chitosan

nanoparticles of a poorly water-soluble drug. *AAPS Pharm SciTech, 24*(6). https://doi.org/10.1208/s12249-023-02609-5 (accessed on 23rd June 2025).
41. Koletti, A. E., Tsarouchi, E., Kapourani, A., Kontogiannopoulos, K. N., Assimopoulou, A. N., & Barmpalexis, P. (2020). Gelatin nanoparticles for NSAID systemic administration: Quality by design and artificial neural networks implementation. *International Journal of Pharmaceutics, 578*, 119118. https://doi.org/10.1016/j.ijpharm.2020.119118 (accessed on 23rd June 2025).
42. Wu, H., He, J., Cheng, H., Liu, Y., Park, H. J., & Li, J. (2022). Development and analysis of machine-learning guided flash nanoprecipitation (FNP) for continuous chitosan nanoparticles production. *International Journal of Biological Macromolecules, 222*, 1229–1237. https://doi.org/10.1016/j.ijbiomac.2022.09.202 (accessed on 23rd June 2025).
43. Smeraldo, A., Ponsiglione, A. M., Netti, P. A., & Torino, E. (2023). Artificial neural network modelling hydro denticity for optimal design by microfluidics of polymer nanoparticles to apply in magnetic resonance imaging. *Acta Biomaterial, 171*, 440–450. https://doi.org/10.1016/j.actbio.2023.09.029 (accessed on 23rd June 2025).
44. Jara, M. O., Landín, M., & Morales, J. (2021). Screening of critical variables in fabricating polycaprolactone nanoparticles using Neuro Fuzzy Logic. *International Journal of Pharmaceutics, 601*, 120558. https://doi.org/10.1016/j.ijpharm.2021.120558 (accessed on 23rd June 2025).
45. Rezvantalab, S., Mihandoost, S., & Rezaiee, M. (2024). Machine learning assisted exploration of the influential parameters on the PLGA nanoparticles. *Scientific Reports, 14*(1). https://doi.org/10.1038/s41598-023-50876-w (accessed on 23rd June 2025).
46. Ma, Z., Li, B., Peng, J., & Gao, D. (2022). Recent development of drug delivery systems through microfluidics: From synthesis to evaluation. *Pharmaceutics, 14*(2), 434. https://doi.org/10.3390/pharmaceutics14020434 (accessed on 23rd June 2025).
47. Ferreira, L. F., Giordano, G. F., Gobbi, Â. L., Piazzetta, M. H. O., Schleder, G. R., & Lima, R. S. (2022). Real-time and *in situ* monitoring of the synthesis of silica nanoparticles. *ACS Sensors, 7*(4), 1045–1057. https://doi.org/10.1021/acssensors.1c02697 (accessed on 23rd June 2025).
48. Martin, Watanabe, R., Hashimoto, K., Higashisaka, K., Haga, Y., Tsutsumi, Y., & Mizuguchi, K. (2023). Evidence-based prediction of cellular toxicity for amorphous silica nanoparticles. *ACS Nano, 17*(11), 9987–9999. https://doi.org/10.1021/acsnano.2c11968 (accessed on 23rd June 2025).
49. Jyakhwo, S., Serov, N., Dmitrenko, A., & Vinogradov, V. V. (2023). Machine learning reinforced genetic algorithm for massive targeted discovery of selectively cytotoxic inorganic nanoparticles. *Small*. https://doi.org/10.1002/smll.202305375 (accessed on 23rd June 2025).
50. Zhang, J., Perrin, M. L., Barba, L., Overbeck, J., Jung, S., Grassy, B., Agal, A., Muff, R., Brönnimann, R., Haluška, M., Roman, C., Hierold, C., Jäggi, M., & Calame, M. (2022). High-speed identification of suspended carbon nanotubes using Raman spectroscopy and deep learning. *Microsystems & Nanoengineering, 8*(1). https://doi.org/10.1038/s41378-022-00350-w (accessed on 23rd June 2025).
51. Kotzabasaki, M., Sotiropoulos, I., Charitidis, C. A., & Sarimveis, H. (2021). Machine learning methods for multi-walled carbon nanotubes (MWCNT) genotoxicity

prediction. *Nanoscale Advances, 3*(11), 3167–3176. https://doi.org/10.1039/d0na00600a (accessed on 23rd June 2025).
52. Ortega-Tenezaca, B., & González-DíAz, H. (2021). IFPTML mapping of nanoparticle antibacterial activity vs. pathogen metabolic networks. *Nanoscale, 13*(2), 1318–1330. https://doi.org/10.1039/d0nr07588d (accessed on 23rd June 2025).
53. Desai, A. S., Ashok, A., Edis, Z., Bloukh, S. H., Gaikwad, M., Patil, R., Pandey, B., & Bhagat, N. (2023). Meta-analysis of cytotoxicity studies using machine learning models on physical properties of plant extract-derived silver nanoparticles. *International Journal of Molecular Sciences, 24*(4), 4220. https://doi.org/10.3390/ijms24044220 (accessed on 23rd June 2025).
54. El-Naggar, N. E., Rabei, N. H., Elmansy, M. F., Elmessiry, O. T., El-Sherbeny, M. K., El-Saidy, M. E., Sarhan, M., & Helal, M. G. (2023). Artificial neural network approach for prediction of AuNPs biosynthesis by *Streptomyces flavolimosus*, characterization, antitumor potency *in-vitro* and *in-vivo* against Ehrlich ascites carcinoma. *Scientific Reports, 13*(1). https://doi.org/10.1038/s41598-023-39177-4 (accessed on 23rd June 2025).
55. Toppo, A. L., Dhagat, S., & Jujjavarapu, S. E. (2022). Comparative study of response surface methodology and artificial neural network for optimization of process parameters for synthesis of gold nanoparticles by *Desmostachya bipinnata* extract. *Preparative Biochemistry & Biotechnology, 53*(2), 195–206. https://doi.org/10.1080/10826068.2022.2062773 (accessed on 23rd June 2025).
56. Suhail, M., Khan, A., Rahim, M. A., Naeem, A., Fahad, M., Badshah, S. F., Jabar, A., & Janakiraman, A. K. (2021). Micro and nanorobot-based drug delivery: An overview. *Journal of Drug Targeting, 30*(4), 349–358. https://doi.org/10.1080/1061186x.2021.1999962 (accessed on 23rd June 2025).
57. Soto, F., & Chrostowski, R. (2018). Frontiers of medical micro/nanorobotics: *In vivo* applications and commercialization perspectives toward clinical uses. *Frontiers in Bioengineering and Biotechnology, 6*. https://doi.org/10.3389/fbioe.2018.00170 (accessed on 23rd June 2025).
58. Das, K., & Chandra, J. (2023). Nanoparticles and convergence of artificial intelligence for targeted drug delivery for cancer therapy: Current progress and challenges. *Frontiers in Medical Technology, 4*. https://doi.org/10.3389/fmedt.2022.1067144 (accessed on 23rd June 2025).
59. Hortelão, A. C., Simó, C. D., Guix, M., Guallar-Garrido, S., Julián, E., Vilela, D., Rejc, L., Ramos-Cabrer, P., Cossío, U., Gómez-Vallejo, V., Patiño, T., Llop, J., & Sánchez, S. (2021). Swarming behavior and *in vivo* monitoring of enzymatic nanomotors within the bladder. *Science Robotics, 6*(52). https://doi.org/10.1126/scirobotics.abd2823 (accessed on 23rd June 2025).
60. Ntika, M., Kefalas, P., Alonso, J., & Stamatopoulou, I. (2014). Formal modelling and simulation of a multi-agent nano-robotic drug delivery system. *Scalable Computing: Practice and Experience, 15*(3). https://doi.org/10.12694/scpe.v15i3.1017 (accessed on 23rd June 2025).
61. Wang, M., Li, X., He, F., Li, J., Wang, H., & Nie, Z. (2022). Advances in designer DNA nanorobots enabling programmable functions. *ChemBioChem, 23*(18). https://doi.org/10.1002/cbic.202200119 (accessed on 23rd June 2025).

62. Singh, A., Chandrasekar, V., Janapareddy, P., Mathews, D. E., Laux, P., Luch, A., Yang, Y., Garcia-Cañibano, B., Balakrishnan, S., Abinahed, J., Ansari, A. A., & Dakua, S. P. (2021). Emerging application of nanorobotics and artificial intelligence to cross the BBB: Advances in design, controlled maneuvering, and targeting of the barriers. *ACS Chemical Neuroscience, 12*(11), 1835–1853. https://doi.org/10.1021/acschemneuro.1c00087 (accessed on 23rd June 2025).
63. Bhabad, S., Lamkhade, D., Koyate, S., Karanjkhele, K., Kale, V., & Doke, R. (2023). Transformative trends: A comprehensive review on role of artificial intelligence in healthcare and pharmaceutical research. *IP International Journal of Comprehensive and Advanced Pharmacology, 8*(4), 210–219. https://doi.org/10.18231/j.ijcaap.2023.034 (accessed on 23rd June 2025).
64. Norori, N., Hu, Q., Aellen, F. M., Faraci, F. D., & Tzovara, A. (2021). Addressing bias in big data and AI for health care: A call for open science. *Patterns, 2*(10), 100347. https://doi.org/10.1016/j.patter.2021.100347 (accessed on 23rd June 2025).
65. Kiseleva, A., Kotzinos, D., & De Hert, P. (2022). Transparency of AI in healthcare as a multilayered system of accountabilities: Between legal requirements and technical limitations. *Frontiers in Artificial Intelligence, 5*. https://doi.org/10.3389/frai.2022.879603 (accessed on 23rd June 2025).
66. Johnson, K. B., Wei, W., Weeraratne, D., Frisse, M. E., Misulis, K. E., Rhee, K., Zhao, J., & Snowdon, J. L. (2020). Precision medicine, AI, and the future of personalized health care. *Clinical and Translational Science, 14*(1), 86–93. https://doi.org/10.1111/cts.12884 (accessed on 23rd June 2025).

CHAPTER 8

Future Possibilities for Integrating AI with Nano-Carrier Technology

MAHAVEER SINGH,[1] ANASUYA PATIL,[2] RAVINDRA SINGH TOMAR,[3] GYANENDRA KUMAR SHARMA,[4] K. LAKSHMI,[5] P. K. ANJALI,[6] and VAIBHAV DAGAJI AHER[7,*]

[1]*Department of Pharmaceutics, Dr Karigowda College of Pharmacy, Hassan, Karnataka, India*

[2]*Department of Pharmaceutics, KLE College of Pharmacy, Rajajinagar, Bangalore, Karnataka, India*

[3]*Department of Electronics and Computer Engineering, Anand School of Engineering and Technology, Sharda University, Agra, Uttar Pradesh, India*

[4]*Sharda School of Pharmacy, Sharda University, Agra, Uttar Pradesh, India*

[5]*Department of Pharmacy, Chettinad School of Pharmaceutical Sciences, Chettinad Hospital and Research Institute, Chettinad Academy of Research and Education, Kelambakkam, Tamil Nadu, India*

[6]*Department of Economics, CHRIST (Deemed to Be University), Bangalore, Karnataka, India*

[7]*Department of Pharmaceutical Medicine, Maharashtra University of Health Sciences, Nashik, Maharashtra, India*

*Corresponding author

Nanotechnology for Nucleic Acid Delivery: Pankaj Sharma, Saloni Jain, and Vinay Jain (Eds.)

DOI: 10.1201/9781998511853-8

ABSTRACT

The convergence of artificial intelligence (AI) and nanotechnology presents exciting prospects for advancing drug delivery systems. This review explores the potential synergies between AI and nanocarrier technology to enhance drug delivery efficiency and therapeutic outcomes. We examine current developments in both fields and propose future directions for integrating AI algorithms with nanocarrier design, optimization, and personalized medicine approaches. AI can play a pivotal role in guiding the rational design of nanocarriers, optimizing drug loading and release kinetics, predicting *in vivo* behavior, and tailoring treatments to individual patient needs. Challenges such as regulatory hurdles, data privacy concerns, and the need for interdisciplinary collaboration are also discussed. Overall, the integration of AI with nanocarrier technology offers unprecedented opportunities to revolutionize drug delivery and improve patient care in the years to come.

8.1 INTRODUCTION

Over the past 30 years, there has been a great deal of advancement in the fast-expanding field of nano-carrier technological advances, which integrates physical, chemical, biological, and digital factors. It has an impact on many medical specialties and is a versatile instrument for creating vaccines, biomaterials, nanotherapeutics, medicinal imaging, and therapies. A number of medical fields, particularly medication delivery, imaging, and implants, might undergo advancement if artificial intelligence (AI) and nanotechnology are combined to create nano-carriers. AI algorithms can analyze large datasets and identify intricate trends, which can help in designing of nanotechnologies. AI can be used to address certain of the challenges associated with targeted medication delivery and manufacture for cancer therapy. High throughput, automation, AI, and data science have all contributed to the development of nano-carrier. The healthcare sector might undergo an upheaval through the application of AI in the development of products that utilize nanotechnology [1]. Once introduced, AI has shown to be a straightforward and effective approach in the field of nanotechnology. Integrating AI and nanotechnology leads to more creative solutions since AI quickly explores data and generates decisions. While the expected combinations of biology, AI, and nanotechnologies have yet to be materialized, the combination is causing a revolution in science and technology [2]. Since AI and nanotechnology have been combined, the field of nanomedicine has experienced a remarkable transformation. AI may be used to build and improve nanotechnologies for treatment and diagnostics. AI can additionally be used to anticipate interactions between substances and biological fluids, the vasculature, the immune system, and cell membranes in order to optimize the curative effectiveness of materials [3]. AI in nano-carrier can help to solve a number of the challenges associated with tailored pharmaceutical delivery and production for cancer therapy. AI systems can identify connections and trends in cell processes and relationships to predict the behavior of individual cells under different settings. Combining AI with nanotechnology might lead to more innovative technologies. Nanoinformatics uses AI and other computational resources to develop and put into practice nanomaterials.

Nanotechnology designers can enhance the development of medical diagnostic and therapeutic devices by leveraging AI algorithms' ability to analyze large datasets and identify intricate patterns. The effectiveness of drug encapsulation and release kinetics, as well as predictions of interactions between nanoparticles and target drugs, biological media, and cell membranes, can all be used to improve nano-formulations [4]. Additionally, patients may be classified according to their health status, and the effectiveness of their medications can be predicted using pattern recognition and classification algorithms [5, 6]. Due to the extreme complexity of cancer, these analytical capabilities are particularly critical.

AI algorithms may be used to analyze large volumes of biological data to identify existing drugs that could be repurposed as treatments for a range of illnesses. AI can reduce the cost and time required for medical research by repurposing drugs that have already received approval [7]. By leveraging the power of AI algorithms and methodologies, the goal is to integrate AI into nanomedicine to enhance various aspects of the field. This chapter aims to explore the potential applications of AI integration in data science, large-scale processing, precision cancer therapy, targeted drug delivery, and automation in nanomedicine. The study's findings led to the discussion of several key areas: the use of AI in nanomedicine; AI-based drug discovery and diagnosis in nanotechnology; AI-assisted drug delivery and nanoparticle synthesis; AI-powered visualization and testing in nanotechnology; AI integration with nanorobotics for therapeutic applications; ethical and safety considerations in AI-enabled nanomedicine; and future directions and implications of AI in nanotechnology for medical research [8–10].

8.1.1 THE FUNDAMENTAL IDEA BEHIND ARTIFICIAL INTELLIGENCE (AI) IN PHARMACEUTICALS

Regarding advancements in AI, there are two main categories. The first category consists of software and technical approaches, including expert systems that simulate human experience and make decisions based on predetermined rules. Artificial neural networks (ANNs), which are systems that emulate brain function, fall into the second category. One of the most advantageous features of ANNs is their ability to generalize. These characteristics make them particularly well-suited for addressing challenges related to nanoformulation optimization in pharmaceutical development [16] (Table 8.1).

TABLE 8.1 Recent Research on Artificial Intelligence (AI) in Pharmaceuticals

Study Title	Authors	Journal/Conference
AI in Drug Discovery and Development: A Review	Xu et al. [11]	Frontiers in Pharmacology
Applications of AI in Pharmaceutical Industry	Zhang et al. [12]	Current Pharmaceutical Biotechnology
Advances in AI for Drug Discovery and Development	Wang and Li [13]	Expert Opinion on Drug Discovery
AI-driven Drug Discovery: Progress, Challenges, and Future Directions	Chen and Smith [14]	Drug Discovery Today
Machine Learning in Drug Discovery and Development	Lee and Kim [15]	Archives of Pharmacal Research

8.1.2 HOW ARTIFICIAL INTELLIGENCE (AI) FUNCTIONS

Constructing an AI system entails meticulously emulating human traits and abilities in a computer, then harnessing the machine's computational power to surpass human capabilities. A deep understanding of the subject is required to comprehend the various subdomains of AI and how they may be applicable across multiple industries, such as:

1. **Machine Learning (ML):** A computer may learn to infer relationships and make judgments from past data thanks to ML. It finds patterns and looks at past data to determine the importance of these data points and reach a possible result without depending on individual experiences [17, 18].

2. **Deep Learning (DL):** It is an approach to machine learning. In the 2000s, DL revitalized neural networks by enabling their training through DL techniques. DL trains a machine using multiple layers of input interpretation to categorize, infer, and predict outcomes. By traversing deep levels of activation vectors and identifying relational patterns—such as recognizing stochastic gradients—it aids in understanding the complex internal representations required for interpreting challenging language or analyzing objects [19].
3. **Neural Networks (NN):** These systems function similarly to brain cells in humans. They are a collection of algorithms that, by recording the connection between several fundamental variables, imitate the functioning of the human brain [17].
4. **Natural Language Processing (NLP):** It is the study of how a machine can read, understand, and understand a language. When a computer understands what the user is trying to say, it will respond correctly [17].
5. **Computer Vision:** Algorithms for computer vision try to understand a picture by breaking it down and looking at different parts of the object. This helps the computer identify and gain knowledge from a set of images, allowing it to generate better outcomes based on earlier discoveries [20].
6. **Cognitive Computing:** Artificial intelligence algorithms aim to mimic the way the human brain functions and produce the intended outcomes by evaluating text, voice, picture, and other inputs in a manner similar to that of humans [21].

8.1.3 FUNDAMENTALS OF NANO-CARRIER TECHNOLOGY

The creation of nanocarriers with a wide range of capabilities targeting various illnesses has become increasingly in demand. Compared to traditional drug dosage forms, nanocarriers offer enhanced stability, reduced adverse effects, and optimal effectiveness due to their minuscule size, large surface area, and practicality. For drug delivery purposes, a variety of nanocarriers have been developed, including micelles, nanospheres, nanoemulsions, nanoshells, nanocapsules, carbon nanotubes, polymersomes, solid lipid nanoparticles, polymer–drug conjugates, peptide nanoparticles, polymeric nanoparticles, and gold nanoparticles. Over the past few years, a number of characterization approaches have been devised and applied to monitor and predict the behavior of nanocarriers in both *in vitro* and *in vivo* settings.

This chapter outlines some basic *in vitro*, *in situ*, *ex vivo*, and *in vivo* characterization techniques for the majority of nanocarriers. We highlight the advantages and limitations of these techniques, as well as the manufacturing, safety, and regulatory challenges that hinder the transition of nanocarriers from the laboratory to clinical application. Additionally, future perspectives are discussed, including the benefits and limitations of AI in the development and enhancement of nanocarriers, along with the integration of AI and nanotechnology [22, 23].

8.2 THE ROLE OF AI IN NANO-CARRIER DESIGN AND DRUG DISCOVERY

AI methods are continually being introduced to address various challenges in nanotechnology (Figure 8.1). With a primary focus on minimizing computational time and achieving efficient parameter estimation, forecasting, and system simulations, key areas in the development of nanoscale modeling include the design of nanosystems, the advancement of nanocomputing, and the refinement of AI techniques [24]. To ensure greater therapeutic efficacy, drug delivery incorporates multiple strategies, including drug composition, manufacturing processes, bioactive ingredient preservation, and targeted transportation to specific sites. To improve the physicochemical properties of medications and address the instability of bioactive compounds—which can significantly impair pharmacokinetic performance—it is essential to optimize drug delivery processes [25].

In an effort to enhance drug delivery, AI techniques have recently been applied to the design, characterization, and production of pharmaceutical delivery nanotechnology. The analysis and interpretation of biological and genetic data remain primary applications of AI technologies. Additionally, this integrated approach has facilitated the acceleration of the drug discovery process by accurately predicting the activities of small molecules and identifying their multiple roles [25]. For example, several AI-based methods have been developed to predict the efficacy of drug combinations by considering their synergistic interactions. In this context, feasible paths toward AI-guided optimization are being explored for multimodal drug

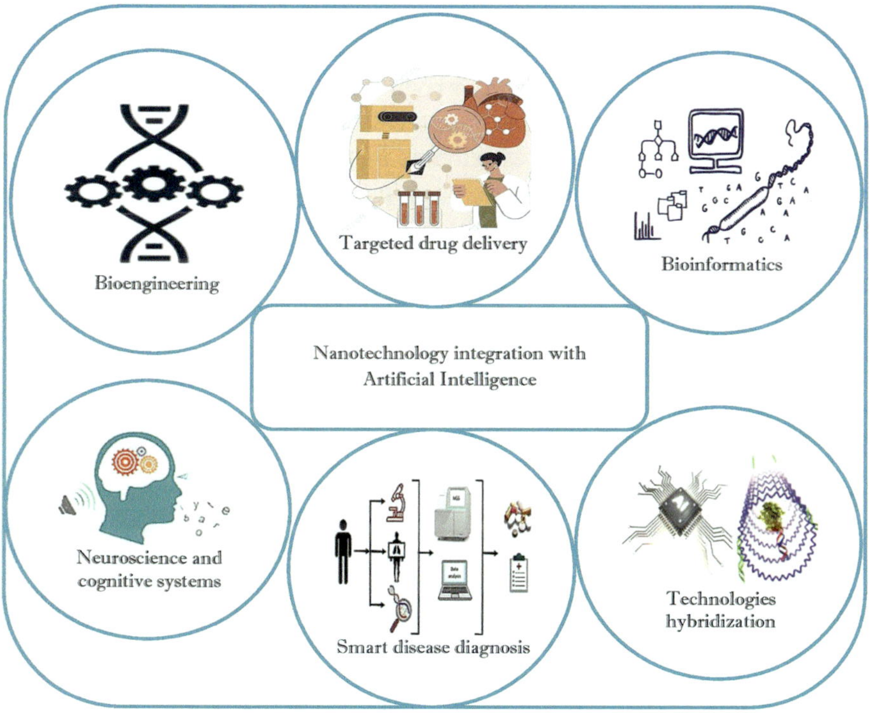

FIGURE 8.1 The potential impact of integrated artificial intelligence and nanotechnologies in scientific domains.

delivery, using various types of nanoparticles to enhance drug localization at the tumor site [26].

Physicians often treat cancer patients with varying genetic characteristics, which may include multiple molecular abnormalities. In cancer treatment, both the properties of the drug and the biological features of the patient are considered simultaneously during drug administration. Given the presence of numerous molecular characteristics for drugs alone, optimizing prescription combinations for individual patients is a significant challenge. Massive databases are generated when these molecular descriptors are combined with patient information such as genetic, metabolic, proteomic, histological, and clinical records. In this context, AI has shown promising results for the industry [27]. The various biological membranes that make up the human body's distinct biological compartments each possess unique physicochemical properties, which contribute to the complexity of the human organism. These segmented systems are often simplified for the purpose of drug delivery. In specific drug delivery systems, a variety of factors—including the proper administration route—must be considered to ensure transport, penetration, and arrival at the target site, which is represented by tissues or membranes within cells. A thorough understanding of the biological environment is essential to identify the relationships between a drug's molecular characteristics and its biological context. Predictive computation becomes increasingly complex as pharmaceutical delivery systems integrate a growing number of diverse factors [28].

Artificial intelligence (AI) has shown great potential in pharmacokinetic evaluations by helping to understand the biological interactions affecting membranes. It utilizes complex inputs—including drug interactions, phenotypic data, chemical reactions, and even genetic information—to optimize drug distribution [29, 30].

8.3 ARTIFICIAL INTELLIGENCE (AI)-POWERED DRUG DELIVERY SYSTEMS

8.3.1 ARTIFICIAL INTELLIGENCE (AI)-ASSISTED DRUG DELIVERY AND NANOPARTICLE SYNTHESIS

The creation of nanoparticles and medication delivery are essential elements of contemporary biotechnology and medicine. Because of their special qualities, nanoparticles—which are frequently between 1 and 100 nm in size—are useful in systems for delivering drugs. Their precise encapsulation and release of pharmaceuticals, as well as their substantial surface area-to-volume ratios and adjustable surface chemistry, are some of these characteristics. Nanoparticle manufacturing, nevertheless, may be an expensive, time-consuming, and complicated process, especially when used in medication delivery systems. The design, synthesis, and application of nanoparticles for medication administration have all been transformed by AI, which has established itself as a game-changing technology in several fields [31].

8.3.2 PHYSIOLOGICAL CUES-RESPONDING SMART DRUG DELIVERY SYSTEMS

Intelligent medication delivery systems are engineered to detect and react to certain physiological signals or medical situations within the body.

AI systems are able to identify alterations in the target location or the patient's physiological condition by analyzing real-time data via biomarkers, sensors, or imaging methods. The term "smart drug delivery systems" describes nanotechnologies with drug payloads that only release the drugs at specific locations determined by either passive or active targeting techniques, preventing the drugs from being released into the bloodstream randomly. As shown in Figure 8.2, these painstakingly designed smart or stimulus-responsive nanoplatforms may respond to both internal and external stimuli [32].

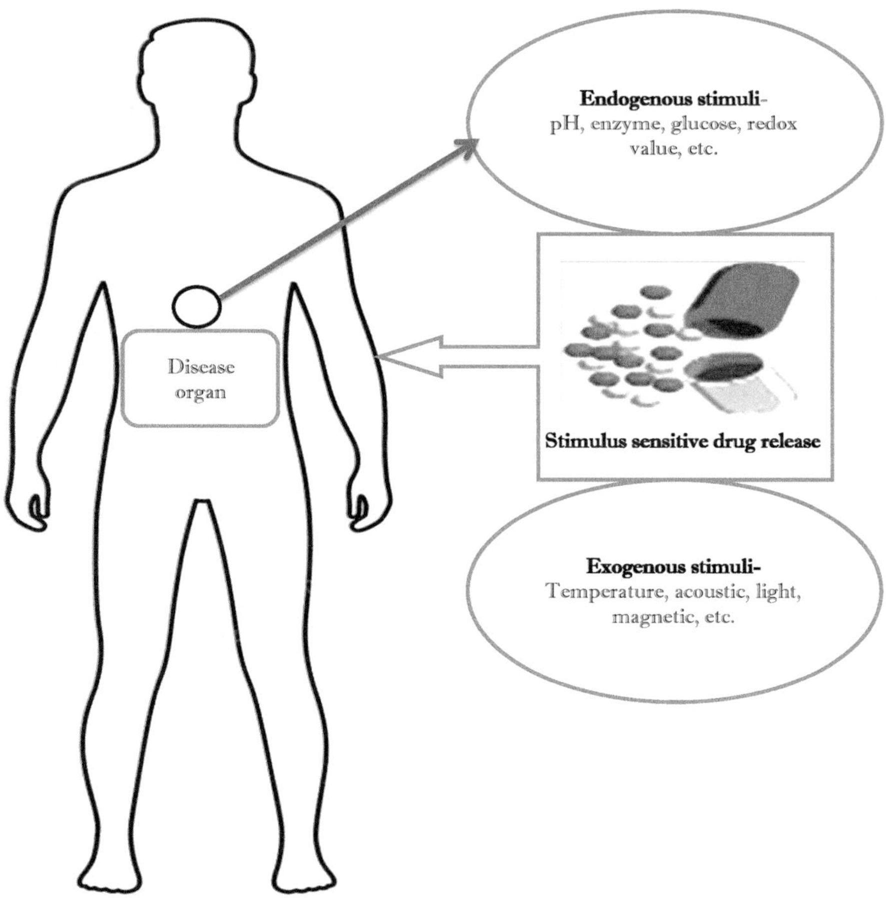

FIGURE 8.2 Nanoplatforms that respond to stimuli in smart medication delivery systems.

A disease's particular clinical features are associated with a variety of internal triggers, including levels of hormones, blood sugar levels, redox gradients, pH variations, and enzyme levels. On the other hand, external triggers can also be used to improve or initiate medication release in the afflicted areas, including temperature, electric pulses, magnetic fields, light, ultrasound, and high-energy radiation [32, 33]. When it comes to cancer treatment, for instance, AI systems are able to evaluate information about biomarkers, metabolism, and tumor size to determine the state of the illness. In order to better target the tumor, the drug delivery mechanism can react to this data by modifying dosage, timing drug release, or activating specific drug delivery processes [32].

8.3.3 ARTIFICIAL INTELLIGENCE (AI)-DRIVEN NANO-CARRIERS

According to Neubert [34], nanocarriers are colloidal drug carrier systems with submicron particle sizes, usually less than 500 nm. AI techniques are steadily emerging as solutions to a variety of nanotechnology-related problems. These include the creation of nanotechnology, nanocomputing, and the incorporation of AI methods into the design of simulation approaches at the nanoscale. The focus is on improving computing effectiveness, optimizing variable estimates, modeling predictions, and facilitating system simulation. Artificial intelligence techniques have recently been applied to the development, characterization, and manufacturing of pharmaceutical delivery nanosystems with the goal of improving drug administration. A large fraction of AI methods are focused on the comprehension and investigation of biological and genetic data.

The process of creating drugs has been considerably accelerated by this well-coordinated method, which has also improved predictive capacities and allowed for the identification of several small molecule properties [17]. Several AI-driven approaches, for example, are being proposed to predict the efficacy of pharmacological combinations based on the synergies between individual treatments. Using different kinds of nanoparticles to improve drug localization at tumor locations, prospective pathways for AI-guided optimization alongside drug delivery are being studied in this context [18]. AI algorithms may significantly improve the effectiveness of nanocarriers designed and optimized for targeted medication delivery, which is an exciting area of drug delivery research.

8.3.4 DEVELOPING AND IMPROVING NANO-CARRIERS FOR PERSONALIZED DRUG DELIVERY

Therapeutic drugs may now be delivered to particular target areas via nanocarriers, including nanoparticles, liposomes, and polymeric micelles [37, 38]. By examining the intricate connections between a nanocarrier's efficiency and attributes, AI algorithms can assist in nanocarrier development and optimization. Investigators may create predictive models that take into account a variety of elements, such as the physicochemical features of nanocarriers, pharmacological properties, and biological factors, by using AI algorithms [38]. For optimal drug delivery, such models can help identify the appropriate nanocarrier materials, sizes, surface modifications, and other formulation characteristics. As seen in Figure 8.3 [39, 40], the AI-based Feedback System Control (FSC) platform is utilized to optimize multimodal drug design, particularly in cancer treatment with nanocarriers.

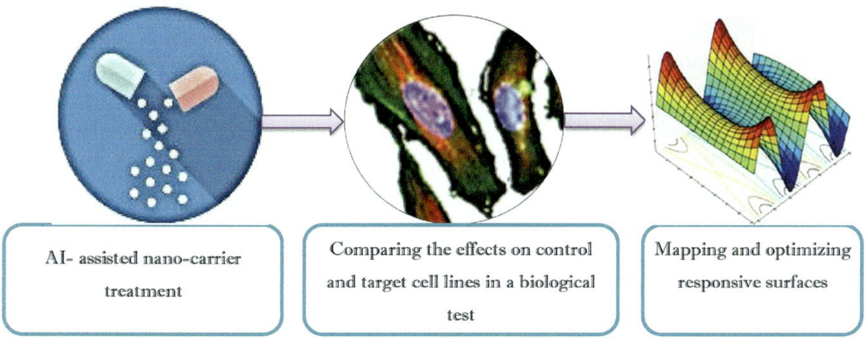

FIGURE 8.3 An illustration of the Feedback System Control (FSC) schematic used to optimize nanocarrier combination treatment.

By developing associations between medications and their corresponding therapeutic windows, the Feedback System Control (FSC) system is utilized to create phenotypic response surfaces. Given the differences in viability tests between cancer and control cell lines, these windows provide information on both efficacy and toxicity. With this methodology, FSC efficiently produces comprehensive combinatorial therapy plans for individual cancer cell lines, guided by the validated phenotypic response surface that determines the globally optimal complex combinations [39].

8.3.5 IMPROVING DRUG RELEASE PROFILES AND ENCAPSULATION EFFICACY

The amount of medicine contained in a nanocarrier is known as encapsulation efficacy, and it has a major impact on the drug delivery system's therapeutic effectiveness [41]. By evaluating information on the relationships between medications and nanocarrier components, AI systems can help increase encapsulation efficiency. Data collected during investigations and comprehensive evaluations may be analyzed using AI and machine learning technologies. To create models for prediction, exploratory data analysis (EDA) is carried out using various techniques. These models are designed to help scientists produce highly precise and repeatable results in the future. The loading of drugs and release variables can be identified using AI systems. This includes the optimization of formulation characteristics such as drug loading schedules, encapsulation methods, and polymer–drug ratios. AI algorithms may guide the drug design process to achieve improved encapsulation efficiency and control drug release kinetics by predicting and simulating drug–nanocarrier interactions [42].

8.4 NANOTECHNOLOGY AND ARTIFICIAL INTELLIGENCE (AI) IN DISEASE DIAGNOSIS

The discipline of nanotechnology has undergone a considerable transformation through the integration of artificial intelligence (AI) and advanced imaging methods. Nanotechnology employs materials at the nanoscale and nanoparticles to identify, treat, and monitor illnesses with unprecedented precision. AI plays a crucial role in enhancing patient outcomes, therapeutic effectiveness, and timely diagnosis when combined with state-of-the-art imaging techniques [43]. Although conventional medical imaging methods such as computed tomography (CT), magnetic resonance imaging (MRI), and X-rays provide valuable data, they have limitations in terms of resolution, specificity, and sensitivity. These limitations may hinder targeted drug delivery and early disease detection.

8.4.1 HERE ARE A FEW WAYS ARTIFICIAL INTELLIGENCE (AI) IS TRANSFORMING MEDICAL IMAGING

1. **Improved Image Analysis:** AI systems are able to handle and analyze massive datasets, which makes it possible to identify

pathological and anatomical modifications that are subtle and may be missed by human radiologists [44, 45].

2. **Image Improvement:** To help see nanoscale structures and substances, machine learning methods can boost contrast, lower artefacts, and boost image quality [46].
3. **Multi-Modal Imaging Integration:** Artificial intelligence has the ability to combine data from many different types of imaging to provide a more complete picture of the body's nanoscale relationships, enhancing diagnostic and therapeutic planning precision.
4. **Real-Time Imaging:** AI systems provide real-time nanoparticle tracking, which enables treatment regimens and medication distribution to be dynamically altered.

8.4.2 NANOMEDICINE DIAGNOSTICS

1. **Typical Diagnostic Procedures:** Conventional diagnostic techniques, such as biopsy of tissue and blood testing, are intrusive, time consuming, and might not give results right away. Nanomedicine aims to replace or enhance current methods by providing extremely precise, less invasive diagnoses.
2. **AI-Augmented Diagnostics:** The following are some ways that AI is changing nanomedicine diagnostics:
   - **Biomarker Recognition:** By analyzing sizable databases of clinical and genomic data, AI can find and verify novel biomarkers for a range of illnesses [47, 48].
   - **Proactive disease Diagnosis:** By using models based on machine learning to analyze patient information, prompt treatment can be made possible, increasing the likelihood of a good outcome [49]. This process predicts illness risk.
   - **Point-of-Care Diagnostics:** By enabling quick on-site diagnosis, AI-powered nanosensors and gadgets minimize the requirement for centralized testing in laboratories [50].

8.4.3 COMBINING ARTIFICIAL INTELLIGENCE (AI) WITH NANOROBOTICS FOR MEDICAL PURPOSES

The intersection of two cutting-edge technology fields—AI and nanorobotics—for medical use is both fascinating and highly promising. This combination has the potential to transform medicine by offering targeted, easily administered, and precise treatments. AI encompasses several technological domains, including machine learning, deep learning, and natural language processing. AI systems can analyze and process enormous volumes of data. They may also identify patterns in the data and make decisions or predictions based on those findings. Nanorobots are tiny devices or machines with nanoscale dimensions, often less than 100 nanometers [51]. These nanoscale robots can be used for surgery, tissue repair, drug delivery, and other applications. Medical applications may benefit significantly from the integration of AI and nanorobotics. When combined, these two fields can offer precise, customized, and minimally invasive treatments that significantly improve patient outcomes. To realize this potential, it will be necessary to address associated challenges, including security, regulatory oversight, and ethical concerns. Ongoing research and development in the fields of nanorobotics and AI are anticipated to lead to exciting advances in healthcare [52, 53].

When AI and nanorobotics are combined, pharmaceutical applications—particularly targeted drug delivery and precision medicine—have the potential to be transformed. Current developments in bio-nanotechnology and engineering offer promising progress toward integrating power sources, intelligent sensors, and AI into nanorobots, despite the challenges that remain. This integration minimizes damage to healthy tissue while providing unparalleled therapeutic and diagnostic precision. Once AI has analyzed an individual's genetic and medical data, nanorobots may deliver personalized treatments. By eliminating the need for large incisions, nanorobots can perform functions that reduce patient discomfort and expedite recovery [54, 55].

8.4.4 THERAPEUTIC USES OF ARTIFICIAL INTELLIGENCE (AI)-NANOROBOTICS

1. **Drug Delivery:** The drugs may be carried and administered to specified body areas using nanorobots. AI can direct them to the

correct spot, enabling accurate and efficient medication delivery [56, 57].

2. **Cancer Therapy:** Highly targeted cancer treatments are achievable through the combination of AI and nanorobots. AI can analyze imaging data to detect cancer cells, whereas nanorobots deliver drugs straight to cancer cells.
3. **Surgery:** AI can assist in the planning and direction of less-invasive surgical operations to improve accuracy. These treatments can be performed by nanorobots.
4. **Tissue Repair:** AI can track the recuperation processes as nanorobots help restore tissue damage at the level of the cell.
5. **Diagnostics and Imaging:** AI can analyze medical pictures to identify abnormalities, and nanorobots can provide contrasting chemicals for medical imaging or conduct on-site diagnostic tests [59].

8.5 OBSTACLES AND PROSPECTIVE VIEWS

8.5.1 REGULATORY AND ETHICAL CONSIDERATIONS

To guarantee the safe and accountable application of these advances, it is imperative to address the ethical implications of AI-driven medication delivery systems. Here are some important considerations:

8.5.1.1 FAIRNESS, ACCOUNTABILITY, AND TRANSPARENCY IN DECISION-MAKING ALGORITHMS

The decision-making procedures and underlying criteria of AI algorithms employed in medication delivery systems ought to be transparent, meaning they should be comprehensible and explainable. By ensuring that individuals, regulators, and physicians can understand exactly how the algorithms arrive at their results, transparency promotes accountability and trust. Another important factor is fairness. To ensure equitable use of medication delivery systems and treatments, AI algorithms must be designed and trained in a manner that prevents bias and discrimination. Existing healthcare inequities based on age and other factors should not be reinforced or exacerbated by these algorithms [59, 60].

8.5.1.2 REGULATORY STRUCTURES FOR RESPONSIBLE AND SAFE APPLICATION

The safe and ethical application of AI in medication delivery systems is heavily dependent on laws and regulations. Safety, effectiveness, and ethical considerations should all be addressed when creating frameworks for evaluating and approving AI algorithms. The U.S. Food and Drug Administration's (FDA) discussion paper, "Utilizing Artificial Intelligence and Machine Learning in Drug and Biological Product Development," is a key step toward addressing the ethical and legal challenges surrounding AI in drug research. Along with proposed guidelines for the use of AI and machine learning, this paper provides insights into the role of AI in drug development, nonclinical studies, and clinical studies. With this initiative, the FDA has taken a major step toward regulating the use of AI in healthcare and has opened new pathways for growth within the industry. It lays the foundation for future regulatory developments in this area by acknowledging both the potential benefits and the challenges associated with AI in drug development [61, 62].

8.5.1.3 AUTONOMY OF THE PATIENT AND INFORMED APPROVAL

A major ethical concern in AI-driven medication delivery systems is obtaining informed consent. Patients should be informed in a clear and understandable manner about how AI algorithms are used in their care and how this may affect them. This empowers patients to make informed decisions regarding their treatment, with an understanding of the benefits, limitations, and risks of AI-driven medication delivery systems. Supporting patient autonomy in decision-making requires effective communication from healthcare providers, who should also address patients' questions and clarify the role of AI [63, 64].

8.5.1.4 STANDARDIZED PROCEDURES FOR DATA GATHERING AND EXCHANGE

For AI-driven medication delivery studies to be consistent, comparable, and reproducible, standardized data collection and sharing procedures must be established. To reliably gather relevant data across research and healthcare settings, standardized data elements, methods, and metadata standards must be defined. Professional organizations and international collaborations can guide these efforts by establishing criteria for data collection. Promoting adherence to these guidelines encourages data sharing, which benefits the scientific community. Where ethically permissible, transparency is enhanced by supporting open data initiatives. Encouraging the release of study results and making anonymized datasets publicly available supports scientific progress and the validation of AI algorithms. To advance personalized healthcare and the field of AI-driven medication delivery, it is essential to address data-related challenges through collaborative, standardized, and ethical approaches that utilize diverse and reliable datasets for effective algorithm design [65–69].

8.6 CONCLUSION

The use of AI in nanotechnology represents a significant advancement at the intersection of modern science and healthcare. As we move toward a period of unprecedented medical opportunities and challenges, the convergence of AI and nanotechnology holds great potential. This combination has the capacity to transform several fields, including diagnostics, drug delivery, therapy customization, and our understanding of complex biological systems. Large datasets can be rapidly analyzed by AI-driven algorithms to uncover new drug candidates, provide insights into disease mechanisms, and develop individualized treatment regimens. Conversely, nanomedicine introduces novel materials and methods at the nanoscale that can precisely target disease sites, enhance drug delivery, and minimize adverse effects. The field of nanotechnology is poised for a revolution through the integration of AI. AI can quickly mine data and make decisions, helping to overcome challenges related to personalized drug delivery and manufacturing for cancer treatment. The fusion of biology, AI, and nanotechnology is driving forward scientific and technological progress. AI algorithms can optimize material properties based on interactions with target drugs, bodily fluids, immune responses, and cell membranes, thereby enhancing the development of nanotechnologies for diagnosis and therapy. As we advance, it will be imperative to promote interdisciplinary collaboration, uphold ethical standards, and address potential concerns with care. The application of AI to nanotechnology represents not only a scientific breakthrough but also a profound commitment to improving human health and well-being. With careful oversight and the continued dedication of researchers and healthcare professionals, humanity stands on the threshold of a healthier and more promising future.

ACKNOWLEDGMENT

None

CONFLICT OF INTEREST

The authors declare no conflict of interest.

FUNDING

None

KEYWORDS

- **artificial intelligence**
- **nanotechnology**
- **nanocarriers**
- **drug delivery**
- **optimization**
- **personalized medicine**

REFERENCES

1. Gessner, I., & Neundorf, I. (2020). Applications of AI-enabled nanomedicines in cancer management and their application in diagnosis, monitoring and therapy. *AJCSIT, 11*(5).
2. Li, F., Chen, Z., & Chen, X. (2023). Integrating artificial intelligence and nanotechnology for precision cancer medicine. *Frontiers in Bioengineering and Biotechnology, 11*, 909525.

3. Sharma, A., Sharma, M., & Kumar, P. (2023). AI powered identification of drug targets and pathways for diagnosis and treatment planning: A review. *NNOA, 8*, 000232.
4. Shamay, Y., Shah, J., Işık, M., Mizrachi, A., Leibold, J., Tschaharganeh, D. F., Roxbury, D., Budhathoki-Uprety, J., Nawaly, K., Sugarman, J. L., & Baut, E. (2018). Quantitative self-assembly prediction yields targeted nanomedicines. *Nature Materials, 17*(4), 361–368.
5. Altomare, D., Di Lena, M., Porcelli, F., Trizio, L., Travaglio, E., Tutino, M., Dragonieri, S., Memeo, V., & De Gennaro, G. (2013). Exhaled volatile organic compounds identify patients with colorectal cancer. *British Journal of Surgery, 100*(1), 144–150.
6. Rubio-Perez, C., Tamborero, D., Schroeder, M. P., Antolín, A. A., Deu-Pons, J., Perez-Llamas, C., Mestres, J., Gonzalez-Perez, A., & Lopez-Bigas, N. (2015). Comprehensive identification of mutational cancer driver genes across 12 tumor types. *Cancer Cell, 27*, 382.
7. Vijayan, R. S. K., Kihlberg, J., Cross, J. B., & Poongavanam, V. (2022). Enhancing preclinical drug discovery with artificial intelligence. *Drug Discovery Today, 27*, 967.
8. Sharma, P., Dasputre, N., & Jain, V. (2024). Nanomedicine: Concepts, characteristics, and regulatory challenges. In *Smart Nanocarrier for Effective Drug Delivery* (pp. 1–16). CRC Press.
9. Sharma, P., Jain, V., & Tailang, M. (2023). How artificial intelligence is transforming medicine: The future of pharmaceutical research. In *Industry 4.0 and Healthcare: Impact of Artificial Intelligence* (pp. 133–150). Singapore: Springer Nature Singapore.
10. Sharma, P. (2023). Nanostructured biomaterials in drug delivery: Current trends and upcoming possibilities. In *Engineered Biomaterials: Synthesis and Applications* (pp. 261–280). Singapore: Springer Nature Singapore.
11. Blanco-Gonzalez, A., Cabezon, A., Seco-Gonzalez, A., Conde-Torres, D., Antelo-Riveiro, P., Pineiro, A., & Garcia-Fandino, R. (2023). The role of AI in drug discovery: Challenges, opportunities, and strategies. *Pharmaceuticals, 16*(6), 891.
12. Thakur, A., Mishra, A. P., Panda, B., Rodríguez, D., Gaurav, I., & Majhi, B. (2020). Application of artificial intelligence in pharmaceutical and biomedical studies. *Current Pharmaceutical Design, 26*(29), 3569–3578.
13. Wang, H., & Li, J. (2024). Advances in AI for drug discovery and development. *Expert Opinion on Drug Discovery, 19*(1), 1–14.
14. Chen, X., & Smith, A. (2023). AI-driven drug discovery: Progress, challenges, and future directions. *Drug Discovery Today, 29*(5), 705–712.
15. Lee, S., & Kim, K. (2022). Machine learning in drug discovery and development. *Archives of Pharmacal Research, 45*(2), 108–120.
16. Agatonovic-Kustrin, S., & Beresford, R. (2022). Basic concepts of artificial neural network (ANN) modeling and its application in pharmaceutical research. *Journal of Pharmaceutical and Biomedical Analysis, 22*(5), 717–727.
17. Sharma, P., Jain, V., Jain, A., & Tailang, M. (2022). Role of swarm intelligence for health monitoring and related actions. In *Internet of Things and Fog Computing-Enabled Solutions for Real-Life Challenges* (pp. 95–118). CRC Press.

18. Sharma, P., Jain, V., & Tailang, M. (2022). Swarm intelligence and machine learning algorithms for cancer diagnosis. In *Swarm Intelligence and Machine Learning* (pp. 34–50). CRC Press.
19. Ciallella, H. L., & Zhu, H. (2019). Advancing computational toxicology in the big data era by artificial intelligence: Data-driven and mechanism-driven modeling for chemical toxicity. *Chemical Research in Toxicology, 32*(4), 536–547.
20. Kakani, V., Nguyen, V. H., Kumar, B. P., Kim, H., & Pasupuleti, V. R. (2020). A critical review on computer vision and artificial intelligence in food industry. *Journal of Agriculture and Food Research, 2*, 100033.
21. Bini, S. A. (2018). Artificial intelligence, machine learning, deep learning, and cognitive computing: What do these terms mean and how will they impact health care? *The Journal of Arthroplasty, 33*(8), 2358–2361.
22. Alshawwa, S. Z., Kassem, A. A., Farid, R. M., Mostafa, S. K., & Labib, G. S. (2022). Nanocarrier drug delivery systems: Characterization, limitations, future perspectives and implementation of artificial intelligence. *Pharmaceutics, 14*, 883. https://doi.org/10.3390/pharmaceutics14040883 (accessed on 23rd June 2025).
23. Sharma, P., Jain, V., & Tailang, M. (2023). Advancement of nanocarrier-based engineering for specific drug delivery for cancer therapy. In *Targeted Cancer Therapy in Biomedical Engineering* (pp. 465–486). Singapore: Springer Nature Singapore.
24. Sacha, G. M., & Varona, P. (2013). Artificial intelligence in nanotechnology. *Nanotechnology, 24*(45), 452002. https://doi.org/10.1088/0957-4484/24/45/452002 (accessed on 23rd June 2025).
25. Tyagi, S., Pathak, A., Rao, N. R., Nehra, S., Asthana, A., Sharma, V., Katyal, G., Bhardwaj, A., Sharma, L., Prakash, S., & Katiyar, D. (2023). AI-assisted formulation design for improved drug delivery and bioavailability. *PHJ, 56*(3), 149–162.
26. Ho, D., Wang, P., & Kee, T. (2019). Artificial intelligence in nanomedicine. *Nanoscale Horizons, 4*(2), 365–377. https://doi.org/10.1039/C8NH00233A (accessed on 23rd June 2025).
27. Tsigelny, I. F. (2019). Artificial intelligence in drug combination therapy. *Briefings in Bioinformatics, 20*(4), 1434–1448. https://doi.org/10.1093/bib/bby004 (accessed on 23rd June 2025).
28. Bhhatarai, B., Walters, W. P., Hop, C. E. C. A., Lanza, G., & Ekins, S. (2019). Opportunities and challenges using artificial intelligence in ADME/Tox. *Nature Materials, 18*(5), 418–422. https://doi.org/10.1038/s41563-019-0332-5 (accessed on 23rd June 2025).
29. Cheng, F., & Zhao, Z. (2014). Machine learning-based prediction of drug–drug interactions by integrating drug phenotypic, therapeutic, chemical, and genomic properties. *Journal of the American Medical Informatics Association, 21*(e2), e278–e286. https://doi.org/10.1136/amiajnl-2013-002512 (accessed on 23rd June 2025).
30. Sharma, P. (2023). Validated ultraviolet spectrophotometric method for simultaneous estimation of Olmesartan medroxalol in marketed formulation. *Asian Journal of Pharmaceutics, 17*(3).
31. Lombardo, D., Kiselev, M. A., & Caccamo, M. T. (2019). Smart nanoparticles for drug delivery application: Development of versatile nanocarrier platforms in biotechnology and nanomedicine. *Journal of Nanomaterials, 2019*.

32. Liu, D., Yang, F., Xiong, F., & Gu, N. (2016). The smart drug delivery system and its clinical potential. *Theragnostic, 6*, 1306–1323. https://doi.org/10.7150/thno.14858 (accessed on 23rd June 2025).
33. Dixit, A., Jain, A. K., Sharma, N., Saluja, G. S., Acharya, M., Rathore, D., Joshi, R., Sharma, P., & Singh, Y. (2015). Hepatoprotective activity of *Wrightia tinctoria* leaves against D-galactosamine induced hepatotoxicity in rats. *Indo-American Journal of Pharmaceutical Research, 5*(1).
34. Neubert, R. H. (2011). Potentials of new nanocarriers for dermal and transdermal drug delivery. *European Journal of Pharmaceutics and Biopharmaceutics, 77*, 1–2. https://doi.org/10.1016/j.ejpb.2010.11.003 (accessed on 23rd June 2025).
35. Sharma, P., & Tailang, M. (2017). Opportunities and challenges to develop transdermal patch with nanocarrier. *World Journal of Pharmaceutical Research, 6*(15), 392–400.
36. Ho, D., Wang, P., & Kee, T. (2019). Artificial intelligence in nanomedicine. *Nanoscale Horizons, 4*, 365–377.
37. Sharma, P., Bhargava, S., Parashar, D., & Mangal, A. (2017). Formulation and evaluation of nanoparticles containing cyclophosphamide. *World Journal of Pharmaceutical Research, 7*(1), 785–798.
38. Zeb, A., Qureshi, O. S., Kim, H. S., Kim, M. S., Kang, J. H., Park, J. S., & Kim, J. K. (2017). High payload itraconazole-incorporated lipid nanoparticles with modulated release property for oral and parenteral administration. *Journal of Pharmacy and Pharmacology, 69*, 955–966.
39. Khong, J., Wang, P., Gan, T. R., Ng, J., Anh, T. T. L., Blasiak, A., Kee, T., & Ho, D. (2019). The role of artificial intelligence in scaling nanomedicine toward broad clinical impact. In Chung, E. J., Leon, L., & Rinaldi, C. (Eds.), *Nanoparticles for Biomedical Applications: Fundamental Concepts, Biological Interactions and Clinical Applications* (pp. 371–400). Amsterdam: Elsevier. https://doi.org/10.1016/C2017-0-04750-X (accessed on 23rd June 2025).
40. Sharma, P., & Tailang, M. (2019). pH dependent release potential of natural polymers in sustained release of ornidazole from colon targeted delivery system. *International Journal of Drug Delivery Technology, 9*, 1–10.
41. Sharma, P., & Tailang, M. (2020). Design, optimization, and evaluation of hydrogel of primaquine loaded nano emulsion for malaria therapy. *FJPS*, *6*, 1–1.
42. Ganju, E., & Gupta, B. K. (2023). Artificial intelligence and machine learning applied interpretation and analysis of optimization study and *in-vitro* release of formulated curcumin loaded nanoparticles. *Journal of Coastal Life Medicine*, *11*, 660–674.
43. Mohammadi, A. T., Sanjarian, S., Tehrany, P. M., Khorram, R., Vafadar, R., Mohseni, H., Arzi, B., Madady, A., Shabbak, A., & Vaseghi, S. (2023). *Cutting-Edge Advances in Surgery*. Nobel Sciences.
44. Esteva, A., Kuprel, B., Novoa, R. A., Ko, J., Swetter, S. M., Blau, H. M., & Thrun, S. (2017). Dermatologist-level classification of skin cancer with deep neural networks. *Nature*, *542*, 115.
45. Sharma, P., & Tailang, M. (2022). Primaquine-loaded transdermal patch for treating malaria: Design, development, and characterization. *FJPS*, *8*(1), 43.
46. Litjens, G., Kooi, T., Bejnordi, B. E., Setio, A. A. A., Ciompi, F., Ghafoorian, M., Van Der Laak, J. A., Van Ginneken, B., & Sánchez, C. I. (2017). A survey on deep learning in medical image analysis. *Medical Image Analysis*, *42*, 60.

47. Huang, S., Yang, J., Fong, S., & Zhao, Q. (2020). Artificial intelligence in cancer diagnosis and prognosis: Opportunities and challenges. *Cancer Letters*, *471*, 61.
48. Sharma, P. (2022). Applications of statistical tools for optimization and development of smart drug delivery system. In *Smart Drug Delivery* (p. 183). Intech Open.
49. Sujatha, R., Chatterjee, J. M., Jhanjhi, N. Z., & Brohi, S. N. (2021). Performance of deep learning vs machine learning in plant leaf disease detection. *Microprocessors and Microsystems*, *80*, 103615.
50. Gao, A., Murphy, R. R., Chen, W., Dagnino, G., Fischer, P., Gutierrez, M. G., Kundrat, D., Nelson, B. J., Shamsudhin, N., Su, H., & Xia, J. (2021). Progress in robotics for combating infectious diseases. *Science Robotics*, *6*, 1462.
51. Nguyen, T., & Sirichokcharoenkun, Y. (2023). *The Limitations and Potential of ChatGPT in Chemistry Education*.
52. Adir, O., Poley, M., Chen, G., Froim, S., Krinsky, N., Shklover, J., Shainsky-Roitman, J., Lammers, T., & Schroeder, A. (2020). Integrating artificial intelligence and nanotechnology for precision cancer medicine. *Advanced Materials*, *32*, 1901989.
53. Sharma, P., Jain, V., & Jain, S. (2021). Fabrication, optimization and evaluation of chronotropic drug delivery system of captopril. *International Journal of Pharmaceutical Sciences and Research*, *12*, 2203–2210.
54. Egorov, E., Pieters, C., Korach-Rechtman, H., Shklover, J., & Schroeder, A. (2021). Robotics, microfluidics, nanotechnology and AI in the synthesis and evaluation of liposomes and polymeric drug delivery systems. *Drug Delivery and Translational Research*, *11*, 345.
55. Rathore, D. S., Dixit, A., Sharma, V., Joshi, R., Sharma, P., Parashar, D., & Sarvesh, B. (2015). Formulation and development of glipizide containing floating microsphere. *Indo American Journal of Pharmaceutical Research*, *5*(8), 2564–2570.
56. Das, K. P. (2023). Nanoparticles and convergence of artificial intelligence for targeted drug delivery for cancer therapy: Current progress and challenges. *Frontiers in Medical Technology*, *4*, 1067144.
57. Sharma, P., Jain, V., & Tailang, M. (2022). *Selection and Role of Polymers for Designing of a Drug Carrier*. IntechOpen.
58. Singh, A. V., Chandrasekar, V., Janapareddy, P., Mathews, D. E., Laux, P., Luch, A., Yang, Y., Garcia-Canibano, B., Balakrishnan, S., Abinahed, J., & Al Ansari, A. (2021). Emerging application of nanorobotics and artificial intelligence to cross the BBB: Advances in design, controlled maneuvering, and targeting of the barriers. *ACS Chemical Neuroscience*, *12*, 1835.
59. Gerke, S., Minssen, T., & Cohen, G. (2020). Ethical and legal challenges of artificial intelligence-driven healthcare. In *Artificial Intelligence in Healthcare* (pp. 295–336). Academic Press, Cambridge.
60. Sharma, P. (2021). Modification of human behavior due to coronavirus outbreak: A brief study on current scenario. *AJP*, *15*(3).
61. Sarkar, B., Das, B., Rawat, V. S., Wahlang, J. B., Nongpiur, A., Tiewsoh, I., Lyngdoh, N. M., Das, D., Bidarolli, M., & Sony, H. T. (2023). Artificial intelligence and machine learning technology driven modern drug discovery and development. *International Journal of Molecular Sciences*, *24*(3), 2026.

62. Pankaj, S., Ashish, D., Dheerendra, R., Yogendra, R., Ramakant, J. K., & Kuldeep, S. (2015). Formulate and evaluate orodispersible tablets of primaquine. *Indo American Journal of Pharmaceutical Research*, *5*(5), 1625–1632.
63. Klugman, C. M., Dunn, L. B., Schwartz, J., & Cohen, I. G. (2018). The ethics of smart pills and self-acting devices: Autonomy, truth-telling, and trust at the dawn of digital medicine. *American Journal of Bioethics*, *18*, 38–47. https://doi.org/10.1080/15265161.2018.1498933
64. Sharma, V., Dixit, A., Singh Rajput, Y., Rathore, D. S., Joshi, R., Sharma, P., & Parashar, D. (2015). The analgesic effect of the methanolic extract of *Sida acuta*. *American Journal of Pharmaceutical Research*, *5*(09).
65. Rodrigues, T. (2019). The good, the bad, and the ugly in chemical and biological data for machine learning. *Drug Discovery Today: Technologies*, *32*, 33–38. https://doi.org/10.1016/j.ddtec.2020.07.001
66. Sharma, P., & Tailang, M. (2018). *In-vivo* study of orodispersible tablet of primaquine. *International Journal of Pharmaceutical Sciences and Research*, *9*(8), 3506–3510.
67. Sharma, P., & Tailang, M. (2020). Design, optimization and evaluation of buccal drug delivery system of propranolol for hypertension treatment. *International Journal of Pharmaceutical Sciences and Research*, *11*(1), 301–311.
68. Sharma, P., & Jain, V. (2023). An overview of current advances and pharmaceutical uses of 3D and 4D printing. *Exploration of Medicine*, *4*, 560–575.
69. Sharma, P., & Tailang, M. (2016). Role & future aspects of primaquine in malaria therapy. *World Journal of Pharmaceutical Research*, *5*(11), 573–581.

CHAPTER 9

Case Studies and Success Stories of AI-Driven Approaches for Nucleic Acid Delivery

SAILESH KUMAR GHATUARY,[1] ANJU SINGH,[2]
HANISH SINGH JAYASINGH CHELLAMMAL,[3] MANISH PAL SINGH,[4]
SHWETA MISHRA,[5] BHUPINDER BHYAN,[6] and
N. G. RAGHAVENDRA RAO[7,*]

[1]*Department of Pharmacy, Shri R. L. T. Institute of Pharmaceutical Science and Technology, Etawah, Uttar Pradesh, India*

[2]*Department of Pharmacy, School of Pharmaceutical Sciences, Chhatrapati Shahu Ji Maharaj University, Kanpur, Uttar Pradesh, India*

[3]*Department of Pharmacology and Pharmaceutical Chemistry, Faculty of Pharmacy, Universiti Teknologi MARA (UiTM), Puncak Alam, Selangor, Malaysia*

[4]*Department of Pharmacy, Sharda School of Pharmacy, Sharda University, Agra, Uttar Pradesh, India*

[5]*Department of Pharmacy, Dr. D. Y. Patil Institute of Pharmaceutical Sciences and Research, Pimpri, Pune, Maharashtra, India*

[6]*School of Pharmaceutical Sciences, RIMT University, Gobindgarh, Punjab, India*

[7]*Department of Pharmaceutics, KIET School of Pharmacy, KIET Group of Institutions, Delhi-NCR, Muradnagar, Ghaziabad, Uttar Pradesh, India*

*Corresponding author

Nanotechnology for Nucleic Acid Delivery: Pankaj Sharma, Saloni Jain, and Vinay Jain (Eds.)

DOI: 10.1201/9781998511853-9

ABSTRACT

This chapter explores the innovative intersection of artificial intelligence (AI) and nucleic acid delivery, presenting case studies and success stories that highlight the transformative potential of this interdisciplinary approach. Nucleic acid delivery holds immense promise for therapeutic applications, offering targeted treatment options for various diseases, including cancer and genetic disorders. However, the effective delivery of nucleic acids faces numerous challenges, including cellular uptake, intracellular trafficking, and immunogenicity. By leveraging AI-driven approaches, researchers have developed novel strategies to overcome these hurdles and enhance the efficiency and specificity of nucleic acid delivery systems. Through a comprehensive review of case studies and success stories, this chapter demonstrates how AI algorithms optimize delivery vehicles, predict potential off-target effects, and personalize treatment regimens based on patient-specific factors. Moreover, it elucidates how machine learning algorithms analyze large datasets to identify novel biomarkers and therapeutic targets, accelerating the discovery and development of nucleic acid-based therapies. The chapter underscores the diverse applications of AI in nucleic acid delivery, ranging from drug discovery and development to clinical translation. By showcasing real-world examples of AI-driven innovations in this field, this chapter aims to inspire future research endeavors and foster collaboration between AI experts and nucleic acid delivery specialists.

9.1 INTRODUCTION

Nucleic acids are essential for all fundamental biological activities, such as cell function, metabolism, development, and reproduction in every living organism. They are the fundamental building blocks of the genetic code. The controlled alteration of nucleic acids for medicinal purposes forms the foundation of gene therapy. Nucleic acid-based therapeutics are being researched to treat or prevent hereditary and acquired conditions by restoring or substituting damaged or missing genetic components. Gene therapy has emerged as a form of medicine to achieve this goal by the transfection of foreign or endogenous nucleic acids into host cells [1, 2]. Administration of various nucleic acid-based agents, including messenger ribonucleic acid (mRNA), deoxyribonucleic acid (DNA), CRISPR/Cas systems, and oligonucleotides, can modify a cell's genetic code.

Some benefits of naked nucleic acid delivery include low immunogenicity—allowing for multiple administrations—ease of quality control, and long-term stability in a lyophilized state. However, the limited use of naked nucleic acids is due to several major drawbacks, such as poor *in vivo* stability, a non-negligible risk of insertional mutagenesis, low transcription and delivery efficiency, and the potential to induce oncogenesis by activating oncogenes [3].

Numerous delivery techniques have been developed, but additional approaches are still needed to enable highly effective transfection with minimal damage for gene therapy. Several virus species, including adeno-associated viruses, adenoviruses, herpes simplex viruses, and retroviruses, possess the inherent capacity to introduce their genetic material into host cells and replicate it, resulting in highly targeted gene delivery to specific cells through strong transduction [4, 5]. However, alternative methods must be developed, as viruses are highly immunogenic and have limited capacity for transgene DNA insertion. Non-viral delivery methods include magnetofection, sonoporation, photoporation, hydroporation, ballistic DNA injection, and needle injection. Alternatively, chemical methods—such as the use of polymers and cationic lipids—are also employed [6, 7]. The concept of stimuli-responsive vectors, which activate only upon reaching the target cells or organ of interest, has also been explored in recent years for non-viral gene delivery [8]. Replacing costly, time-consuming, and labor-intensive conventional scientific methods with more modern techniques, such as AI-based computational modeling, could be advantageous for improving the development of effective and safe gene delivery vectors. Artificial intelligence (AI) uses a computer or robot controlled by a computer to perform highly complex analytical tasks, utilizing machine-based intelligence as opposed to the natural intelligence exhibited by humans. Table 9.1 provides a brief summary of AI and its associated case studies, which include the ability to accurately simulate biological responses related to nucleic acid delivery, assess the efficacy of therapeutic agents and delivery vehicles, regulate drug and gene delivery parameters, and simulate cells and their organelles to develop highly efficient and non-toxic gene delivery systems (Figure 9.1) [9–12]. Since there is currently no chapter addressing how AI could enhance the engineering of nucleic acid delivery vectors, we will discuss AI's role in the development of genetic material delivery systems, mRNA vaccines, and CRISPR/Cas technologies in this chapter.

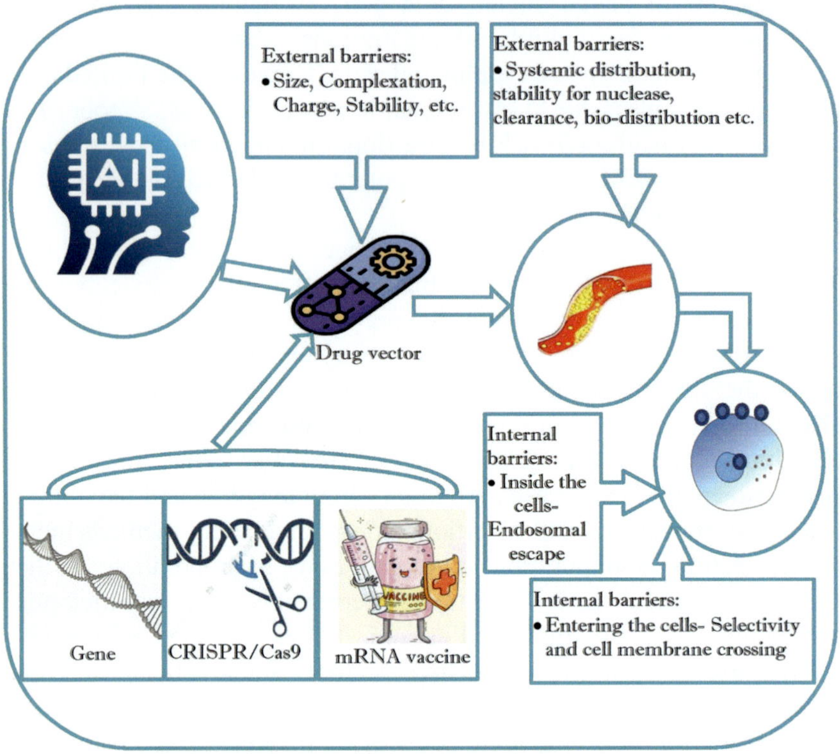

FIGURE 9.1 Diagram illustrating how artificial intelligence is being used to create new nanovectors that effectively penetrate both internal and extracellular barriers.

TABLE 9.1 Summarized Table for Case Studies and Success Stories of Artificial Intelligence (AI)-Driven Approaches for Nucleic Acid Delivery

Case Study/Success Story	Description	AI Approach
NanoFlare: AI-guided nanoparticle delivery system for cancer therapy [67]	NanoFlare utilizes machine learning algorithms to predict optimal nanoparticle characteristics for efficient nucleic acid delivery in cancer cells.	Machine learning algorithms analyze nanoparticle properties and cellular uptake data to predict effective delivery systems.
AI-driven liposomal delivery platform for mRNA vaccines [68]	This case study demonstrates how AI algorithms optimize liposomal formulations for mRNA vaccine delivery, improving stability and efficacy.	Deep learning models analyze lipid composition and structural properties to design liposomes with enhanced mRNA delivery capabilities.

TABLE 9.1 *(Continued)*

Case Study/Success Story	Description	AI Approach
SmartRNA: AI-powered RNA-targeting nanoparticles for gene editing [69]	SmartRNA utilizes artificial intelligence to design nanoparticles capable of targeted delivery of CRISPR-Cas9 components for precise gene editing.	AI algorithms predict RNA sequence motifs and guide nanoparticle design for efficient targeting and delivery.
AI-guided exosome-based delivery system for siRNA therapeutics [70]	This success story showcases how AI algorithms analyze patient-specific data to tailor exosome-based delivery systems for siRNA therapeutics, improving treatment efficacy and reducing side effects.	Machine learning models integrate patient data, including genetic profiles and disease characteristics, to optimize exosome cargo and surface modifications for targeted siRNA delivery.
Deep learning-based optimization of viral vectors for gene therapy [71]	Deep learning algorithms are employed to predict optimal viral vector properties for efficient gene delivery, minimizing off-target effects and enhancing therapeutic outcomes.	Convolutional neural networks analyze viral vector structure-function relationships and predict modifications for improved gene delivery specificity and efficiency.
AI-driven design of peptide-based carriers for nucleic acid delivery [72]	Artificial intelligence algorithms are used to design peptide-based carriers capable of efficient nucleic acid delivery across cell membranes, enabling targeted gene therapy and RNA interference.	Machine learning models predict peptide sequences with high cell-penetrating and nucleic acid-binding properties, facilitating the development of effective delivery vehicles.

9.2 FUNDAMENTALS OF NUCLEIC ACID DELIVERY

In order to modify the expression of proteins in lesions, foreign nucleic acids are delivered, offering a unique therapeutic approach for both congenital and inherited diseases [13–15]. The rapid development timeline, broad range of targeting options, and exceptional therapeutic efficacy of nucleic acid therapies distinguish them from traditional small-molecule and antibody treatments [16, 17]. Nucleic acid medications also provide a way to overcome the limitations associated with undruggable targets [18]. For diseases that were once considered incurable, these advancements offer viable therapeutic options. The field of nucleic acid therapeutics has experienced tremendous progress in both the prevention and treatment of various diseases due to the rapid development of molecular biology techniques such as CRISPR–Cas gene delivery and *in vitro* transcription [19, 20].

In vivo administration of naked nucleic acids presents many obstacles. Selection of delivery vectors is critical to obtaining full therapeutic benefits from nucleic acid medicines. The most suitable vectors would shield nucleic acids from enzyme destruction, aid in cellular absorption and endosomal escape, and be as safe as possible. Effective cellular absorption has been made possible by the development of viral vectors, including adenovirus, lentivirus, and adeno-associated virus [21]. The U.S. Food and Drug Administration has approved Luxturna R and Zolgensma R, two nucleic acid medications administered by viral vector platforms [22, 23]. The majority of the time, nucleic acid therapies based on viral vectors are more effective than traditional treatments over an extended period of time; nevertheless, these pharmaceuticals only require a single injection to be therapeutically effective. However, repetitive delivery of viral vectors is complicated by the possibility of inducing antiviral immune reactions [24]. Furthermore, in several cases of therapeutic usage of viral vector nucleic acid medications, severe events including aberrant blood clots occurred [25]. In the past few years, there has been an increasing interest in the structure of nonviral carriers. Non-viral vectors are easier to produce on a large scale and have lower immunogenicity than viral vectors without the danger of insertional mutations. Traditional non-viral vectors often have restricted tissue selectivity and poor transfection effectiveness [26]. Thankfully, novel substances have surfaced that possess enhanced cell transfection and effective tissue-targeted properties [27]. As demonstrated by a number of preclinical and clinical investigations, lipid nanoparticles (LNPs) have demonstrated considerable promise in the delivery of nucleic acids as drugs [28–30]. The Food and Drug Administration approved Onpattro® (Patisiran), an siRNA–LNP medication that has shown promise in addressing hereditary transthyretin-mediated amyloidosis using just one dosage every three weeks, in 2018 [31]. More than 200 siRNA treatments are presently being developed, and five siRNA-based medications have hit the market after Onpattro's authorization.

Lately, the global SARS-CoV-2 pandemic has led to the remarkable rise of mRNA-based vaccinations against infectious diseases. The two therapies that have shown the most efficacy in preventing and controlling SARS-CoV-2 are BNT162b2 (Comirnaty®) by BioNTech/Pfizer and mRNA-1273 (Spikevax®) by Moderna [31, 32]. Because mRNA vaccines are highly effective, simple to produce, adaptable, and have demonstrated excellent clinical trial efficacy, they hold tremendous potential for both preventing and curing pandemics [33]. China launched its first indigenous COVID-19 mRNA vaccine for emergency use, SYS6006, in March 2023. The vaccine was developed by CSPC Pharmaceuticals Corporation. Nucleic acid-based vaccines account for approximately 20% of the 966 vaccine candidates currently under investigation worldwide, according to a recent study [34, 35]. These vaccines may usher in a new era of pandemic prevention and control and open new avenues for drug development and discovery. Nucleic acid medicines have already made significant strides in the treatment of heart, liver, and eye diseases [36, 37].

9.3 ROLE OF ARTIFICIAL INTELLIGENCE (AI) IN DRUG DELIVERY

AI can improve nanosystem design by allowing for a deeper comprehension of the biological milieu, which can then be used to generate medicinal products through nanoengineering. The human body is a complex system that, for medication delivery purposes, is often simplified into compartments separated by biological barriers. The concept of biological membranes refers to the physicochemical properties of the barriers that divide various biological compartments, thereby encompassing a wide range of epithelia and environments. For instance, an orally administered medication undergoes gastric transit and must pass through the intestinal or stomach epithelium to enter the circulation. It must then reach its target, which may be a tissue, a cellular membrane component, or even an intracellular substance. Biological barriers may be permeated in two ways: passively or actively. Passive diffusion across membranes is governed by physicochemical gradients and typically depends on the molecular properties of the drug. The interaction between the drug and the biological milieu continuously affects its molecular characteristics, influencing *in silico* drug distribution predictions. Furthermore, passive permeation is often ineffective for biologics and certain small molecules unless facilitated by specific drug delivery systems. Active diffusion is carried out by energy-dependent cellular mechanisms, including membrane transport; therefore, it often involves complex biological interactions and substantially higher energy consumption. This may necessitate expanding system simulations to include a greater number of specific variables for computation [38].

The quality by design (QbD) layout of a delivery system is optimized to take advantage of one or more transport processes identified as bottlenecks influencing the pharmacokinetics of the drug, thereby streamlining the system under investigation. For instance, the development of an oral insulin formulation places significant emphasis on the drug's transit across the intestinal wall into the circulation, as nearly the entire API administered orally is lost during this process. The predictability of preclinical models represents one of the limitations at this stage of research and development. For cognitively demanding and complex *in silico* models, accurate parameterization is often the foundation of reliable prediction [39]. Characteristics and models are frequently computed using theoretical information (e.g., physical principles) and empirically validated.

The effort to uncover, create, and define processes, such as membrane contacts, in the modelled human milieu might benefit substantially from the use of AI capable of researching and analyzing multi-layered data. A smart search of literature for variables and comparisons of models has become one of its most important strategies, although it is typically left to the study units' unique expertise and expertise. A computerized system able to investigating, modelling, netting, and improving searching might substantially help to improve the organized assessment of models and parameters. Thus, the capacity to make an accurate prediction and systematically enhance it using findings from *in silico* or clinical studies would represent an ongoing advance, allowing for methodical choice of models and grading [38]. Systemic biology databases are close to becoming able to serve AI applications and provide strong knowledge for AI training. Several instances of neural network software and application vendors, such as those used in pharmacokinetics assessment, have recently established a good foundation for the use of this kind of technology [40]. Additional instances of sophisticated AI systems are developing as instruments to include into the model's complicated inputs, such as medication conversations, phenotypic, chemical, and genetic databases, paving the door for customized medicine [41].

The model is subsequently employed to assess the potential influence of the drug delivery method on the pharmacokinetics of the drug, which includes accumulation and toxicity. A vital decision-making step is deciding which components and modeling should be examined and mimicked, whether to design the system's superior characteristics prior to the empirical trial or to determine the essential qualities that cause what is seen in results from the experiment [42]. For example, a business that owns a medication drug delivery system (a liposome) wants to simulate the influence of their technology on the long-term market circulation of a variety of prospective medicaments. For each of the aforementioned APIs, the algorithm should reflect the most significant absorption, distribution, metabolism, and excretion (ADME) characteristic relative to the drugs in the liposome, forecasting the permeability of the barriers for every drug relative to all of them in the liposome. This may need researching a complex system using combined empirical and *in silico* modeling. An artificial intelligence tool might assist in combining data from various sources and provide recommendations for these medications, considerably benefiting the drug delivery system. For example, examining cellular, pharmaceutical kinetics, and patient data might reveal the most significant obstacles in advancing the creation of a certain medicine system.

A passive AI might assist in incorporating novel molecular property traits that are comparable to recognized substances while also proposing delivery strategies that are expected to be successful for producing a therapy. Given that even a slight boost to the bioavailability or local concentration of a potent drug can result in a significant therapeutic benefit, the results of precise pharmacological modeling can have a substantial influence on the future production of new pharmaceuticals. Drug reuse, or the application of known therapies to new diseases, may benefit immediately from AI adoption in the initial phases of drug discovery [40]. Yet, in many circumstances, medication development through new composition or enhanced drug delivery may be necessary to tailor the medicine's pharmacokinetics or stability to the needs of individual patients. The availability of reliable, information-rich databases remains a barrier to AI adoption. Given the possibility that a large portion of today's results are insufficiently comparable to allow for impartial assessment of algorithms and variables, a proactive AI capable of recognizing and performing to generate or confirm current knowledge may aid in the consolidation of the data required for eventual AI application. This would therefore allow for the creation of a passive AI application that can absorb facts and guide researchers in overcoming the lack of specialized expertise necessary for the logical design of a product.

The impact of active AI, collecting variables, and self-supervising results from experiments may allow for stricter result coding in an understanding database. To give an instance, an AI managing a liquid controller, a UV probe, and a pump runs a series of micronized tests—that is, microfluidic lab-on-chip tests for membrane penetration, biological or biochemical relationships, and potentially even an organ-on-chip study [43, 44]. The AI gathers knowledge on medicines and their distribution mechanisms from relevant literature. It may retest leakage characteristics over an actual or mimicked biomembrane, such as the standard system. In this way, it may combine previous findings into a logical and recorded database; at some point, the AI will perform a comparative study using a new medicine. Another AI in a different lab simulates glomerular filtration or controlled dissolution, whereas enzymatic affinities are evaluated on a chip in a third lab. The outcomes are organized into a database. A development firm researching medication delivery methods can conduct an investigation for an API that could be useful based on their ADME and model the effect of medication delivery systems using more specific variables. In the meantime, an AI bot may use the information to propose a delivery method to a researcher looking to improve insulin absorption in the digestive tract. Once the medication's mechanisms of behavior, metabolism, obstacles, and delivery method have been determined, a foundation for the development and research of the product is created [45, 46].

9.4 CASE STUDY 1: PREDICTIVE MODELING FOR LIPID NANOPARTICLES (LNPS) FORMULATION

LNPs are frequently utilized to deliver mRNA vaccinations. At present, LNP optimization is based mostly on evaluating ionizable lipids using standard methods, which are costly and time-consuming. The current work seeks to use computational techniques to speed the creation of LNPs for mRNA vaccines. Initially, 325 data points of mRNA vaccine LNP compositions having IgG titer were collected. LightGBM, a method based on machine learning, was utilized to create a high-performing prediction model. More significantly, the method discovered key substructures of ionizable lipids in LNPs that were consistent with previously reported findings. The animal study findings revealed that LNP with DLin-MC3-DMA (MC3) as an ionizable lipid and an N/P ratio of 6:1 caused greater efficacy in mice over LNP with SM-102, which was in accordance with the model predictions. Molecular dynamic simulation was employed to study the molecular workings of the LNPs used in the study. The findings revealed that molecules of lipid accumulated to form LNPs, whereas molecules of mRNA were bound within the LNPs. To summarize, the machine learning prediction algorithm for LNP-based mRNA vaccines was initially built, confirmed through tests, and then combined with molecular simulation. In the not-too-distant future, the method of prediction might be utilized to perform a virtual evaluation of LNP compositions [47].

LNPs are nanocarriers made up of four different lipids that can be utilized for gene therapy, protein replacement, and vaccine production. Nevertheless, LNPs confront a number of challenges, including toxicity, immunological activation, and limited effectiveness in delivery. To address these issues, artificial intelligence may be utilized to improve LNP design and composition, as well as to predict their attributes and performance. Furthermore, antibody-targeted ligation can be employed to enhance the selectivity and specificity of LNPs by linking an antibody that detects a specific antigen on the outer layer of the cell to the LNP [48].

9.5 CASE STUDY 2: MACHINE LEARNING FOR TARGETED DELIVERY SYSTEMS

Nanoparticles, liposomes, and polymeric micelles are examples of nanocarriers that have proven successful in delivering therapeutic medicines to specific target areas (Table 9.1) [49]. AI algorithms can aid in nanocarrier development and optimization by analyzing complex correlations between their attributes and efficiency. Scientists may use AI algorithms to construct forecasting models that take into account a variety of criteria, such as nanocarrier physicochemical properties, pharmacological features, and biological aspects [49, 50]. These simulations can help determine the best nanocarrier materials, size, surface modifications, and other formulation characteristics for optimal medication delivery.

Shahiwala et al. [51] present a machine learning technique for creating optimal medication compositions. The recommended reporting materials for systematic reviews and meta-analyses approach was used for screening literature, yielding 114 niosome compositions. Eleven features (input factors) of pharmaceuticals and niosomes that influence the size of particles and drug entrapment (output variables) were carefully identified and employed in network development. The model was trained using the hyperbolic tangent of the sigmoid transfer function, in addition to Levenberg–Marquardt backpropagation. The network achieved a maximum prediction accuracy of 93.76% and 91.79% for percent drug entrapment and particle size, respectively. Sensitivity analysis revealed that the drug/lipid ratio and cholesterol/surfactant ratios were the most important parameters influencing percent drug entrapment and particle size of niosomes. To verify the established model, nine Donepezil hydrochloride niosome batches were created using a 3×3 factorial design with components including drug/lipid proportion and cholesterol/surfactant ratio. The model achieved a prediction accuracy of greater than 97% for experimental batches. Lastly, global artificial neural networks (ANN) outperformed local response surface methodologies for Donepezil niosome compositions. Although the ANN accurately identified the characteristics of Donepezil niosomes, various medications with diverse physical and chemical characteristics must be evaluated to prove the reliability of the model and its utility for developing novel drug niosomal compositions [51].

9.6 CASE STUDY 3: DEEP LEARNING FOR ENHANCING INTRACELLULAR DELIVERY EFFICIENCY

Kumar et al. [52] investigate the possibility of laser-induced nano-photonporation as a non-invasive approach for intracellular administration of micro/macromolecules at the individual cell level. This study suggests using gold-coated spiky nanoparticles of polymers (Au-PNPs) and gold nanorods (GNRs) to accomplish effective intracellular micro/macromolecule delivery at the single-cell scale. The effectiveness and survivability of Au-PNP-mediated photon-poration are compared to those of GNR-mediated intracellular delivery by shifting the wavelength of operation to the near-infrared (NIR) region. Au-PNPs are used as mediators in combination with nanosecond-pulsed lasers to provide highly effective delivery into cells while maintaining excellent cell viability. Laser pulses aimed at Au-PNPs produce more than 100 hot spots per particle due to plasmon resonance, enabling the development of photothermal vapor nanobubbles (PVNBs). Such PVNBs form transient pores, allowing cargo to be transferred from the extracellular to the intracellular environment without damaging the cells. Optimizing wavelengths in the NIR region, in addition to low laser intensity (27 mJ/cm^2) and nanoparticle concentration (34 μg/mL), results in 96% delivery efficacy and up to 99% cell survival across multiple cell types, notably cancer and neurons. Additionally, significant cell viability (90%–95%) is maintained 48 hours after laser irradiation. This new breakthrough has great potential for a variety of applications, including the administration of medications, gene therapy, and regenerative healthcare. This work highlights the proposed technique's effectiveness and adaptability, establishing it as a vital tool for improving intracellular delivery techniques in medical fields [52].

A lack of knowledge regarding intracellular delivery and targeting impedes the growth of nucleic acid-based therapies delivered by nanoparticles. Using an siRNA-targeting and small-molecule profiling technique in conjunction with sophisticated imaging and machine learning, scientific insights on the process of mRNA distribution by lipid nanoparticles (MC3-LNP) are provided. This procedure is known as Enhanced Cellular and Endocytic Characterization for Inside of Cells Delivery (ACE-ID). To determine the impact on effective mRNA delivery, a cell-based scanning experiment and disruption of 178 intracellular trafficking sites were utilized. Targets that improve delivery are identified by collecting data-rich phenotypic characteristics from images using modern image analysis methods. Machine learning is utilized to discover critical traits associated with increased delivery, revealing fluid-phase endocytosis as a fruitful cellular entry pathway. With this new understanding, MC3-LNP is re-engineered to focus on macropinocytosis, which increases the delivery of mRNA both *in vitro* and *in vivo*. The ACE-ID technique is useful for improving nanomedicine-based intracellular methods of administration and has the potential to accelerate the development of nucleic acid-based therapeutic delivery systems [53].

9.7 CASE STUDY 4: ARTIFICIAL INTELLIGENCE (AI)-GUIDED DESIGN OF NOVEL DELIVERY VEHICLES

Around the world, researchers are seeking viable therapeutic agents against SARS-CoV-2. While computer simulations of docking continue to be widely used for *in silico* ligand design and high-throughput evaluation of medicinal drugs, they have significant limitations in the development of novel potential ligands due to their substantial computational cost and the vastness of chemical space. We describe a *de novo* molecular design technique that uses AI to uncover novel anti-SARS-CoV-2 therapeutics. A recurrent search and retrain technique employs a Monte Carlo tree search algorithm, a multitask neural network surrogate model, and recurrent neural networks for computationally expensive docking modeling and rollouts, respectively. The authors generate multiple (~100) novel drug candidates that outperform both Food and Drug Administration (FDA)-approved (~1,000) and non-FDA molecules (~1 million) in terms of binding to either the isolated spike protein (S-protein) at the host receptor interface or the S-protein/angiotensin-converting enzyme 2 (ACE2) receptor complex, using Vina scores as the evaluation metric. This AI approach may be broadly applicable for the rapid development and identification of chemical compounds with specified capabilities [54].

Exscientia [55], a UK-based company, collaborated with Evotec to create an AI-designed small-molecule blocker for the A2A receptor for the 2020 clinical trial EXS-21546 as immunotherapy for cancer. Protein kinase C theta, another putative first-in-class small-molecule inhibitor developed by Exscientia, is intended for use in immunological and inflammatory conditions. In a move currently undergoing clinical validation, another UK-based company adapted baricitinib for the treatment of COVID-19 [55].

A Phase II clinical trial (INS018_055) involving individuals suffering from idiopathic pulmonary fibrosis (IPF) saw the successful administration of the first dose of an AI-developed "first-in-class" anti-fibrotic small-molecule antagonist in 2023 by the Hong Kong-based AI company *in-silico* Medicine [55]. The ISM3312 [55] clinical study was shown to reduce viral load in lung tissue in COVID-19 patients in a separate preclinical investigation conducted by *in-silico* Medicine.

9.8 SUCCESS STORIES IN CLINICAL TRANSLATION

9.8.1 OVERVIEW OF SUCCESSFUL AI-DRIVEN APPROACHES IN CLINICAL TRIALS

The most important evaluation method for the secure, dependable, and successful development of medicines is clinical trials. AI is being used more and more in medical and healthcare organizations due to data-related limitations, labor-intensive manual processes, remote patient monitoring, and the complexity of conventional clinical trials on individuals. A tailored artificial intelligence solution is the most effective approach for conducting quick and efficient clinical trials. By using AI solutions, potential issues are eliminated, clinical trial execution times are shortened, and the procedure becomes more precise and efficient [56].

Holoscan MGX enables the development and implementation of real-time AI applications. By providing an all-in-one, healthcare-grade conventional layout and long-term software support, Clara Holoscan MGX broadens the Clara Holoscan platform and accelerates development in the healthcare industry [57]. This benefits the corporation by enhancing the AI it employs for medication discovery, diagnosis, and therapy. AstraZeneca selected an additional novel candidate for idiopathic pulmonary fibrosis (IPF) for its medicinal product pipeline, according to a May 2022 announcement from BenevolentAI, a leading clinical-stage AI-enabled drug discovery company [58]. The Compassionate Platform for IPF and chronic kidney disease (CKD) was used to identify the candidate. AstraZeneca then evaluated and selected it for inclusion in its pipeline. This builds upon the agreement reached in January 2022 to expand the collaboration with AstraZeneca to cover two additional disease areas: heart failure and systemic lupus erythematosus. The company's collaborative relationships have improved as a result of this (Table 9.1).

9.8.2 CASE EXAMPLES OF NUCLEIC ACID DELIVERY SYSTEMS REACHING CLINICAL STAGES

A few of these advancements have even made it to the clinical stage. For example, the initial clinical use of siRNA delivery was made possible by the natural polymer cyclodextrin [59, 60]. The natural macrocyclic oligosaccharide cyclodextrin has a hydrophobic interior and hydrophilic exterior, which can interact and increase the stability of NAs. However, its relatively high toxicity presents a significant obstacle to widespread translation into healthcare applications [61]. In addition to cyclodextrin, a number of other naturally occurring polymers have been thoroughly investigated as potential options for nucleic acid delivery methods. These include chitosan, dextran, hyaluronic acid, and gelatin [62, 63].

This issue has been effectively resolved by the German company CureVac through the development of the RNA active system. Protamine functions as a TLR7/8 blocker in this protamine–mRNA combination to trigger a Th1 cell reaction, while the mRNA expressing the desired protein is delivered to antigen-presenting cells (APCs) to trigger an adaptive immune response [64]. In a Phase I/II trial, CV9103, a self-adjuvanted mRNA vaccine that targeted prostate cancer antigens, was shown to be immunogenic and tolerable. In a clinical trial involving individuals with stage IV non-small-cell lung cancer, 21 out of the 25 participants (84%) and 12 out of 26 patients (46.2%) showed evidence of stable disease [65]. A Phase I/II clinical study combining the CV9202 vaccine with either anti-PD-L1 durvalumab or anti-CTLA-4 tremelimumab is being conducted; the results have not yet been released.

For instance, the FixVac (cancer antigen) mRNA–lipid nanoparticle (LNP) vaccine is being assessed in a number of active clinical studies. BNT111 is the first mRNA–LNP vaccine in a series that incorporates a common tumor-associated antigen (TAA) by sharing FixVac (cancer antigen) preset combinations. Of the four melanoma-associated proteins that exhibit significant immunogenicity and frequency in melanoma, BNT111 expresses at least one of them. BNT111 demonstrated the ability to elicit CD4- and CD8-positive T cell responses in 39 out of 50 patients (75%) who exhibited an immunological reaction to one or more TAAs, according to a Phase I dose-escalation study (NCT02410733) that assessed its safety and efficacy. Six individuals (35%) and two patients (12%) with stable disease were among the 17 individuals who underwent combination treatment with BNT111 and anti-PD-1. Three patients (12%) experienced partial recovery, and seven patients (28%) had stable disease out of the 25 patients who received BNT111 alone. FixVac BNT111 is currently being investigated in a randomized Phase II clinical trial (NCT04526899) for the management of stage III and IV melanoma that is recurrent and incurable or unresponsive to anti-PD-1 antibodies. BNT111 can be used alone or in combination with cemiplimab, an anti-PD-1 antibody. The efficacy of the cancer vaccine BNT112, which contains five TAAs, as a treatment for individuals with metastatic prostate cancer, either in isolation or in conjunction with cemiplimab, is currently being evaluated in a Phase I/II clinical study (NCT04382898) [66].

9.9 ETHICAL AND REGULATORY CONSIDERATIONS

A major ethical problem in AI-driven medication systems for distribution is obtaining informed permission. Patients should be informed in an understandable manner about how AI algorithms are used in their care and how this might affect them.

9.9.1 ETHICAL IMPLICATIONS OF AI-DRIVEN HEALTHCARE FACILITIES

The healthcare industry must navigate a complicated web of ethical issues as it explores the transformational potential of robots and AI. Although robots and AI have great promise to improve patient treatment and expedite procedures, they also bring unique ethical issues that need to be carefully considered and addressed. This section explores the moral implications of deploying robots and AI in healthcare, emphasizing key areas of concern.

9.9.1.1 DATA SAFETY AND CONFIDENTIALITY

- **Data Protection for Patients:** The use of robots and AI in healthcare produces a significant quantity of private patient information. The safety and confidentiality of this data must be guaranteed, as any compromise might seriously harm patient confidence and the accuracy of the data [73].

9.9.1.2 APPROPRIATE DATA MANAGEMENT AND STORAGE

- **The Handling of Data Procedures:** Healthcare facilities need to have acceptable procedures for gathering, preserving, and using patient data. To protect information about patients, this comprises strong data anonymization methods, encoding, and safe data-sharing procedures [74].

9.9.1.3 DISPARITIES AND PREJUDICE

- **Taking Care of Algorithmic Bias:** AI systems may unintentionally reinforce prejudices found in past medical records, which might result in discrepancies in diagnosis and course of treatment.

Algorithms that reduce prejudice and advance equity in healthcare choices must be developed [75].

9.9.1.4 SAFEGUARDING IMPARTIALITY IN ARTIFICIAL INTELLIGENCE (AI)-DRIVEN JUDGMENT

- **The Ability to Explain and Honesty:** In healthcare AI, clear decision-making procedures are essential. To promote responsibility and trust, both patients and medical professionals need to comprehend the reasoning underlying AI-driven suggestions [76].

9.9.1.5 RESPONSIBILITY AND TRANSPARENCY

Determining who is clearly responsible for the behavior of AI systems is difficult yet necessary when it comes to robotic and AI systems. Ethical usage requires identifying the person accountable for mistakes or unfavorable outcomes [77–80].

9.10 IMPLICATIONS OF AI FOR THE DELIVERY OF NUCLEIC ACIDS

Artificial intelligence is capable of quickly and accurately analyzing a wide range of tasks. By using AI to transport genes, cutting-edge delivery devices with remarkable features including programmability, accountability, little toxicity, robust effectiveness, and tailored distribution might be created. Yet, using AI for delivering genes will present a number of difficulties, including ethical issues, environmental adaptation, lost code retrieval, loss of information risk, high maintenance and repair expenses, and continual software upgrades. Before AI applications become commonplace, these obstacles must be understood and addressed [81–83]. The first problem to be solved would be the costly and laborious procedure of gathering a sizable amount of high-quality data to produce an AI model with adequate reliability and precision [84, 85]. In contrast with the aforementioned cases, where AI-based models have primarily been used to address specific problems—such as cell binding for a limited the library of delivery vehicle formulations—algorithms and networks must become more potent and versatile in the not-too-distant future in order to foresee multiple outcomes from a broad range of compositions and biological inputs. The organization and analysis of these AI-based methods and data provide another difficulty, and it looks like computer scientists, biologists, and material scientists must work together on this project concurrently. By utilizing AI and its subsets (ML and DL, for example) in different stages of clinical research with humans, extremely effective and customized delivery methods may be created. This requires the collection of sophisticated and precise pathophysiology data from target patient populations, in addition to a solid grasp of the biology of the final goal and its constituent organs and cells. Genotype-to-phenotype forecasting, phenotype-to-genotype visualization, patient hiring, cohort identification, and choosing would all be required. Clinical studies might be more precisely planned with the use of knowledge from past reported trials, comparisons of intricate multiple factors, and millions of observation points. These objectives would be more easily attained if data silos were eliminated, third-party data was used, big and diverse data sources were managed, complicated and concealed trends were found, and complex consequences were predicted. There is an inherent bias in the information that is currently accessible due to a number of factors, such as the difficulty of applying AI to produce new sets of data due to the various formats and quality levels of health record information coming from numerous nations with varying rules (e.g., genetic records primarily concentrate on individuals of European descent). Enabling collaborative decision-making while safeguarding autonomy for patients and confidentiality of data is also essential [86–89].

9.11 CONCLUSIONS

Cutting-edge contemporary methods, such as AI-based computer simulations, may eventually replace the use of conventional experiments for improving new gene carriers in terms of characterization, synthesis methodologies, transfection effectiveness, specific delivery, and cytotoxicity. When compared with trial-and-error methods, this might result in significantly less money and time, as well as better outcomes. By using a light-sensitive microscope with AI capabilities, AI might make it easier to see organelles within cells and cell contents precisely. AI has the potential to reduce the negative consequences of CRISPR/Cas techniques and to follow the advancement of gene delivery vehicles throughout intracellular movement. AI-driven computer simulations and algorithms are also capable of simulating organelles within cell membranes and the ways in which they communicate with the gene delivery vehicles. Creating a gene/mRNA vaccine delivery carrier that can pass through extracellular and intracellular obstructions, leading to strong transfection efficacy and minimal toxicity, could be easier than in the past. The design of ideal gene delivery vehicles may be improved by combining big data from the aforementioned artificial intelligence models with understanding of viral cell entrance processes.

ACKNOWLEDGMENT

None

CONFLICT OF INTEREST

The authors declare no conflict of interest

FUNDING

None

KEYWORDS

- **artificial intelligence**
- **case studies**
- **drug delivery**
- **gene therapy**
- **lipid nanoparticles**
- **nanocarriers**
- **nucleic acid delivery**
- **personalized medicine**

REFERENCES

1. Dunbar, C. E., High, K. A., Joung, J. K., Kohn, D. B., Ozawa, K., & Sadelain, M. (2018). Gene therapy comes of age. *Science*, *359*(6372), eaan4672.
2. Verma, I. M., Naldini, L., Kafri, T., Miyoshi, H., Takahashi, M., Blömer, U., Somia, L., Wang, F., & Gage, F. (2000). Gene therapy: Promises, problems and prospects. In *Genes and Resistance to Disease* (pp. 147–157). Springer: Singapore.
3. Herweijer, H., & Wolff, J. (2003). Progress and prospects: Naked DNA gene transfer and therapy. *Gene Therapy*, *10*(6), 453–458.
4. Challis, R. C., Ravindra, Kumar, S., Chan, K. Y., Challis, C., Beadle, K., Jang, M. J., Kim, H. M., Rajendran, P. S., Tompkins, J. D., Shivkumar, K., & Deverman, B. E. (2019). Systemic AAV vectors for widespread and targeted gene delivery in rodents. *Nature Protocols*, *14*(2), 379–414.
5. Colella, P., Trapani, I., Cesi, G., Sommella, A., Manfredi, A., Puppo, A., Iodice, C., Rossi, S., Simonelli, F., Giunti, M., & Bacci, M. L. (2014). Efficient gene delivery to the cone-enriched pig retina by dual AAV vectors. *Gene Therapy*, *21*(4), 450–456.
6. Trentin, D., Hubbell, J., & Hall, H. (2005). Non-viral gene delivery for local and controlled DNA release. *Journal of Controlled Release*, *102*(1), 263–275.
7. Mehier-Humbert, S., & Guy, R. H. (2005). Physical methods for gene transfer: Improving the kinetics of gene delivery into cells. *Advanced Drug Delivery Reviews*, *57*(5), 733–753.
8. Karimi, M., Ghasemi, A., Zangabad, P. S., Rahighi, R., Basri, S. M. M., Mirshekari, H., Amiri, M., Pishabad, Z. S., Aslani, A., Bozorgomid, M., & Ghosh, D. (2016). Smart micro/nanoparticles in stimulus-responsive drug/gene delivery systems. *Chemical Society Reviews*, *45*(5), 1457–1501.
9. Hassanzadeh, P., Atyabi, F., & Dinarvand, R. (2019). The significance of artificial intelligence in drug delivery system design. *Advanced Drug Delivery Reviews*, *151*, 169–190.
10. He, S., Leanse, L. G., & Feng, Y. (2021). Artificial intelligence and machine learning assisted drug delivery for effective treatment of infectious diseases. *Advanced Drug Delivery Reviews*, *178*, 113922.
11. Ho, D., Wang, P., & Kee, T. (2019). Artificial intelligence in nanomedicine. *Nanoscale Horizons*, *4*(2), 365–377.
12. Castro, B. M., Elbadawi, M., Ong, J. J., Pollard, T., Song, Z., Gaisford, S., Pérez, G., Basit, A. W., Cabalar, P., & Goyanes, A. (2021). Machine learning predicts 3D printing performance of over 900 drug delivery systems. *Journal of Controlled Release*, *337*, 530–545.
13. Zhao, Y. X., Shu, R., & Liu, J. (2021). The development and improvement of ribonucleic acid therapy strategies. *Molecular Therapy–Nucleic Acids*, *26*, 997–1013. https://doi.org/10.1016/j.omtn.2021.09.002 (accessed on 23rd June 2025).
14. Sarli, S. L., & Watts, J. K. (2022). Harnessing nucleic acid technologies for human health on Earth and in space. *Life Sciences in Space Research*, *35*, 113–126. https://doi.org/10.1016/j.lssr.2022.08.006 (accessed on 23rd June 2025).
15. Sharma, P., Dasputre, N., & Jain, V. (2024). Nanomedicine: Concepts, characteristics, and regulatory challenges. In *Smart Nanocarrier for Effective Drug Delivery* (pp. 1–16). CRC Press.

16. Chen, J. X., Zhu, D. D., Lian, B. P., Shi, K., Chen, P., Li, Y., Lin, W., Ding, L., Long, Q., Wang, Y., & Laurini, E. (2023). Cargo-selective and adaptive delivery of nucleic acid therapeutics by bola-amphiphilic dendrimers. *Proceedings of the National Academy of Sciences of the United States of America*, *120*(21), 11. https://doi.org/10.1073/pnas.2220787120 (accessed on 23rd June 2025).
17. Sharma, P., Jain, V., Jain, A., & Tailang, M. (2022). Role of swarm intelligence for health monitoring and related actions. In *Internet of Things and Fog Computing-Enabled Solutions for Real-Life Challenges* (pp. 95–118). CRC Press.
18. Finan, C., Gaulton, A., Kruger, F. A., Lumbers, R. T., Shah, T., Engmann, J., Galver, L., Kelley, R., Karlsson, A., Santos, R., & Overington, J. P. (2017). The druggable genome and support for target identification and validation in drug development. *Science Translational Medicine*, *9*(383), 15. https://doi.org/10.1126/scitranslmed.aag1166 (accessed on 23rd June 2025).
19. Kazemian, P., Yu, S. Y., Thomson, S. B., Birkenshaw, A., Leavitt, B. R., & Ross, C. J. (2022). Lipid-nanoparticle-based delivery of CRISPR/Cas9 genome-editing components. *Molecular Pharmaceutics*, *19*(6), 1669–1686. https://doi.org/10.1021/acs.molpharmaceut.1c00916 (accessed on 23rd June 2025).
20. Sharma, P., Jain, V., & Tailang, M. (2023). Advancement of nanocarrier-based engineering for specific drug delivery for cancer therapy. In *Targeted Cancer Therapy in Biomedical Engineering* (pp. 465–486). Springer Nature Singapore.
21. Dogbey, D. M., Torres, V. E., Fajemisin, E., Mpondo, L., Ngwenya, T., Akinrinmade, O. A., Perriman, A. W., & Barth, S. (2023). Technological advances in the use of viral and non-viral vectors for delivering genetic and non-genetic cargos for cancer therapy. *Drug Delivery and Translational Research*, *13*(11), 2719–2738. https://doi.org/10.1007/s13346-023-01362-3 (accessed on 23rd June 2025).
22. Zhao, Z. M., Anselmo, A. C., & Mitragotri, S. (2022). Viral vector-based gene therapies in the clinic. *Bioengineering & Translational Medicine*, *7*(1), 20. https://doi.org/10.1002/btm2.10258 (accessed on 23rd June 2025).
23. Sharma, P., Jain, V., & Tailang, M. (2023). How artificial intelligence is transforming medicine: The future of pharmaceutical research. In *Industry 4.0 and Healthcare: Impact of Artificial Intelligence* (pp. 133–150). Springer Nature Singapore.
24. Ertl, H. C. J. (2022). Immunogenicity and toxicity of AAV gene therapy. *Frontiers in Immunology*, *13*, 9. https://doi.org/10.3389/fimmu.2022.975803 (accessed on 23rd June 2025).
25. Gresele, P., Momi, S., Marcucci, R., Ramundo, F., De Stefano, V., & Tripodi, A. (2021). Interactions of adenoviruses with platelets immune thrombotic thrombocytopenia syndrome. *Hematological*, *106*(12), 3034–3045. https://doi.org/10.3324/haematol.2021.279289 (accessed on 23rd June 2025).
26. Ferreras, L. A. B., Chan, S. Y., Reina, S. V., Vazquez Reina, S., & Dixon, J. E. (2021). Rapidly transducing and spatially localized magnetofection using peptide-mediated non-viral gene delivery based on iron oxide nanoparticles. *ACS Applied Nano Materials*, *4*(1), 167–181. https://doi.org/10.1021/acsanm.0c02465 (accessed on 23rd June 2025).
27. Shukla, A., & Maiti, P. (2022). Nanomedicine and versatile therapies for cancer treatment. *MedComm*, *3*(3), e163. https://doi.org/10.1002/mco2.163 (accessed on 23rd June 2025).

28. Paunovska, K., Loughrey, D., & Dahlman, J. E. (2022). Drug delivery systems for RNA therapeutics. *Nature Reviews Genetics*, *23*(5), 265–280. https://doi.org/10.1038/s41576-021-00439-4 (accessed on 23rd June 2025).
29. Tenchov, R., Bird, R., Curtze, A. E., & Zhou, Q. (2021). Lipid nanoparticles—from liposomes to mRNA vaccine delivery, a landscape of research diversity and advancement. *ACS Nano*, *15*(11), 16982–17015. https://doi.org/10.1021/acsnano.1c04996 (accessed on 23rd June 2025).
30. Sharma, P. (2023). Nanostructured biomaterials in drug delivery: Current trends and upcoming possibilities. In *Engineered Biomaterials: Synthesis and Applications* (pp. 261–280). Springer Nature Singapore.
31. Polack, F. P., Thomas, S. J., Kitchin, N., Absalon, J., Gurtman, A., Lockhart, S., Perez, J. L., Pérez Marc, G., Moreira, E. D., Zerbini, C., & Bailey, R. (2020). Safety and efficacy of the BNT162b2 mRNA COVID-19 vaccine. *The New England Journal of Medicine*, *383*(27), 2603–2615. https://doi.org/10.1056/NEJMoa2034577 (accessed on 23rd June 2025).
32. Teo, S. P. (2022). Review of COVID-19 mRNA vaccines: BNT162b2 and mRNA-1273. *Journal of Pharmacy Practice*, *35*(6), 947–951. https://doi.org/10.1177/08971900211009650 (accessed on 23rd June 2025).
33. Wang, Y., Zhang, Z., Luo, J., Han, X., Wei, Y., & Wei, X. (2021). mRNA vaccine: A potential therapeutic strategy. *Molecular Cancer*, *20*(1), 33. https://doi.org/10.1186/s12943-021-01311-z (accessed on 23rd June 2025).
34. Yue, J., Liu, Y., Zhao, M., Bi, X., Li, G., & Liang, W. (2023). The R&D landscape for infectious disease vaccines. *Nature Reviews Drug Discovery*. https://doi.org/10.1038/d41573-023-00119-4 (accessed on 23rd June 2025).
35. Sharma, P. (2021). Modification of human behavior due to coronavirus outbreak: A brief study on current scenario. *AJP*, *15*(3).
36. Huang, Y., Zhu, X., Guo, X., Zhou, Y., Liu, D., Mao, J., Xiong, Y., Deng, Y., & Gao, X. (2023). Advances in mRNA vaccines for viral diseases. *Journal of Medical Virology*, *95*(7), 20. https://doi.org/10.1002/jmv.28924 (accessed on 23rd June 2025).
37. Sharma, P., Jain, V., & Tailang, M. (2022). Swarm intelligence and machine learning algorithms for cancer diagnosis. In *Swarm Intelligence and Machine Learning* (pp. 34–50). CRC Press.
38. Bhhatarai, B., Walters, W. P., Hop, C. E. C. A., Lanza, G., & Ekins, S. (2019). Opportunities and challenges using artificial intelligence in ADME/Tox. *Nature Materials*, *18*, 418–422.
39. Sharma, P., & Tailang, M. (2020). Design, optimization, and evaluation of hydrogel of primaquine loaded nano emulsion for malaria therapy. *FJPS*, *6*, 1–1.
40. Mak, K. K., & Pichika, M. R. (2019). Artificial intelligence in drug development: Present status and future prospects. *Drug Discovery Today*, *24*, 773–780.
41. Ryu, J. Y., Kim, H. U., & Lee, S. Y. (2018). Deep learning improves prediction of drug-drug and drug-food interactions. *Proceedings of the National Academy of Sciences of the United States of America*, *115*, E4304–E4311.
42. Sharma, P., & Jain, V. (2023). An overview of current advances and pharmaceutical uses of 3D and 4D printing. *Exploration of Medicine*, *4*, 560–575.

43. Cui, P., & Wang, S. (2018). Application of microfluidic chip technology in pharmaceutical analysis: A review. *Journal of Pharmaceutical Analysis*, *9*. https://doi.org/10.1016/J.JPHA.2018.12.001 (accessed on 23rd June 2025).
44. Sharma, P. (2023). Validated ultraviolet spectrophotometric method for simultaneous estimation of olmesartan medoxomil in marketed formulation. *AJP*, *17*(03).
45. Balogh, G. T., Müller, J., & Könczöl, A. (2013). pH-gradient PAMPA-based *in vitro* model assay for drug-induced phospholipids in early stage of drug discovery. *European Journal of Pharmaceutical Sciences*, *49*, 81–89.
46. Sharma, P., & Tailang, M. (2017). Opportunities and challenges to develop transdermal patch with nanocarrier. *World Journal of Pharmaceutical Research*, *6*(15), 392–400.
47. Wang, W., Feng, S., Ye, Z., Gao, H., Lin, J., & Ouyang, D. (2022). Prediction of lipid nanoparticles for mRNA vaccines by the machine learning algorithm. *Acta Pharmaceutica Sinica B*, *12*(6), 2950–2962.
48. Yuan, Y., Wu, Y., Cheng, J., Yang, K., Xia, Y., Wu, H., & Pan, X. (2024). Applications of artificial intelligence to lipid nanoparticle delivery. *Particuology*, *90*, 88–97.
49. Zeb, A., Qureshi, O. S., Kim, H. S., Kim, M. S., Kang, J. H., Park, J. S., & Kim, J. K. (2017). High payload itraconazole-incorporated lipid nanoparticles with modulated release property for oral and parenteral administration. *Journal of Pharmacy and Pharmacology*, *6*, 955–966.
50. Sharma, P., Bhargava, S., Parashar, D., & Mangal, A. (2017). Formulation and evaluation of nanoparticles containing cyclophosphamide. *World Journal of Pharmaceutical Research*, *7*(1), 785–798.
51. Shahiwala, A. F., Qawoogha, S. S., & Faruqui, N. (2023). Designing optimum drug delivery systems using machine learning approaches: A prototype study of niosomes. *AAPS PharmSciTech*, *24*(4), 94.
52. Kumar, A., Nahak, B. K., Gupta, P., Santra, T. S., & Tseng, F. G. (2024). Laser-induced intracellular delivery: Exploiting gold-coated spiky polymeric nanoparticles and gold nanorods under near-infrared pulses for single-cell nano-photon-poration. *Micromachines*, *15*(2), 168.
53. Hunter, M. R., Cui, L., Porebski, B. T., Pereira, S., Sonzini, S., Odunze, U., Iyer, P., Engkvist, O., Lloyd, R. L., Peel, S., & Sabirsh, A. (2023). Understanding intracellular biology to improve mRNA delivery by lipid nanoparticles. *Small Methods*, *7*(9), 2201695.
54. Srinivasan, S., Batra, R., Chan, H., Kamath, G., Cherukara, M. J., & Sankaranarayanan, S. K. (2021). Artificial intelligence-guided *de novo* molecular design targeting COVID-19. *ACS Omega*, *6*(19), 12557–12566.
55. Singh, S., Gupta, H., Sharma, P., & Sahi, S. (2024). Advances in artificial intelligence (AI)-assisted approaches in drug screening. *Artificial Intelligence Chemistry*, *2*(1), 100039.
56. Chopra, H., Shin, D. K., Munjal, K., Dhama, K., & Emran, T. B. (2023). Revolutionizing clinical trials: The role of AI in accelerating medical breakthroughs. *International Surgery Journal*, *109*(12), 4211–4220.
57. AuntMinnie.com. (2024). Nvidia unveils Clara Holoscan MGX at GTC 2022. https://www.auntminnie.com/index.aspx?sec=log&itemid=135326 (accessed on 23rd June 2025).
58. BenevolentAI. (2024). BenevolentAI achieves further milestones in AI-enabled target identification collaboration with AstraZeneca. https://www.benevolent.

com/news-and-media/press-releases-and-in-media/benevolentai-achieves-further-milestones-ai-enabled-target-identification-collaboration-astrazeneca/ (accessed on 23rd June 2025).

59. Yin, H., Kanasty, R. L., Eltoukhy, A. A., Vegas, A. J., Dorkin, J. R., & Anderson, D. G. (2014). Non-viral vectors for gene-based therapy. *Nature Reviews Genetics*, *15*, 541–555. https://doi.org/10.1038/nrg3763 (accessed on 23rd June 2025).
60. Pankaj, S., Ashish, D., Dheerendra, R., Yogendra, R., Ramakant, J. K., & Kuldeep, S. (2015). Formulate and evaluate orodispersible tablets of primaquine. *Indo American Journal of Pharmaceutical Research*, *5*(5), 1625–1632.
61. Barata, P., Sood, A. K., & Hong, D. S. (2016). RNA-targeted therapeutics in cancer clinical trials: Current status and future directions. *Cancer Treatment Reviews*, *50*, 35–47. https://doi.org/10.1016/j.ctrv.2016.08.004 (accessed on 23rd June 2025).
62. Xiao, Y., Shi, K., Qu, Y., Chu, B., & Qian, Z. (2019). Engineering nanoparticles for targeted delivery of nucleic acid therapeutics in tumor. *Molecular Therapy–Methods & Clinical Development*, *12*, 1–18. https://doi.org/10.1016/j.omtm.2018.09.002 (accessed on 23rd June 2025).
63. Sharma, P., & Tailang, M. (2019). pH dependent release potential of natural polymers in sustained release of ornidazole from colon targeted delivery system. *International Journal of Drug Delivery Technology*, *9*, 1–10.
64. Kowalczyk, A., Doener, F., Zanzinger, K., Noth, J., Baumhof, P., Fotin, M., & Heidenreich, R. (2016). *Vaccine*, *34*, 3882.
65. Kübler, H., Scheel, B., Gnad-Vogt, U., Miller, K., Schultze-Seemann, W., Vom Dorp, F., Parmiani, G., Hampel, C., Wedel, S., Trojan, L., & Jocham, D. (2015). Self-adjuvanted mRNA vaccination in advanced prostate cancer patients: A first-in-man phase I/IIa study. *Journal for Immunotherapy of Cancer, 3, 26.*
66. Lorentzen, C. L., Haanen, J. B., Met, Ø., & Svane, I. M. (2022). Clinical advances and ongoing trials of mRNA vaccines for cancer treatment. *The Lancet Oncology*, *23*(10), e450–e458.
67. Fujita, H., Ohta, S., Nakamura, N., Somiya, M., & Horie, M. (2023). Progress of endogenous and exogenous nanoparticles for cancer therapy and diagnostics. *Genes*, *14*(2), 259.
68. Lopes, C., Cristóvão, J., Silvério, V., Lino, P. R., & Fonte, P. (2022). Microfluidic production of mRNA-loaded lipid nanoparticles for vaccine applications. *Expert Opinion on Drug Delivery*, *19*(10), 1381–1395.
69. Mollé, L. M., Smyth, C. H., Yuen, D., & Johnston, A. P. (2022). Nanoparticles for vaccine and gene therapy: Overcoming the barriers to nucleic acid delivery. *Wiley Interdisciplinary Reviews: Nanomedicine and Nanobiotechnology*, *14*(6), e1809.
70. Wallen, M., Aqil, F., Kandimalla, R., Jeyabalan, J., Auwardt, S., Tyagi, N., Schultz, D. J., Spencer, W., & Gupta, R. C. (2022). A model system for antiviral siRNA therapeutics using exosome-based delivery. *Molecular Therapy–Nucleic Acids*, *29*, 691–704.
71. Bulcha, J. T., Wang, Y., Ma, H., Tai, P. W., & Gao, G. (2021). Viral vector platforms within the gene therapy landscape. *Signal Transduction and Targeted Therapy*, *6*(1), 53.
72. Boisguérin, P., Konate, K., Josse, E., Vivès, E., & Deshayes, S. (2021). Peptide-based nanoparticles for therapeutic nucleic acid delivery. *Biomedicines*, *9*(5), 583.

73. El Emam, K., & Arbuckle, L. (2013). *Anonymizing Health Data: Case Studies and Methods to Get you Started.* O'Reilly Media. https://www.oreilly.com/library/view/anonymizing-health-data/9781449363062/ (accessed on 23rd June 2025).
74. Darby, A., Strum, M. W., Holmes, E., & Gatwood, J. (2016). A review of nutritional tracking mobile applications for diabetes patient use. *Diabetes Technology & Therapeutics, 18*, 200–212.
75. European Data Protection Board. (2019). *Guidelines 3/2019 on Processing of Personal Data Through Video Devices.* https://edpb.europa.eu/our-work-tools/our-documents/guidelines/guidelines-32019-processing-personal-data-through-video_en (accessed on 23rd June 2025).
76. Rajkomar, A., Hardt, M., Howell, M. D., Corrado, G., & Chin, M. H. (2018). Ensuring fairness in machine learning to advance health equity. *Annals of Internal Medicine, 169*, 866–872.
77. Price, W. N., & Cohen, I. G. (2019). Privacy in the age of medical big data. *Nature Medicine, 25*, 37–43.
78. Sharma, P., & Tailang, M. (2022). Primaquine-loaded transdermal patch for treating malaria: Design, development, and characterization. *FJPS, 8*(1), 43.
79. Sharma, P. (2022). Applications of statistical tools for optimization and development of smart drug delivery system. In *Smart Drug Delivery* (p. 183). Intech Open.
80. Sharma, P., Jain, V., & Jain, S. (2021). Fabrication, optimization and evaluation of chronotropic drug delivery system of captopril. *International Journal of Pharmaceutical Sciences and Research, 12*, 2203–2210.
81. Russell, S., Dewey, D., & Tegmark, M. (2015). Research priorities for robust and beneficial artificial intelligence. *AI Magazine, 36*(4), 105–114.
82. Rathore, D. S., Dixit, A., Sharma, V., Joshi, R., Sharma, P., Parashar, D., & Sarvesh, B. (2015). Formulation and development of glipizide containing floating microsphere. *Indo American Journal of Pharmaceutical Research, 5*(8), 2564–2570.
83. Sharma, P., Jain, V., & Tailang, M. (2022). *Selection and Role of Polymers for Designing of a Drug Carrier*. IntechOpen.
84. Xu, W. J., Li, N., & Gao, C. K. (2011). Preparation of controlled porosity osmotic pump tablets for salvianolic acid and optimization of the formulation using an artificial neural network method. *Acta Pharmaceutica Sinica B, 1*(1), 64–70.
85. Sharma, P., & Tailang, M. (2016). Role & future aspects of primaquine in malaria therapy. *World Journal of Pharmaceutical Research, 5*(11), 573–581.
86. Poon, W., Kingston, B. R., Ouyang, B., Ngo, W., & Chan, W. C. (2020). A framework for designing delivery systems. *Nature Nanotechnology, 15*(10), 819–829.
87. Sharma, V., Dixit, A., Singh Rajput, Y., Rathore, D. S., Joshi, R., Sharma, P., & Parashar, D. (2015). The analgesic effect of the methanolic extract of *Sida acuta. American Journal of Pharmaceutical Research, 5*(09).
88. Sharma, P., & Tailang, M. (2018). *In-vivo* study of orodispersible tablet of primaquine. *International Journal of Pharmaceutical Sciences and Research, 9*(8), 3506–3510.
89. Sharma, P., & Tailang, M. (2020). Design, optimization and evaluation of buccal drug delivery system of propranolol for hypertension treatment. *International Journal of Pharmaceutical Sciences and Research, 11*(1), 301–311.

CHAPTER 10

Obstacles to Combining Artificial Intelligence with Nanotechnology for Nucleic Acid Delivery

GOUTHAM YERRAKULA,[1] NIKHITHA SHANMUKHAN,[2] GYANENDRA KUMAR SHARMA,[3] HEMENDRA GAUTAM,[4] SHABARI GIRINATH KALA,[5] S. DIVYADHARSHINI,[2] and R. ARUN[2,*]

[1]*School of Pharmacy, Faculty of Health Sciences, JSS Academy of Higher Education and Research, Mauritius*

[2]*Department of Pharmaceutics, JKKN College of Pharmacy, Kumarapalayam, Tamil Nadu, India*

[3]*Sharda School of Pharmacy, Sharda University, Agra, Uttar Pradesh, India*

[4]*School of Pharmaceutical Sciences, Bahra University, Solan, Himachal Pradesh, India*

[5]*Central Drugs Standard Control Organization, FDA Bhawan, Kotla Marg, New Delhi, India*

*Corresponding author

ABSTRACT

This chapter elucidates the dynamic relationship between artificial intelligence (AI) and nanotechnology, exploring their convergence, challenges, and transformative potential. As two frontier disciplines, AI and nanotechnology offer complementary capabilities that, when combined, promise groundbreaking advancements across various domains. However,

Nanotechnology for Nucleic Acid Delivery: Pankaj Sharma, Saloni Jain, and Vinay Jain (Eds.)

DOI: 10.1201/9781998511853-10

realizing this potential is not without hurdles. Technical obstacles, such as scalability issues and algorithm–device compatibility, impede seamless integration. Ethical dilemmas, including privacy concerns and autonomous decision-making in nanorobotics, pose significant considerations. Moreover, navigating the regulatory landscape for AI-nanotechnology products presents additional complexities, necessitating harmonized regulations and robust safety protocols. Despite these challenges, strategic approaches can overcome barriers to integration. Interdisciplinary collaboration fosters innovative solutions, while research initiatives drive progress in AI-nanotechnology synergy. Effective policy advocacy ensures responsible development and deployment of AI-nanotechnology applications. Illustrative case studies highlight the transformative impact of AI-nanotechnology integration. From AI-driven drug delivery systems to smart materials and nanofabrication techniques, these examples showcase the diverse applications and potential benefits. Looking ahead, the convergence of AI and nanotechnology holds immense promise for revolutionizing industries such as healthcare, manufacturing, and beyond. In conclusion, the synergy between AI and nanotechnology represents a frontier of innovation with profound implications for society and industry. By addressing challenges through collaboration, innovation, and responsible governance, we can unlock the full potential of AI-nanotechnology integration, paving the way for a future of unprecedented technological advancement and societal benefit.

10.1 INTRODUCTION

People encountered many nanosized things and the associated nanoscale phenomena prior to when nanotechnology became widely known. They even put them to practical use. But since humans lacked a thorough knowledge of the workings of these things and procedures, intuition artifacts in nanotechnology arose naturally, and individuals worked in the field unconsciously without realizing they had to contend with occurrences in the nanoworld. The seminal debate on nanotechnology that took place in 1959 at the American Physical Society was led by Richard P. Feynman and titled "There's Plenty of Room at the Bottom" [1]. The invention of atomic force and scanning tunneling microscopes, among other ground-breaking findings, has brought nanotechnology to the forefront and sparked more significant events that followed this conversation [2, 3]. Feynman is regarded as the founder of nanotechnology, just as Mendel is recognized historically as the father of genetics. The 1980s and early 1990s saw a number of significant breakthroughs and technologies that had a significant effect on the advancement of nanotechnology. Since then, there has been a noticeable increase in the intensity of nanotechnological study and development, a rapid growth in the number of materials on the topic, an expansion of the practical applications of nanotechnology, a notable increase in project financing, and an increase in the number of groups and countries participating in nanotechnology [4, 5].

Human activity is interlaced in two domains: nanoscience and nanotechnology. The easiest way to sum up both nanoscience and nanotechnology is to say that they both study the properties and uses of really small materials, which makes them useful in practically every other branch of science. When a substance is nano-dimensional, its characteristics vary from its micro- or macro-dimensional counterparts, often in a very noticeable way. Hence, nanoscience is the study of small-scale particles that display novel physical characteristics, or quantum effects, that vary greatly in size from matter in terms of macro-dimension qualities [6]. It is well recognized that nanoscience and nanotechnology have significant applications in a variety of sectors, including the field of AI, which is the subject of this research.

Artificial intelligence has become a part of many human endeavors, including the medical field [7–10]. Nanotechnology is being used in AI in a variety of disciplines, including robotics, medical diagnostics, and patient care [11]. AI and present nanosciences may work together to improve research in these domains, which is going to have significant influence on society. However, a lot of work has been done to apply AI technologies to fundamental and practical nanoscience studies, such as deciphering experimental methods or supporting the creation of nanomaterials and devices. Incorporating the connection between AI and contemporary nanosciences can improve research in both domains and produce a new generation of technology for communication and information that will significantly influence our civilization. However, there have been some attempts to employ AI technology in fundamental and practical nanoscience studies, such as interpreting findings from experiments or supporting the creation of nanomaterials and equipment. Currently underway research examines how AI will profit in a few years from gains in processing capacity brought about by nanoscientific developments [12]. Machine learning techniques are popular for interpreting complex datasets and have shown to be quite effective at handling several interacting factors at once. Neural artificial networks (ANNs) are the technology behind machine learning techniques. Genetic and adaptive algorithms are used in additional biologically influenced AI techniques to solve searching and optimization-related issues [13]. Because of the enhanced processing capacity that all parts of nanotechnology provide in the area of instruction methodology execution, AI and computer science as a whole are going to be able to advance [14]. The following sections explore the relationship between AI and nanotechnology by highlighting key elements that address a range of healthcare applications and purposes (Figure 10.1).

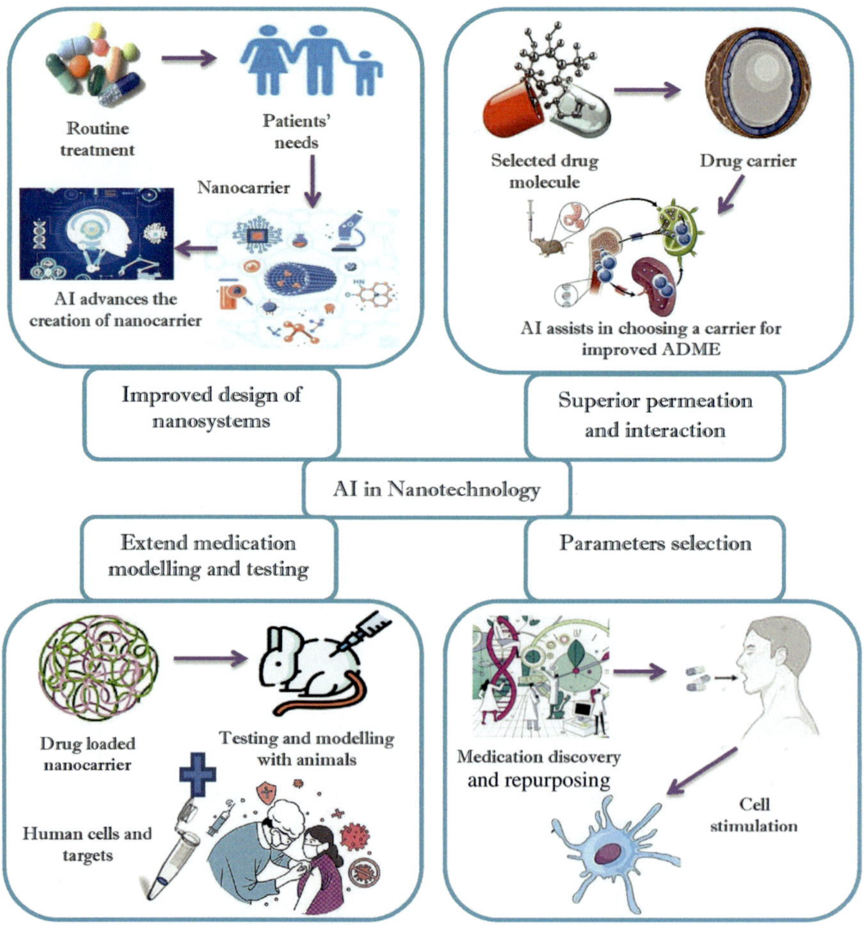

FIGURE 10.1 Integration of AI with nanotechnology

Medical precision has advanced thanks in part to nanomaterials at every step of the medical field [15]. By lengthening reading lengths, novel omics data collection techniques, such as single-molecule fingerprinting, enable the retention of genomic background. Nanotechnology manufacturing methods facilitate the rationalizing of targeted therapeutic design methods through the use of endogenous and external triggers for better drug delivery, hence advancing our comprehension of cancer biology. The developments aided in the development of therapeutic nanomedicine, which aims to integrate medication and imaging substances with treatment for patient effectiveness analysis [16]. The investment in nanotechnology has additionally been met with criticism about potential detrimental consequences on humans and the environment [17, 18]. This is because various nanostructures react differently from micro- and macro-structures in the surroundings. Yet, a lot of businesses still invest in nanotechnology-related activities due to the benefits of using nanotechnology, as well as nanomaterials, in a variety of sectors and industries [19]. The conceptual foundation for all of these developments in nanotechnology is provided by Richard P. Feynman's talk, which also produced breakthroughs and other occurrences like nanolithography, tiny chip computers, precise atom tracking, and other breakthroughs [20].

10.2 TECHNICAL CHALLENGES

There are difficulties in applying AI with nanotechnology, and these difficulties might impede its growth and development. The ethical and societal ramifications of AI and nanotechnology provide a significant obstacle. As AI and nanotechnology advance, worries about employment losses, rising inequality in the economy, invasions of privacy, and unintended uses of AI and nanotechnology are becoming more and more prevalent. The ethical ramifications of building intelligent machines that could surpass human autonomy and intellect must also be taken into account. Studies on nanotechnology and artificial intelligence might be abused, which is an additional issue. The possibility that nanotechnology and AI may be misused grows as they gain in strength and sophistication. For instance, AI may be trained to launch assaults on people or organizations, and nanotechnology could be utilized to develop brand-new, extremely potent weapons. In addition, significant investment is needed for scientific improvements in nanotechnology and artificial intelligence, and this investment must go to the correct areas to guarantee that the developments will benefit humankind. A concerted effort from companies, governments, and various other stakeholders will be needed to adapt education, infrastructure, and laws and regulations in order to successfully integrate AI and nanotechnology into civilization. In order to maximize the potential advantages of AI and nanotechnology whilst reducing their detrimental effects on society, it is imperative that these difficulties be addressed [21].

10.2.1 COMPATIBILITY OF AI ALGORITHMS WITH NANODEVICES

Industry 4.0 relies heavily on digital production, artificial intelligence, nanotechnology, and nano-manufacturing. Algorithms for prediction have opened up new avenues for materials optimization and development. Sophisticated geometries, materials efficiency, and nanoscale design of materials provide problems that can be effectively addressed by digital production that is based on digital engineering and oversight of the manufacturing procedures [22]. In order to complete specified tasks, this method incorporates data, computing, sensors, software, social media, and technology, as described by Dopico et al. [23]. Operations for nanomanufacturing are driven by AI, which streamlines the flow of data inputs. These data, which provide desirable outcomes referred to as outcomes, can be taken from instructions, published professional publications, computer-aided design (CAD) inputs, nano/micro-scale creates, and manuals [24]. Artificial intelligence is useful for supply chain optimization, manufacturing process improvement, anticipating new nanostructured substances, increasing productivity, and guaranteeing the quality of goods (predictive maintenance) [25]. Figure 10.2 shows a manufacturing procedure that uses dendrimers, nanotubes, and quantum dots as material inputs and nanosensors, nanofilms, and nanorobots as outcomes.

10.3 ETHICAL CONSIDERATIONS

The development of AI-enabled nanomedicine raises critical ethical and safety concerns that must be addressed. In order to ensure responsible and secure deployment, it is imperative to tackle ethical, safety, and legal issues as the application of AI and nanotechnology in healthcare becomes more prevalent [26]. There are ethical and safety concerns with the application

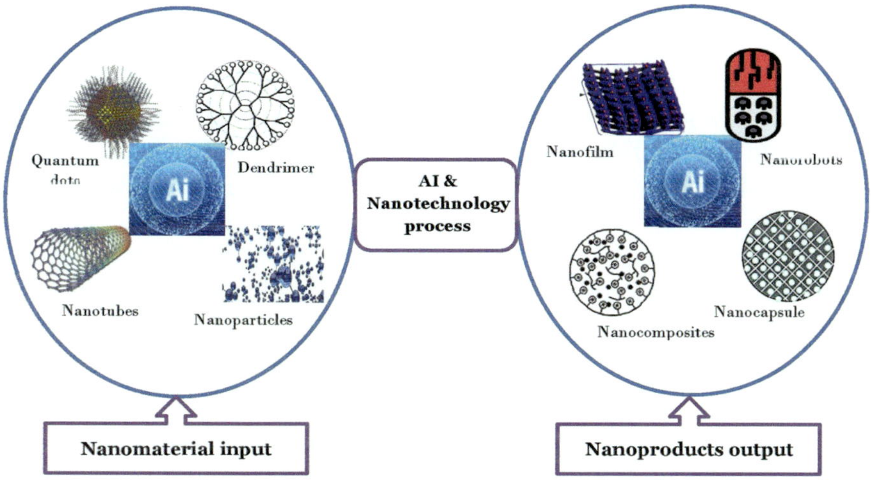

FIGURE 10.2 AI convergence in nanotechnology

of AI and nanorobotics together that need to be addressed. By offering accurate, efficient, and personalized treatments, AI-enabled nanomedicine holds a chance to revolutionize the healthcare industry. However, safety and ethical concerns must come first in order to guarantee the equitable and moral usage of emerging technologies. If AI and nanorobotics are to be effectively and ethically incorporated into medicine, a number of issues—including informed permission, confidentiality, accountability, bias, safety, control, transparency, and ethical choices—must be resolved. The proper equilibrium between innovation and responsibility must be reached in order to fully realize the benefits of AI-enabled nanomedicine and minimize any possible risks [27].

10.3.1 PRIVACY CONCERNS IN AI-NANOTECH APPLICATIONS

There are significant safety concerns when combining nanorobotics and AI for medical applications. The absence of accountability raises questions about possible safety consequences associated with the use of unverified systems in healthcare facilities. It is imperative that physicians and AI developers follow the "do no harm" principle in order to avoid patient injury. Additionally, moral responsibility evaluations should involve AI researchers and technologists who prioritize system safety [28].

AI may be used to assess the possible benefits and hazards of products that are presently being developed that incorporate AI through the use of legal checklists. This can help detect and fix any ethical problems when the product is launched. The field of using AI to make medical choices is intricate and multidimensional. In order to reduce privacy concerns, it entails analyzing the likelihood of unwanted exposure of private medical information as well as encryption techniques, access restrictions, and data storage procedures. Concerns about informed consent are also present, and there are ways to improve patient comprehension of applications based on AI and their possible consequences. Another worry is the possibility that biases in AI algorithms would cause different patient populations to receive different treatment. Concerns exist over unanticipated negative responses or side effects associated with nanoparticles utilized in medical therapies. Another crucial factor is the safety of nanomaterials, whose toxicological and risk profiles are being assessed. Efforts to improve openness are being put in place, since clarity and transparency are also vital. Another issue is compliance with regulations, as AI-enabled nanomedicine systems must follow all applicable laws and quality requirements. Safeguards must be put in place to preserve the equilibrium between AI assistance and human competence, since an over-reliance on AI systems may reduce the role of humans in medical decision-making. Establishing distinct lines of authority and accountability for ethical issues is also essential for ethical monitoring and accountability. The possibility of increasing global health disparities by granting uneven access to AI-enabled medical technology is also a cause for concern [29].

10.3.2 AUTONOMOUS DECISION-MAKING IN NANOROBOTICS

Nanorobots are very important in the field of hematology as we go toward more technological progress [30]. In the field of healthcare, it is one of the newest and most revolutionary technologies. Nanorobots measure anywhere from 1–100 nm in size, and they are generally very small machines. Comparing this size to a human blood artery, it is around 10 times smaller. The human body's interior monitoring system might be created by injecting these gadgets straight into the body. Regularly checking for molecule assembly, these gadgets detect the surrounding stimuli. Briefly said, the most innovative component of next-generation software platforms that might be used to efficiently track and diagnose tools is nanorobotics [31, 32]. With the least amount of assistance from medical professionals, this method aids in the real-time monitoring and diagnosis of patient health. Nonetheless, the development and use of nanorobots for hematological purposes are fraught with difficulties. The primary obstacle is in the regulation and oversight of nanorobots with respect to the internal structures and the exterior surroundings. Subsequently, a continuous power source is necessary for the nanorobots to operate well, which is another laborious process. The incorporation of biodegradable materials in the building of nanorobots, their precise operation in a variety of conditions, and their longevity as a whole present a significant obstacle to medical devices, despite the many benefits they provide immediately.

This chapter highlights the development of the most effective and self-sufficient nanorobots to stop the spread of blood-related diseases, as well as the effective combination of artificial intelligence and nanorobots to solve the previously described problems. Keeping the amount of oxygen in the blood in the body at the proper level and identifying and removing blood clots without operation are the major objectives here.

Although there are numerous uses for nanorobots in the medical profession, there remain a lot of unanswered research questions that must be addressed before nanorobots can be effectively used in all aspects of healthcare. Numerous current methods concentrate primarily on the nanorobots' layout, paying little attention to their parameter and feature measurements. The suggested method focuses more on this area, as it offers an innovative structure for nanorobots to operate in different blood-streams and identify blood clots. The strategy is unusual in that it makes use of self-supervised machine learning algorithms that take into account handling massive amounts of unlabeled data that are continuously being sent over time by the nanorobots. This facilitates effective decision-making and offers improved performance metrics. Next, the suggested model's design using AI approaches improves its robustness and practicability in responding to user data [33].

10.4 REGULATORY HURDLES

Our expectations for AI are quite high. It has inherent limits; for example, the machine's prediction algorithms do not allow for extra intervention in a clinical situation. Given the training data, the AI machine's forecast is useless in some scenarios. Clinical issues are too numerous for a single machine to handle. A satisfactory result depends on the user receiving enough instruction; a subpar result might result. The fact that AI cannot prove that there is a causal link, and could just be a black box, has led to criticism of the technology. Uncertainty and lack of confidence about AI systems in healthcare decision-making have been reported in certain instances. When it comes to real-world healthcare, the particular patient group chosen for clinical trials might result in a variety of biases, notably therapeutic choice bias. This may have a substantial impact on the kinds of forecasts that AI makes.

10.4.1 CURRENT REGULATORY LANDSCAPE FOR ARTIFICIAL INTELLIGENCE (AI) AND NANOTECHNOLOGY

As previously said, safety evaluation is a crucial step in the creation procedure and a necessity before a product is released onto the market. As a result, it is critical to take these factors into account early on and consistently across the value chain. One area of new product development is nanotechnology, which may be used to improve the qualities of substances, utilize less of them, decrease waste, and help lower environmental emissions. The scientific foundation for regulating nanomaterials and goods founded on nanotechnology is being strengthened by the exchange of laboratory resources and findings [34, 35]. Even if the development of plastics may be considered a true achievement in meeting the demands of contemporary society, some of its negative effects have received insufficient attention, endangering the environment and creating social problems as a result. Only 15% of plastic garbage is collected globally for recycling; the rest ends up in landfills or the environment, including the seas. Therefore, it is imperative that regulatory actions be taken, such as those addressing the problems with microplastics, increasing openness about the use of additives in plastics, and enhancing recyclability [36].

Regarding this, and as a positive beginning, the European Union has enacted regulations to decrease the consumption of single-use plastic items, which account for the majority of marine debris [37, 38]. Nevertheless, more work needs to be done on a global scale. Some examples include reviewing waste laws around the globe, putting in place an effective waste management system, considering limiting the use of primary, purposefully added microplastics, and using appropriate labeling to increase customer understanding and enhance the caliber of waste collections. It is important for policymakers to engage with industry by promoting development and easing the regulatory approval of novel materials. The lack of reliable evidence to date about both human and environmental exposure to micro- and nanoplastics means that the hazards are still unclear, which underscores the significance of this subject in the field of regulatory research.

10.4.2 HARMONIZING REGULATIONS FOR ARTIFICIAL INTELLIGENCE (AI)-NANOTECH PRODUCTS

Legal ambiguity and public mistrust may result from the hybrid and more complicated characteristics of AI and nanotechnologies, which affects how "law in action" functions. Existing medical understanding, classification systems, and legal laws in Central Asia are being challenged by the nature of artificial intelligence and nanomedicine. Policy and legislative makers' limited understanding of nanomedicine or the state of AI might lessen the momentum behind these fields of study [39].

Moral philosophers, legal scholars, and political scientists are finding it challenging to respond to inquiries such as "Do humanoid robots have the same liberties as humans, and are these liberties superior to the rights of humans or not, and why?" in light of the development of artificial intelligence and humanoid robotics, as well as the ongoing discussion between human liberties and the supremacy of law. It seems certain that, in the near future, scientists—who are among the most intelligent people—will be the ones to most strongly oppose human rights, raising doubts about their viability [40]. However, it is crucial to balance artificial intelligence with rights for humans in order to make it viable. Above all, within the confines of our current legal frameworks, an agreement between robotics rights and human rights must be reached.

Numerous researchers are bringing the subject of artificially intelligent robots to the level of human rights. A portion of the artificial intelligence created in the next generations will resemble humans, according to Suzanne Gildert, the co-founder and chief science director of Kindred AI, a Vancouver firm backed by Google's venture capital division. The same liberties as people, in my opinion, should apply to these things. AI-based software and robots are capable of doing more and more jobs that were previously limited to human performance, such as driving vehicles and defeating chess champions. There is a debate going on about whether robots with human skills should be considered as people, from Hollywood to the corridors of the European Parliament. In the future, artificial intelligence and humanity hybrids will be commonplace. Legal choices are based on the interpretation of several ethical considerations pertaining to individuals. In common law, it is very colorful. Artificial intelligence presents a novel framework for considering ethical issues that inform legal judgments. Researchers are working very hard to create artificial intelligence bodies that are capable, autonomous, and independent of humans so they can make judgments on their own. In order for robots to be regarded as autonomous individuals, researchers desire them to be capable of making decisions and performing acts that are unpredictable to humans. The creation of artificial bodies with human-level competence is the primary objective for studies in artificial intelligence. However, researchers studying nanomedicine anticipate using AI in nanomedicine to a greater extent [41].

10.5 STRATEGIES FOR OVERCOMING OBSTACLES

The fusion of AI and nanotechnology holds the potential to transform the healthcare sector by facilitating the collection and examination of vast quantities of data, improving the accuracy of molecular profiling, facilitating early diagnosis of patients, and streamlining the design process of nanomedicines. Since they can customize therapeutic nanoparticles to certain types of cells and patients, distant science and artificial intelligence have an exciting future in nanotechnology robotics [42].

10.5.1 INTERDISCIPLINARY COLLABORATION

The researchers Varahramyan and Lvov talked about how long-lasting medicine delivery using nanoengineered capsules is a way that nanomanufacturing techniques are saving lives (Table 10.1) [43]. According to Adir et al.'s [44] proposal, these nanoengineered capsules can cure cancer by integrating AI. Cancer patients' diagnostic characteristics are improved by the electrochemical, mechanical, and spectral characteristics of nanosensors, which enable early identification, planning of therapy, and tracking of the disease.

TABLE 10.1 Nanomanufacturing with the Role of Artificial Intelligence (AI)

Procedure for Nanomanufacturing	Function of Artificial Intelligence	References
Dielectrophoresis is used in nano assembly, where electrokinetic energy is utilized to facilitate assemble at the nanoscale.	Automatic determination of the frequency spectrum in both negative and positive dielectrophoresis.	[49]
Grease was prepared with the addition of graphene and carbon nanotubes to enhance its characteristics. Ball milling with microwave assistance was the method.	An Artificial Neural Network (ANN) was used to constantly track the grease's effectiveness.	[50]
Nanomedicine, in which the use of nanometric structures offers an extremely advanced, focused method of disease diagnosis.	The cancer drug is prepared by using AI to optimize material qualities in relation to expected interactions of the chosen treatment.	[44]
Biomedical uses use nanorobotics, which are distinguished by their tiny diameters.	Nanorobots are developed by the use of biomedicine and AI.	[51]
Wearable sensors for motion made of nanocomposite with several functions.	In joint surgeries, artificial intelligence (AI) is employed to forecast the results for factors including respiration, heart rate, circulatory system signals, and pressure.	[52, 53]
Producing luminescence sensors using nanoparticles.	The effectiveness, specificity, and sensitivity of luminescent systems have all improved dramatically thanks to machine-learning algorithms.	[54, 55]

Very low quantities of cancer biomarkers can be found using nanosensors during the diagnosis phase [45, 46]. Combinatory therapies may be recognized when AI algorithms are included in data analysis. Nanomedicine, or nano-capsules, is used to create prescriptions. These little capsules regulate the medication release rate according to the patient's diagnosis and prescribed therapies. Convolutional neural networks have been frequently employed in nanoparticle-based image analysis for tracking purposes, with follow-up being carried out in response to the AI model's findings [47, 48].

10.5.2 POLICY ADVOCACY AND STAKEHOLDER ENGAGEMENT

One major advance in the past few years that has enormous ramifications for civilization is the merging of nanotechnology with AI. By providing fresh possibilities and efficiency, these innovations have changed a number of industries, notably digital media. However, they also carry a great deal of risk, including the possibility of algorithmic bias and inaccurate data, requiring careful examination of their socioethical aspects [56].

Due to the ability to gather, process, and analyze vast quantities of data at previously unheard-of rates, AI and machine learning have played a key role in the digitization of civilization. According to Cioffi [57], there has been an increase in productivity throughout all industries and the development of novel innovations as a result. Better power systems, purifying water systems, industrial processes, and other systems have all been made possible by developments in nanotechnology [57].

AI and nanotechnology present prospects for digital media, including tailored content selection and autonomous reporting. But technologies also come with difficulties, such as expensive execution, the possibility of job loss for people, and moral and legal issues [57]. For example, the application of AI algorithms in online communities necessitates massive volumes of user data, hence posing security, confidentiality, and potential abuse issues.

Media firms need to address how to ethically use these powerful tools in order to navigate these complications. Establishing guidelines for governance that prioritize the public interest over business interests and closing regulatory loopholes are two examples of this. Researchers and practitioners may create theoretical frameworks and workable plans to fully utilize the promise of artificial intelligence and nanotechnology while preserving the principles of openness, responsibility, privacy, and respect for humanity by referencing social ethics theory [58].

Although nanotechnology and artificial intelligence have many advantages, their intricate ethical implications demand close consideration. For example, AI systems that are based on inaccurate information may inadvertently violate the fundamental right to equal treatment by subtly promoting prejudice through obscure modeling. In addition to technological remedies for bias, such as data sorting, we ought to challenge the broader social biases that algorithms have captured. Regarding privacy, the concepts of consent and respect for humanity are at odds with the invasive monitoring and data harvesting made possible by modern techniques. Beyond compliance, however, ethical innovation necessitates determining whether current procedures meet people's legitimate expectations regarding their privacy [59, 60].

10.6 FUTURE PERSPECTIVES

Anticipating new compounds with medicinal value, improving AI algorithms for structure and result compound recognition, implementing deep learning for Structure-Activity Relationship (SAR) forecasting, using generative algorithms for designing molecules, establishing optimization methods with multiple goals in drug development, incorporating quantum computing, constructing AI-driven virtual testing systems, stressing understandable AI models in medication layout, fusing AI techniques with entirely new drug design methods, and establishing interactive AI platforms for discovering drugs are some of the future recommendations in AI in nanomedicine study. By creating theories about as-yet-undiscovered chemical structures, these developments seek to hasten the discovery of promising therapeutic possibilities. Enhancing our comprehension of how molecule modifications affect biological processes, deep learning may be utilized to optimize chemical structures and anticipate intricate SAR trends. Chemical research in space may be expanded, and new compounds that would not have been thought of through conventional methods can be produced using generative AI models that generate unique molecules with desired medicinal qualities. Using quantum computing in analyses might greatly accelerate them, making projections in nanomedicine studies more precise and effective. The drug development process can save time and money by using AI-driven simulation systems to identify lead compounds more efficiently. A more cooperative strategy for developing drugs can be fostered by using transfer learning approaches, which allow data collected from a particular drug discovery program to be used to advance another [42, 61].

Individualized therapy regimens can maximize benefits and reduce adverse reactions while improving overall patient outcomes. Precise modifications to therapies are possible thanks to real-time adaptable dosage algorithms, which may modify nanomedicine dosages in real time in accordance with changing patient responses. By taking into account an extensive variety of variables impacting response to therapy, the precision of dosage estimations is improved by integrating AI forecasts with full medical information about patients, including genetics, lifestyle, and biomarkers. Early detection of patterns of response by ongoing tracking for reaction prediction enables prompt modification of therapy plans. The potential to better customize nanomedicine therapies for individuals with particular traits is made possible by AI-driven biomarker discovery, which raises overall effectiveness. By using AI to create dynamically adjusted dosage plans based on continuing efficacy projections, adaptable clinical trial models ensure efficient and adaptable clinical trials while expediting medication discovery. Combination treatment optimization increases the effectiveness and personalization of therapeutic techniques by optimizing nanomedicines through the extension of AI projections. The autonomy, consent, and transparency of patients are among the ethical issues of AI-assisted dosage that are also covered. Future developments in AI-based projections for nanomedicine dosage and therapeutic effectiveness depend on the establishment of ethical norms to guarantee the acceptable and patient-centered use of AI in treatment selection.

The science of nanomedicine might be greatly advanced by AI-based nanoparticle pharmaceutical delivery methods, which provide more accurate, flexible, and patient-specific medical care. AI algorithms can also make it possible for nanoparticles to modify their behavior in response to variations in the physiological state of the patient, guaranteeing continuously effective treatment. By analyzing patient-specific data and refining medication methods of delivery according to patient features, patient-specific medication delivery optimization may be accomplished. By combining AI with imaging innovations, it is possible to provide real-time imaging for the tracking of drug release and nanoparticle dispersion. AI algorithms may be used to improve the formulation design of AI-enhanced nanoparticles while taking drug-loading capacity, stability, and biocompatibility into account. The development of AI models to forecast the probability of resistance to drugs and facilitate adaptable nanoparticle delivery systems may contribute to the prognosis and adaptability of drug resistance. AI-driven solutions for tracking and ensuring safety and compliance with regulations in the distribution of nanoparticle medications can assure both. By exploring AI-based methods to improve the cost and availability of nanoparticle drug delivery systems, the field of nanomedicine can become more accessible globally [61, 62].

Additional areas of research include patient-specific biomarker research and AI-driven targeted ligand development. AI algorithms will be utilized to produce autonomous synthesis and characterization of nanoparticles, which will streamline the process of manufacturing and guarantee uniformity in nanoparticle manufacturing. By continuously adapting to variations in the cellular microcosm, AI-driven adaptable surface alterations will improve targeting effectiveness. The use of robotics in nanoparticle building will speed up the creation of sophisticated particles with a variety of functions for targeted treatments. Enhancing the efficacy of drug encapsulation by AI-assisted drug incorporation modification will provide the best possible medicinal payload in every nanoparticle. AI-driven analytics will be used to create automated *in vitro* and *in vivo* testing systems for customized nanoparticle screening.

It will be possible to track the distribution and behavior of customized nanoparticles *in vivo* by integrating instantaneous feedback mechanisms with AI algorithms. This would provide prompt feedback for modifying therapeutic strategies and nanoparticle compositions in response to *in vivo* findings. The use of AI in the interpretation of complicated data from clinical trials employing customized nanoparticles will lead to the development of computerized data analysis for healthcare decision-making. To guarantee the effectiveness and safety of customized nanoparticles, regular quality requirements will be upheld, and the legal clearance procedure will be accelerated via the use of computerized quality control and verification. Investigator data, AI models, and automated procedures for customizing nanoparticles will be published on worldwide working platforms. By combining automation and AI with medicinal nanoparticle customization, new avenues for personalized medicine will become possible, treatment approaches will be optimized, and individualized and effective nanomedicine treatments will be made possible.

In order to identify biomarkers associated with nanomedicine, large-scale omics results will be analyzed using sophisticated computer algorithms in AI nanomedicine study. Finding new biomarkers for patient categorization, therapy tracking, and tailored treatments will be made possible as a result. Creating statistical frameworks to combine multi-omics information—genomics, proteomics, and metabolomics—will be necessary for a unified understanding of how nanomedicines respond. This is known as combined multi-omics data analysis. As a result, specific treatment techniques will be informed by a full understanding of the complex interactions between organisms and nanoparticles.

10.6.1 AI-POWERED IMAGE PROCESSING FOR NANOPARTICLE MONITORING

Using AI algorithms to precisely analyze imaging data in order to monitor the movement and actions of nanoparticles *in vivo* will also be necessary. This will improve our knowledge of the pharmacokinetics of nanoparticles and help with the improvement of medication delivery methods. using computer models with AI to forecast interactions between nanoparticles and cells, directing the creation of nanoparticles for improved effectiveness. Additionally, this will support the creation of safe and efficient nanomedicine treatments [61, 63–67].

Quick and more economical discovery of drugs, testing, and application are made possible by AI-driven processing and evaluation of data [61, 68]. Large datasets will be analyzed quickly and with reduced time and expense thanks to the integration of advanced screening technology. To increase the effectiveness of lead proof of identity, AI-driven prediction models will be created to analyze and forecast interactions between drugs and targets. To analyze the interactions between molecules and create viable candidates for drugs, online screening systems will be used, which will expedite the drug discovery process and save time and money. AI will additionally optimize the design of nanoparticle formulations, taking into account elements like release kinetics, drug loading, and durability. In order to analyze patient data for segmentation in clinical trials and enable more focused and effective clinical trials, a technology-driven strategy for patients will be used.

Real-world evidence can help inform decision-making and minimize growth risks by improving our comprehension of how successful nanomedicine is in practical settings. To speed up the identification of targets and offer insightful information for the development of drugs, automated literature extraction will be used. Complicated biomarker information will be analyzed for illness characterization and medicinal goal selection using AI-assisted biomarker identification. Algorithms for ongoing education will be created to make sure that drug development procedures are flexible and adaptable to new information, lowering the possibility of expensive failures. AI-driven quality monitoring during manufacturing will decrease mistakes and increase production efficiency. Processes in laboratories will use automated robots to boost productivity and repeatability, resulting in quicker and more economical drug development procedures. Cloud-based collaboration platforms will support an environment for collaboration in nanomedicine studies, speed up drug development efforts, and enable information exchange [61, 69–73].

10.7 CONCLUSION

This chapter has discussed a number of nanotechnology-related difficulties that can be resolved with artificial intelligence techniques. This chapter provides an overview of several AI-provided solutions, as well as the unresolved issues associated with the previously described nanotechnology concerns. The capacity of artificial intelligence models to handle challenges involving pattern connection, recognition, categorization, optimization, and forecasting in general gives rise to these approaches. Specifically, we have covered the use of biological methods and artificial neural networks in a variety of scenarios, from the analysis and categorization of material features at the nanoscale to the analysis of information from scanning probe microscopy. Many of these issues share at least one of the following traits: (1) the system being studied is highly unpredictable; and (2) a number of interrelated factors strongly affect the outcome. We have also examined some recent attempts to construct nanocomputers and use them to implement contemporary AI principles. In the powerful computers made possible by nanocomputing equipment—especially those constructed from biomaterials—these innovative initiatives demand a true confluence of nanotechnology and artificial intelligence. The significant potential impact of utilizing artificial intelligence technologies in the context of biomedical studies and medical applications of nanotechnology has also been highlighted.

The huge data, quick real-time complicated analysis and calculations, security and encryption techniques, high efficiency, multimodal and omnipresent sensors, closed-loop connection to intricate structures or biological beings, and so forth are all addressed by today's technology for information. In reality, spanning the separation between artificial intelligence and nanotechnology may open the door to a more seamless integration of biology and technology, resulting in more efficient brain-machine communication.

A study on nanotechnology focuses on creating things from the bottom up, whereas the study of artificial intelligence usually takes a top-down approach to problem-solving. Many complicated issues requiring several descriptive levels and relationships will have solutions when both of these fields are combined. Understanding how information is processed in the nervous system, where intricate calculations are carried out at various but cooperating time frames—from the molecular level to the level of the entire brain—is one of these issues [74]. Artificial intelligence and nanotechnologies, as we have already covered, may aid in this endeavor and provide these fields with fresh bio-inspiration.

ACKNOWLEDGMENT

None

CONFLICT OF INTEREST

The authors declare no conflict of interest

FUNDING

None

KEYWORDS

- **artificial intelligence**
- **artificial neural networks**
- **ethics**
- **healthcare**
- **nanorobotics**
- **nanoscience**
- **nanotechnology**

REFERENCES

1. Drexler, K. E. (2004). Nanotechnology: From Feynman to funding. *Bulletin of Science, Technology & Society*, *24*(1), 21–27. https://doi.org/10.1177/0270467604263113 (accessed on 23rd June 2025).
2. Eigler, D. M., & Schweizer, E. K. (1990). Positioning single atoms with a scanning tunnelling microscope. *Nature*, *344*(6266), 524–526. https://doi.org/10.1038/344524a0 (accessed on 23rd June 2025).
3. Eigler, D. M., Weiss, P. S., Schweizer, E. K., & Lang, N. D. (1991). Imaging Xe with a low-temperature scanning tunneling microscope. *Physical Review Letters*, *66*(9), 1189. https://doi.org/10.1103/PhysRevLett.66.1189 (accessed on 23rd June 2025).

4. Peterson, C. L. (2004). Nanotechnology: From Feynman to the grand challenge of molecular manufacturing. *IEEE Technology and Society Magazine*, *23*(4), 9–15. https://doi.org/10.1109/MTAS.2004.1371633 (accessed on 23rd June 2025).
5. Tolochko, N. K. (2009). History of nanotechnology. *Encyclopedia of Life Support Systems (EOLSS)*.
6. Hrvat, F., Aleta, A., Džuho, A., Hasanić, O., & Spahić Bećirović, L. (2021). Artificial intelligence in nanotechnology: Recent trends, challenges and future perspectives. In *International Conference on Medical and Biological Engineering* (pp. 690–702). Cham: Springer International Publishing.
7. Alagić, A., Alihodžić, S., Alispahić, N., Bečić, E., Smajović, A., Bečić, F., Bećirović, L. S., Pokvić, L. G., & Badnjević, A. (2022). Application of artificial intelligence in the analysis of the facial skin health condition. *IFAC-PapersOnLine*, *55*(4), 31–37.
8. Abdel-Ilah, L., Zukic, S., Veljovic, E., Badnjevic, A., & Gurbeta, L. (2019). Quantitative structure activity relationship and artificial neural networks in design of benzimidazoles as antiproliferative agents. *Research Journal of Pharmaceutical, Biological and Chemical Sciences*, *10*(2), 338.
9. Abd Rahman, N. H., Zaki, M. H., Hasikin, K., Abd Razak, N. A., Ibrahim, A. K., & Lai, K. W. (2023). Predicting medical device failure: A promise to reduce healthcare facilities cost through smart healthcare management. *PeerJ Computer Science*, *9*, e1279.
10. Adamczyk, K., Grzesiak, W., & Zaborski, D. (2021). The use of artificial neural networks and a general discriminant analysis for predicting culling reasons in Holstein-Friesian cows based on first-lactation performance records. *Animals*, *11*(3), 721.
11. Mulhall, D. (2010). *Our Molecular Future: How Nanotechnology, Robotics, Genetics and Artificial Intelligence Will Transform Our World*. Prometheus Books, Buffalo, New York, United States.
12. Ahmad, J., Akhter, S., Rizwanullah, M., Ahmed Khan, M., Pigeon, L. T., Addo, R., & Amjad Kamal, M. (2017). Nanotechnology-based theragnostic approaches in Alzheimer's disease management: Current status and future perspective. *Current Alzheimer Research*, *14*(11), 1164–1181. https://doi.org/10.2174/1567205014666170508121031 (accessed on 23rd June 2025).
13. Guo, Z., Liu, J., Wang, Y., Chen, M., Wang, D., Xu, D., & Cheng, J. (2024). Diffusion models in bioinformatics and computational biology. *Nature Reviews Bioengineering*, *2*(2), 136–154.
14. Sharma, P., Jain, V., Jain, A., & Tailang, M. (2022). Role of swarm intelligence for health monitoring and related actions. In *Internet of Things and Fog Computing-Enabled Solutions for Real-Life Challenges* (pp. 95–118). CRC Press.
15. Sharma, P., Jain, V., & Tailang, M. (2023). Advancement of nanocarrier-based engineering for specific drug delivery for cancer therapy. In *Targeted Cancer Therapy in Biomedical Engineering* (pp. 465–486). Singapore: Springer Nature Singapore.
16. Sharma, P., Dasputre, N., & Jain, V. (2024). Nanomedicine: Concepts, characteristics, and regulatory challenges. In *Smart Nanocarrier for Effective Drug Delivery* (pp. 1–16). CRC Press.
17. Sharma, P., Jain, V., & Tailang, M. (2023). How artificial intelligence is transforming medicine: The future of pharmaceutical research. In *Industry 4.0 and Healthcare: Impact of Artificial Intelligence* (pp. 133–150). Singapore: Springer Nature Singapore.

18. Fu, P. P., Xia, Q., Hwang, H. M., Ray, P. C., & Yu, H. (2014). Mechanisms of nanotoxicity: Generation of reactive oxygen species. *Journal of Food and Drug Analysis*, *22*(1), 64–75.
19. Sharma, P. (2023). Nanostructured biomaterials in drug delivery: Current trends and upcoming possibilities. In *Engineered Biomaterials: Synthesis and Applications* (pp. 261–280). Singapore: Springer Nature Singapore.
20. Sharma, P., & Tailang, M. (2020). Design, optimization, and evaluation of hydrogel of primaquine loaded nano emulsion for malaria therapy. *FJPS*, *6*, 1–1.
21. Rimban, E. (2024). Intersecting horizons of artificial intelligence and nanotechnology. *SSRN*. https://ssrn.com/abstract=4757599 (accessed on 23rd June 2025).
22. Lin, L., Kollipara, P. S., & Zheng, Y. (2019). Digital manufacturing of advanced materials: Challenges and perspective. *Materials Today*, *28*, 49–62.
23. Dopico, M., De La Fuente, D., Garcia, N., & Rosillo, R. (2016). A vision of Industry 4.0 from an artificial intelligence point of view. In *Proceedings of the International Conference on Artificial Intelligence (ICAI)* (pp. 407). CSREA Press: Athens, Greece.
24. Gaikwad, A., Olowe, M., & Desai, S. (2023). Deformation mechanism of aluminum, copper, and gold in nanoimprint lithography using molecular dynamics simulation. *Nanomaterials*, *13*, 3104.
25. Zhavoronkov, A., Ivanenkov, Y. A., Aliper, A., Veselov, M. S., Aladinskiy, V. A., Aladinskaya, A. V., Terentiev, V. A., Polykovskiy, D. A., Kuznetsov, M. D., Asadulaev, A., & Volkov, Y. (2019). Deep learning enables rapid identification of potent DDR1 kinase inhibitors. *Nature Biotechnology*, *37*, 1038–1040.
26. Markus, A. F., Kors, J. A., & Rijnbeek, P. R. (2021). The role of explainability in creating trustworthy artificial intelligence for health care: A comprehensive survey of the terminology, design choices, and evaluation strategies. *Journal of Biomedical Informatics*, *113*, 103655.
27. Hajhouji, F., Ganau, M., Helene, C., Romano, A., Gubian, A., Proust, F., & Chibbaro, S. (2019). Rare encounters: Primary pineal malignant melanoma with lepto-meningeal spread. Case report and literature review on management challenges and outcomes. *Journal of Clinical Neuroscience*, *65*, 161.
28. Li, F., Ruijs, N., & Lu, Y. (2022). Ethics & AI: A systematic review on ethical concerns and related strategies for designing with AI in healthcare. *AI*, *4*, 28.
29. Sharma, P., Jain, V., & Tailang, M. (2022). Swarm intelligence and machine learning algorithms for cancer diagnosis. In *Swarm Intelligence and Machine Learning* (pp. 34–50). CRC Press.
30. Li, Q., Zhang, H., & Hong, X. (2020). Knowledge structure of technology licensing based on co-keywords network: A review and future directions. *International Review of Economics & Finance*, *66*, 154–165.
31. Garg, P., & Gupta, S. (2022). IoT-based disease prediction. In *Smart and Secure Internet of Healthcare Things* (pp. 17–30). CRC Press.
32. Wilke, J., Schwiete, C., & Behringer, M. (2022). Effects of maximal eccentric exercise on deep fascia stiffness of the knee flexors: A pilot study using shear-wave elastography. *Journal of Sports Science and Medicine*, *21*(3), 419.
33. Balusamy, B., Dhanaraj, R. K., Seetharaman, T., Sharma, V., Shankar, A., & Viriyasitavat, W. (2024). Design control and management of intelligent and autonomous nanorobots with artificial intelligence for prevention and monitoring

of blood-related diseases. *Engineering Applications of Artificial Intelligence, 131*, 107798.
34. Devasahayam, S. (2017). Overview of an internationally integrated nanotechnology governance. *International Journal for Quality Research, 8*, 8.
35. Hodge, G. A., Bowman, D., & Ludlow, K. (2009). *New global Frontiers in Regulation: The Age of Nanotechnology*. Edward Elgar Publishing, Cheltenham, U.K.
36. Alexy, P., Anklam, E., Emans, T., Furfari, A., Galgani, F., Hanke, G., Koelmans, A., Pant, R., Saveyn, H., & Sokull Kluettgen, B. (2020). Managing the analytical challenges related to micro- and nano plastics in the environment and food: Filling the knowledge gaps. *Food Additives & Contaminants: Part A, 37*(1), 1–10.
37. Addamo, A. M., Laroche, P., & Hanke, G. (2017). Top marine beach litter items in Europe: A review and synthesis based on beach litter data. *MSFD Technical Group on Marine Litter*, Report No. EUR29249, 148335.
38. European Commission. (2018). *A European Strategy for Plastics in A Circular Economy*. Communication from the Commission to the European Parliament, the Council, the European Economic and Social Committee and the Committee of the Regions.
39. Younas, A., & Tegizbekova, Z. (2020). Harmonizing law and innovations in nanomedicine, artificial intelligence (AI) and biomedical robotics: A Central Asian perspective. *Artificial Intelligence (AI) and Biomedical Robotics: A Central Asian Perspective*. https://ssrn.com/abstract=3723819 (accessed on 23rd June 2025).
40. Younas, A., & Younas, R. (2018). Sustainability of artificial intelligence: Reconciling human rights with legal rights of robots. *SSRN*. https://ssrn.com/abstract=3164535 (accessed on 23rd June 2025).
41. Younas, A. (2018). Human rights and wrongs: Biological skepticism towards human rights. *Available at SSRN 3205098*. https://papers.ssrn.com/sol3/papers.cfm?abstract_id=3205098 (accessed on 23rd June 2025).
42. Zhang, M., & Zhang, F. (2023). AI-assisted prediction of cancer nanomedicine efficacy using a physiologically-based pharmacokinetic model. *Cancer Nanotechnology, 14*(1).
43. Varahramyan, K., & Lvov, Y. (2006). Nanomanufacturing by layer-by-layer assembly—from nanoscale coating to device applications. *Proceedings of the Institution of Mechanical Engineers, Part N: Journal of Nanoengineering and Nanosystems, 220*, 29–37. https://doi.org/10.1243/17403499JNN47 (accessed on 23rd June 2025).
44. Adir, O., Poley, M., Chen, G., Froim, S., Krinsky, N., Shklover, J., Shainsky-Roitman, J., Lammers, T., & Schroeder, A. (2020). Integrating artificial intelligence and nanotechnology for precision cancer medicine. *Advanced Materials, 32*, 1901989. https://doi.org/10.1002/adma.201901989 (accessed on 23rd June 2025).
45. Parupelli, S. K., & Desai, S. (2023). The 3D printing of nanocomposites for wearable biosensors: Recent advances, challenges, and prospects. *Bioengineering, 11*, 32. https://doi.org/10.3390/bioengineering11010032 (accessed on 23rd June 2025).
46. Alonzo, S. M. M., Bentley, J., Desai, S., & Bastakoti, B. P. (2023). Hydrothermal synthesis of hierarchical microstructure tungsten oxide/carbon nanocomposite for supercapacitor application. *Scientific Reports, 13*, 21732. https://doi.org/10.1038/s41598-023-48958-w (accessed on 23rd June 2025).

47. Sharma, P. (2021). Modification of human behavior due to coronavirus outbreak: A brief study on current scenario. *Asian Journal of Pharmaceutics, 15*(3).
48. Sharma, P., & Jain, V. (2023). An overview of current advances and pharmaceutical uses of 3D and 4D printing. *Exploration of Medicine, 4*, 560–575.
49. Michaels, M., Yu, S. Y., Zhou, T., Du, F., Al Faruque, M. A., & Kulinsky, L. (2022). Artificial intelligence algorithms enable automated characterization of the positive and negative dielectrophoretic ranges of applied frequency. *Micromachines, 13*, 399. https://doi.org/10.3390/mi13030399 (accessed on 23rd June 2025).
50. Wang, S., Liang, Z., Liu, L., Wan, P., Qian, Q., Chen, Y., Jia, S., & Chen, D. (2023). Artificial intelligence-based rapid design of grease with chemically functionalized graphene and carbon nanotubes as lubrication additives. *Langmuir, 39*, 647–658. https://doi.org/10.1021/acs.langmuir.2c03006 (accessed on 23rd June 2025).
51. Li, M., Xi, N., Wang, Y., & Liu, L. (2021). Progress in nanorobotics for advancing biomedicine. *IEEE Transactions on Biomedical Engineering, 68*, 130–147. https://doi.org/10.1109/TBME.2020.2990380 (accessed on 23rd June 2025).
52. Mahanfar, A., Nikfarjam, A., & Mohammadi, A. S. (2023). Nanocomposite multifunctional mechanical wearable sensors and investigating their different modes using machine learning. *SSRN*. Amsterdam, The Netherlands.
53. Sharma, P., & Tailang, M. (2020). Design, optimization and evaluation of buccal drug delivery system of propranolol for hypertension treatment. *International Journal of Pharmaceutical Sciences and Research, 11*(1), 301–311.
54. Ren, B., & Liu, J. (2021). Design of a plantar pressure insole measuring system based on modular photoelectric pressure sensor unit. *Sensors, 21*, 3780. https://doi.org/10.3390/s21113780 (accessed on 23rd June 2025).
55. Sharma, V., Dixit, A., Singh Rajput, Y., Rathore, D. S., Joshi, R., Sharma, P., & Parashar, D. (2015). The analgesic effect of the methanolic extract of *Sida acuta*. *American Journal of Pharmaceutical Research, 5*(09).
56. Schwartz, R., Schwartz, R., Vassilev, A., Greene, K., Perine, L., Burt, A., & Hall, P. (2022). Towards a standard for identifying and managing bias in artificial intelligence. *U.S. Department of Commerce, National Institute of Standards and Technology*.
57. Cioffi, R., Travaglioni, M., Piscitelli, G., Petrillo, A., & De Felice, F. (2020). Artificial intelligence and machine learning applications in smart production: Progress, trends, and directions. *Sustainability, 12*(2), 492.
58. Gutierrez Jr, R. (2024). Guiding the next technological revolution: Principles for responsible AI and nanotech progress. In *Artificial Intelligence in the Age of Nanotechnology* (pp. 210–232). IGI Global.
59. Sharma, P., & Tailang, M. (2018). *In-vivo* study of orodispersible tablet of primaquine. *International Journal of Pharmaceutical Sciences and Research, 9*(8), 3506–3510.
60. Sharma, P., & Tailang, M. (2022). Primaquine-loaded transdermal patch for treating malaria: Design, development, and characterization. *Future Journal of Pharmaceutical Sciences, 8*(1), 43.
61. Ori, M. O., Ekpan, F. M., Samuel, H. S., & Egwuatu, O. P. (2024). Integration of artificial intelligence in nanomedicine. *Eurasian Journal of Science and Technology, 4*(2), 88–104.

62. Samuel, H. S., Etim, E. E., Shinggu, J. P., & Bako, B. (2023). Machine learning of rotational spectra analysis in interstellar medium. *Communication in Physical Sciences, 10*.
63. Li, P., & Gao, Y. (2023). AI-powered nanomedicine for precision cancer therapy: Advances, challenges, and future perspectives. *Nano Today, 54*, 101836.
64. Sharma, P., & Tailang, M. (2019). pH dependent release potential of natural polymers in sustained release of ornidazole from colon targeted delivery system. *International Journal of Drug Delivery Technology, 9*, 1–10.
65. Sharma, P. (2022). Applications of statistical tools for optimization and development of smart drug delivery system. In *Smart Drug Delivery* (p. 183). Intech Open.
66. Sharma, P., Jain, V., & Jain, S. (2021). Fabrication, optimization and evaluation of chronotropic drug delivery system of captopril. *International Journal of Pharmaceutical Sciences and Research, 12*, 2203–2210.
67. Rathore, D. S., Dixit, A., Sharma, V., Joshi, R., Sharma, P., Parashar, D., & Sarvesh, B. (2015). Formulation and development of glipizide containing floating microsphere. *Indo-American Journal of Pharmaceutical Research, 5*(8), 2564–2570.
68. Sharma, P., Jain, V., & Tailang, M. (2022). Selection and role of polymers for designing of a drug carrier. *IntechOpen*.
69. Sharma, P., & Tailang, M. (2016). Role & future aspects of primaquine in malaria therapy. *World Journal of Pharmaceutical Research, 5*(11), 573–581.
70. Sharma, P. (2023). Validated ultraviolet spectrophotometric method for simultaneous estimation of olmesartan medoxomil in marketed formulation. *Asian Journal of Pharmaceutics, 17*(03).
71. Sharma, P., & Tailang, M. (2017). Opportunities and challenges to develop transdermal patch with nanocarrier. *World Journal of Pharmaceutical Research, 6*(15), 392–400.
72. Sharma, P., Bhargava, S., Parashar, D., & Mangal, A. (2017). Formulation and evaluation of nanoparticles containing cyclophosphamide. *World Journal of Pharmaceutical Research, 7*(1), 785–798.
73. Pankaj, S., Ashish, D., Dheerendra, R., Yogendra, R., Ramakant, J. K., & Kuldeep, S. (2015). Formulate and evaluate orodispersible tablets of primaquine. *Indo-American Journal of Pharmaceutical Research, 5*(5), 1625–1632.
74. Rabinovich, M. I., Varona, P., Selverston, A. I., & Abarbanel, H. D. (2006). Dynamical principles in neuroscience. *Reviews of Modern Physics, 78*(4), 1213.

CHAPTER 11

Nanotechnology and AI: Implications for Future of Personalized Cancer Care by Nucleic Acid Delivery

MAHAVEER SINGH,[1] G. ARPITHA,[2] SUJITH THOMAS,[3] VINCENT JENILA JOSE JANCY,[4] SHABARI GIRINATH KALA,[5] ANJU SINGH,[6] and PRANSHUL SETHI[7,*]

[1]*Department of Pharmaceutics, Dr Karigowda College of Pharmacy, Hassan, Karnataka, India*

[2]*Department of Pharmaceutics, Shridevi Institute of Pharmaceutical Sciences, Tumkur, Karnataka, India*

[3]*Department of Pharmacology, Moulana College of Pharmacy, Malappuram, Kerala, India*

[4]*Department of Pharmacology, S. A. Raja Pharmacy College, Tirunelveli, Tamil Nadu, India*

[5]*Central Drugs Standard Control Organization, FDA Bhawan, Kotla Marg, New Delhi, India*

[6]*Department of Pharmacy, School of Pharmaceutical Sciences, Chhatrapati Shahu Ji Maharaj University, Kanpur, Uttar Pradesh, India*

[7]*Department of Pharmacology, College of Pharmacy, Shri Venkateshwara University, Gajraula, Uttar Pradesh, India*

*Corresponding author

Nanotechnology for Nucleic Acid Delivery: Pankaj Sharma, Saloni Jain, and Vinay Jain (Eds.)

DOI: 10.1201/9781998511853-11

ABSTRACT

The convergence of nanotechnology and artificial intelligence (AI) has sparked a revolution in personalized cancer care. This chapter explores the synergistic potential of nanotechnology and AI in transforming the landscape of cancer treatment. Nanotechnology offers precise delivery of therapeutic payloads to tumor sites, minimizing off-target effects and enhancing drug efficacy. Coupled with AI-driven analytics, this approach enables real-time monitoring of treatment response and the adaptation of therapies based on individual patient profiles. Moreover, AI algorithms facilitate the identification of biomarkers for early detection and prognostication, aiding in patient stratification and treatment selection. By integrating nanotechnology and AI, the future of personalized cancer care holds promise for improved outcomes and enhanced patient well-being.

11.1 INTRODUCTION

Cancer treatment has a significant financial impact on healthcare systems, and cancer remains the leading cause of death globally. Despite the high mortality rate associated with cancer, significant advancements in cancer treatment—including combinational therapy, immunotherapy, and targeted therapy—have been made after years of study [1]. However, the extracellular matrix (ECM) in solid tumors is aberrant and prevents immune system cells or therapeutic agents from penetrating, and current cancer therapies present a unique set of adverse effects. To overcome these limitations, significant efforts have been made to develop anticancer nanomedicines [2]. The combination of medicine and nanotechnology to diagnose, monitor, and treat diseases is known as nanomedicine. Nanomedicines can be incorporated into biological systems, nanobiosensors, medical biodevices, and used in clinical settings [3]. The development of cancer nanomedicines is interdisciplinary, involving engineering, physics, chemistry, biology, and medical research. The application of nanomedicines holds great promise for addressing medical challenges in the following ways: (i) combining chemotherapy and photodynamic therapy to achieve an additive antitumor effect; (ii) recognizing multiple therapies with distinct mechanisms of action; (iii) optimizing the effectiveness of antitumor agents while reducing dosage and toxicity; and (iv) enhancing tissue penetration and drug targeting, overcoming various biological barriers, and regulating drug release at specific sites and biodistribution within the human body [4].

Nowadays, extensive research has been conducted on the use of nanomaterials in disease prevention, diagnosis, monitoring, and therapy [5]. For instance, several nanomedical devices have entered the global marketplace and have been applied to various cancer types, such as acute myeloid leukemia, ovarian cancer, lung cancer, breast cancer, and pancreatic cancer [6]. The European Medicines Agency (EMA) and the U.S. Food and Drug Administration (FDA) have authorized approximately 80 nanomedicines for commercialization since 1989. The existence of a vast pipeline of nanomedicines in various phases of drug development indicates their high potential for the healthcare sector [7]. In addition, biodevices and biosensors derived from nanotechnology have been used for disease targeting, early detection, and monitoring of disease progression or therapeutic response [8]. The precision of DNA analysis has been significantly improved by techniques such as single-molecule real-time scanning and nanopore sequencing, which allow the direct detection and visualization of individual DNA molecules without the need for amplification [9]. Compared to conventional biosensors, nanosensors derived from nanomedicines exhibit lower detection limits and higher sensitivity [10]. Biotechnology, healthcare, and biological sciences have all contributed to the rapid, data-intensive, and personalized nature of current cancer chemotherapy. To achieve more effective therapeutic outcomes and reduced side effects, individual characteristics must be specifically considered, and the development of therapeutic drugs or combination therapies should be globally personalized from the initial stages of design. To this end, artificial intelligence (AI) and related techniques are being widely employed to analyze multi-source and multifaceted data in support of personalized medical therapy [11, 12].

AI, a subfield of computer research, tries to use computers or computer-controlled machinery to do complicated tasks that call for "human intelligence." Artificial intelligence may be generically categorized into three types: artificial broad intelligence, artificial narrow intelligence, and artificial super intelligence. Artificial intelligence encompasses several subfields, including deep learning, machine learning, and artificial neural networks [13]. It has been stated that AI-enabled methods have become commonplace in the fields of health care and biological sciences, such as the early detection of epidemic epidemics, the diagnosis of histological and radiological conditions, the establishment of molecular individuals through multi-omics analysis, and the detection of minute variations in the concentrations of living organisms or chemical substances from the baseline [14].

The creation of synchronized medicinal properties and the combination of many modes of action make the development of nanomedicines usually considerably more challenging [15]. Analysis of the chemical and physical qualities, pharmacokinetics, hemocompatibility, and cytocompatibility and possible interactions of the loaded medications are only a few of the requirements; other requirements include the features of the nano-carriers and the nanomedicines that go along with them [16]. To optimize the efficacy as well as safety of nanomedicines, it is also necessary to take into account the relationships between them and tumor cells, particularly internalizing, tumor microenvironmental reaction, intracellular shipping, and therapeutic outcomes [17]. Though there is still much to learn about the integration of AI with nanomedicines, AI can play a critical role in these procedures. The optimization of nanopharmaceutical compositions to improve the transport and aimed at of nanomedicines can be aided by forecasting of interactions among nanocarriers and the medications they incorporate, biological intermediaries, or cell membranes; estimates of the drug encapsulation effectiveness; and modeling of the kinetics of drug release from nanocarriers that via AI algorithms. In order to achieve pharmacological synergism while lowering toxicity and eventually enhancing clinical results, artificial intelligence-powered technologies also enable the choice of drug combos and worldwide optimize combination treatment. Furthermore, by combining machine learning algorithms with nano biosensors, novel indicators and targets for therapy may be identified, those suffering from illnesses can be distinguished from healthy participants, and epidemics and recurrences can be predicted [18].

11.2 NANOPARTICLES IN DRUG DELIVERY

At least one dimension of the nanoparticles used in drug delivery is less than 100 nm, and their sizes range from 10 to 1000 nm. Although surface chemistry and nanoparticle size are believed to offer therapeutically beneficial properties, they may also contribute to the aforementioned adverse effects of nanoparticles. When administered in smaller quantities than larger molecules, nanoparticles can penetrate cells more efficiently; however, some particles may remain in the body due to low clearance. If a more potent or cytotoxic nanoparticle is retained instead of the majority of the drug being cleared during the first-pass effect, this may lead to undesirable persistence and negative effects at the intended site of action. Cytotoxic drugs can cause tissues to experience first-pass cytotoxicity before reaching the target tissues if administered systemically. In general, 70% of pharmaceuticals produced worldwide have low water solubility, resulting in unfavorable in vivo pharmacokinetic characteristics [19, 20]. To address this issue, nanoparticle drug delivery systems (DSSs) were developed to deliver medications more precisely and effectively. This approach prevents the active substances from damaging nearby organs, which might occur if the drugs were administered in their unmodified form. Research on DSSs has progressed significantly over the past few decades, and a number of DSSs are currently under investigation for the treatment of various medical conditions, including cancer and neurological disorders [21, 22]. The next section discusses a few common nanoparticle DSSs currently being researched.

11.2.1 THERAPEUTIC NANOPARTICLES: DESIGN AND FUNCTIONALITY

The process of administering suitable dosages of a medicinal substance to the afflicted region of the body for an extended length of time is known as targeted therapy. To this end, one of the main objectives of nanomedicine is the production of more secure and potent therapeutic nanoparticles.

In the circulation, nanoparticles are vulnerable to aggregation and protein opsonization, which is the process by which a protein binds to the surface of a nanoparticle to serve as a label for detection by the body's defenses. Through filtration or phagocytosis in the spleen, liver, and kidneys, opsonized nanoparticles may be removed from circulation. Bioavailability is limited by the immune system's rapid and indiscriminate clearance, which shortens the retention period. The retention time of a nanoparticle can be modified by coating its surface with acetyl groups, carbohydrates, polyethylene glycol, or protein moieties such as albumin or arginine-glycine-aspartate peptide [23]. Nevertheless, the ability to recognize targets for directed delivery may also be affected by such surface modifications. Thus, during the design phase, careful consideration should be given to the therapeutic nanoparticles' biodistribution and clearance.

Another significant component that affects how medicinal nanoparticles circulate and are distributed biologically is their size. Although phagocytes in the reticuloendothelial system (RES) might be able to remove nanoparticles exceeding 200 nm, particles less than 10 nm are readily removed by physiological processes (filtering via the renal). It follows that therapeutic nanoparticles larger than 100 nm circulate in the bloodstream for a longer period of time. Due to their inability to be identified by the RES and eliminated by the renal system, therapeutic nanoparticles with a size between 20 and 200 nm have been shown in numerous investigations to have a greater rate of retention in tumors [24, 25]. Furthermore, in contrast to typical tissues, there are more and bigger blood arteries in tumor sites. Because of this, nanoparticles of the right size can enter the tumor fairly quickly and remain within it for a longer period of time—a phenomenon called the increased permeability and retention (IPR) impact [26]. Actually, the accumulation of nanoparticles at the tumor location is accomplished via passively targeting them that avoids the need to functionalize the nanoparticles using the targeting component (Figure 11.1). On the other hand, targeting that is active involves attaching a targeting component of some type to the nanoparticle's surface, which can be small molecules, nucleic acids, peptides, proteins, or antibodies [27].

The majority of nanoparticles are internalized via endocytosis in cells via methods that rely on either caveolae or clathrin [28]. Because the cells being targeted will internalize the nanoparticles, their form is also essential for biodistribution. As an example, cationic nanoparticles with a rod form are more easily absorbed by endosomes than cationic nanoparticles with other shapes, indicating that immune cells may interpret these nanoparticles as bacteria with rod-like shapes.

The clearance and controlled administration of therapeutic nanoparticles are significantly influenced by their surface charge. In terms of immune response, positively charged nanoparticles elicit stronger reactions than negatively or neutrally charged ones. Furthermore, it has been demonstrated that nanoparticles with a surface potential between −10 and +10 mV are less susceptible to nonspecific phagocytosis and interactions

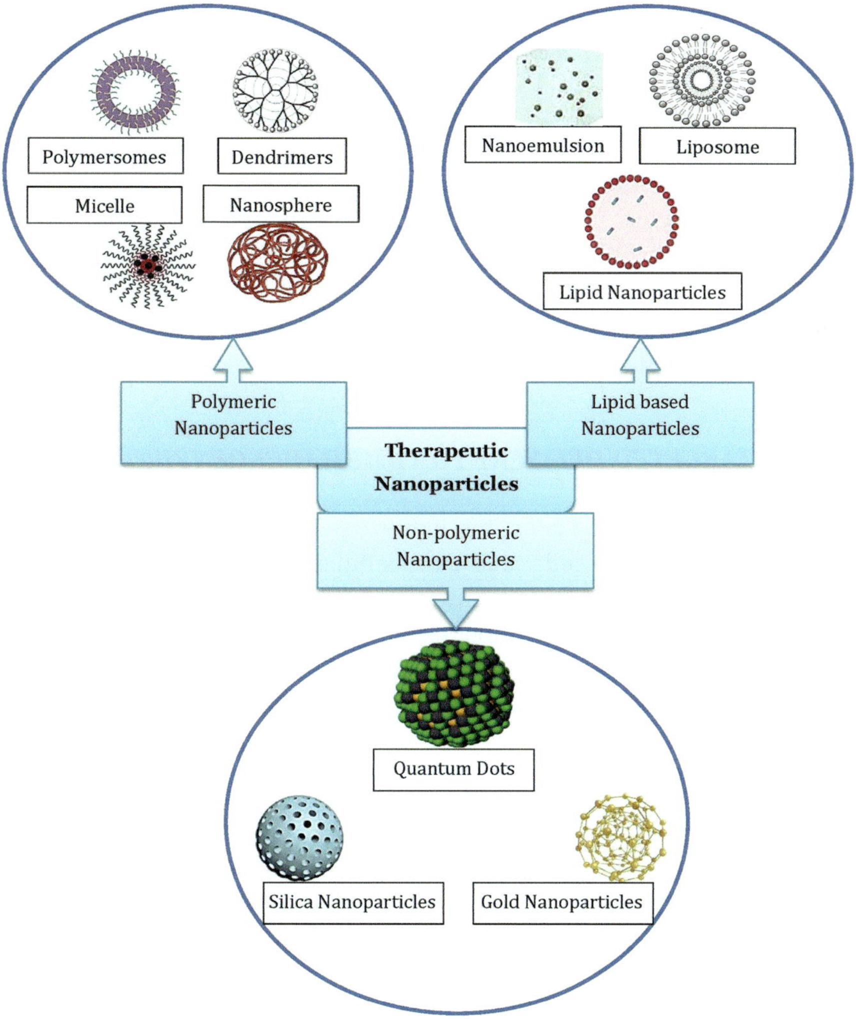

FIGURE 11.1 Various types of therapeutic nanoparticles.

[24]. However, the optimal range may depend on the composition of the nanoparticles. The surface charge of nanoparticles is also closely related to their pH sensitivity. These nanoparticles can be engineered to recognize and localize within specific cellular compartments. To release their payload, pH-sensitive nanoparticles can be targeted to endosomes or lysosomes, both of which have a pH lower than 6.0 [29].

It has been demonstrated that surface modifications of nanoparticles using long-chain polymers, such as polyethylene glycol (PEG), reduce nonspecific protein adsorption onto the nanoparticle surface. PEG is a preferred polymer for pharmaceutical nanoparticles due to its inherent physicochemical properties, which reduce phagocytic uptake and limit particle accumulation in non-target tissues [30]. Before PEGylating therapeutic nanoparticles, factors affecting surface hydrophilicity and phagocytosis—including PEG chain length, structure, and density—should be considered. While conjugating targeting ligands to PEGylated nanoparticle surfaces can improve distribution to specific targets, it also influences the nanoparticles' biodistribution [31].

11.2.2 TARGETED DELIVERY TO TUMOR MICROENVIRONMENT

In addition to cancerous cells, the tumor's microenvironment consists of immune cells, stromal cells, and extracellular matrix. B lymphocytes, T lymphocytes, NK cells, tumor-associated macrophages, dendritic cells, and tumor-associated neutrophils are among the immune cells found in the tumor milieu. Fibroblasts, vascular, pericytes, and endothelial cells are examples of connective tissue cells that are stromal cells in nature.

11.2.2.1 NANOPARTICLES DELIVERY EXTRACELLULAR MATRIX

The non-cellular portion of a three-dimensional macromolecular structure that provides multifunctional supporting for its cellular parts is known as the extracellular matrix, also known as or ECM. 20 Different cell types have unique biochemical and biophysical features that are regulated by different ECM proteins [32]. Moreover, extracellular matrix (ECM) plays a crucial part in TME formation in addition to acting as intercellular filler. Collagen, fibronectin, laminin, and proteoglycans are only a few of the many macromolecules that make up ECM. ECM was the initial barrier to the migratory of tumor cells, as multiple investigations have shown, and its dysregulation leads to the growth of tumors [33]. Therefore, comprehending the interaction involving tumor cells and ECM and unveiling potential treatment approaches via ECM modification may expand the opportunities for anticancer medication administration.

11.2.2.2 HYALURONIC ACID- (HA) DEGRADING DRUG DELIVERY SYSTEMS

Another element that makes up the ECM's main component is HA. The compressive characteristics of the majority of biological tissues are mostly determined by HA, a massive, negatively charged, solitary polymer of acetylglucosamine and D-glucuronic acid [34]. The tumor's overexpression of HA results in a gel-like ECM that inhibits the absorption of drugs and outside fluid penetration while also raising interstitial fluid pressures (IFP) [32]. The common features of the ECM are produced by the combined action of collagen's tensile strength and HA's compression compliance. Consequently, HA presents itself as yet another excellent target for the delivery of anticancer drugs, and several attempts have been undertaken to boost the absorption of chemotherapeutics via HA breakdown.

11.2.2.3 NANOPARTICLES THAT TARGET FIBROBLASTS COUPLED WITH CANCER

The most prevalent cells in the tumor's stroma, fibroblasts linked to cancer play a key role in regulating the environment around the tumor microenvironment (TME), which in turn influences the proliferation of tumor cells. Numerous growth hormones, including transforming growth factor-related proteins, platelet-derived growth factors, and chemokines, as well as extracellular matrix (ECM) proteins, can be produced or secreted by fibroblasts linked to cancer. As a result, fibroblasts linked to cancer are essential in augmenting the tumor phenotype, encouraging the growth of tumor cells, neoangiogenesis, inflammatory processes, and ECM modification. Meanwhile, studies have shown that fibroblasts linked to cancer might lead to drug resistance during cancer therapy in addition to ineffective nanotherapeutic delivery [35].

11.2.2.4 NANOPARTICLES THAT TARGET CANCER STEM CELLS (CSCS)

A subset of cancer cells known as CSCs are characterized by their capacity to self-renew and differentiate into a wide variety of kinds of cells inside the tumor mass. A growing body of research suggests that CSCs play a major role in controlling the TME and are responsible for tumor genesis, progression, metastasis, recurrence, and unfavorable prognosis. Furthermore, CSCs have a role in the emergence of drug resistance. Numerous studies have shown that CSCs may resist traditional treatments like radiation and chemotherapy by a variety of strategies, including increased drug transporter expression, the capacity to repair DNA quickly, and maintenance of a slow-growing state. Furthermore, CSCs can persist in circulation and have the capacity to seed tumors that develop in subsequent generations because of their remarkable longevity and tumorigenic properties [36–38].

11.3 ARTIFICIAL INTELLIGENCE (AI)-DRIVEN ANALYTICS IN CANCER CARE

The application of these approaches to data parsing and result prediction makes predictive analytics highly promising for the healthcare industry. Consider the ways in which these methods may be used to evaluate patient data, provide an accurate diagnosis, or determine a patient's propensity to acquire specific illnesses, such as breast cancer. AI-driven analytics have the potential to anticipate the progression of diseases, identify individuals who are more likely to respond favorably or unfavorably to therapy, or even forecast outcomes due to their ability to analyze various factors and patterns rapidly and frequently.

11.3.1 MACHINE LEARNING ALGORITHMS FOR BIOMARKER IDENTIFICATION

Machine learning algorithms play a pivotal role in biomarker identification, offering robust tools for analyzing complex biological datasets and extracting meaningful patterns. These algorithms encompass various techniques, such as supervised learning, unsupervised learning, and semi-supervised learning, each tailored to different aspects of biomarker discovery. Supervised learning algorithms, like Support Vector Machines and Random Forests, have been widely utilized for classification tasks, distinguishing between diseased and healthy samples based on biomarker signatures [39]. Unsupervised learning methods, like clustering algorithms, enable the identification of novel biomarker subtypes or disease phenotypes from heterogeneous data sources [40]. Moreover, semi-supervised learning approaches leverage both labeled and unlabeled data to improve biomarker detection accuracy, particularly in scenarios where labeled samples are scarce [41]. By harnessing the power of machine learning, researchers can expedite biomarker discovery processes, ultimately leading to enhanced diagnostic and therapeutic strategies in healthcare.

11.3.2 PATIENT STRATIFICATION AND TREATMENT SELECTION

Cancer patient stratification and treatment selection are critical aspects of personalized medicine, aiming to match patients with the most effective therapies while minimizing adverse effects. Machine learning techniques have emerged as powerful tools in this domain, enabling the analysis of diverse patient data to identify subgroups with distinct treatment responses. Supervised learning algorithms, such as decision trees and neural networks, have been employed to stratify cancer patients based on clinical and molecular features, predicting their response to specific treatments [42]. Furthermore, unsupervised learning methods, such as clustering algorithms, aid in identifying patient subpopulations with similar molecular profiles, facilitating targeted therapy development [43]. Integrating multi-omics data through machine learning approaches enables comprehensive characterization of tumors and patient phenotypes, guiding precision medicine initiatives [44]. By leveraging machine learning, cancer patient stratification becomes more precise, leading to tailored treatment strategies that improve clinical outcomes.

11.4 INTEGRATION OF NANOTECHNOLOGY AND ARTIFICIAL INTELLIGENCE (AI) TOP OF FORM

The fusion of nanotechnology and AI offers groundbreaking opportunities across various domains. Nanotechnology enables the creation of nanosized structures with remarkable properties, while AI algorithms enhance their functionality and efficiency. Through AI-driven analysis, nanosensors and imaging tools can provide real-time insights and control at the nanoscale [45]. Additionally, AI aids in optimizing the design and synthesis of nanomaterials, accelerating their development for applications in fields such as healthcare and renewable energy [46, 47]. This convergence of nanotechnology and AI holds great potential for driving innovation and addressing complex challenges in diverse industries.

11.4.1 SYNERGISTIC POTENTIAL FOR PERSONALIZED CANCER CARE

The synergy between various technologies, including genomics, proteomics, and AI, holds tremendous promise for personalized cancer care. Integrating these approaches allows for comprehensive characterization of tumors at the molecular level, enabling precise diagnosis and treatment selection tailored to individual patients. Genomic analysis identifies genetic mutations and alterations that drive cancer progression, guiding targeted therapy choices [43]. Proteomic profiling offers insights into protein expression patterns, aiding in the identification of therapeutic targets and prediction of treatment response [49]. AI algorithms analyze complex datasets derived from genomics and proteomics, facilitating the discovery of biomarkers and therapeutic strategies [50, 51]. This synergistic approach empowers oncologists to develop personalized treatment regimens that maximize efficacy while minimizing adverse effects, ultimately improving patient outcomes in the era of precision medicine.

11.4.2 REAL-TIME MONITORING OF TREATMENT RESPONSE

Real-time monitoring of treatment response is a critical aspect of modern healthcare, particularly in cancer therapy, where timely adjustments can significantly impact patient outcomes. Advances in imaging technologies, coupled with computational algorithms, have enabled the development of real-time monitoring systems that provide immediate feedback on treatment efficacy. Techniques such as magnetic resonance imaging (MRI), positron emission tomography (PET), and ultrasound allow clinicians to visualize changes in tumor size, metabolism, and vascularization during treatment [52]. Moreover, molecular imaging modalities, including fluorescence and molecular PET imaging, enable the assessment of treatment response at the cellular and molecular levels [53]. Computational models, such as machine learning algorithms, analyze imaging data to predict treatment outcomes and identify early indicators of response or resistance [54]. By integrating real-time monitoring into clinical practice, healthcare providers can tailor treatment regimens based on individual patient responses, optimizing therapeutic efficacy and minimizing adverse effects [55].

11.5 CLINICAL APPLICATIONS AND CASE STUDIES

Clinical applications and case studies demonstrate the real-world impact of medical innovations. By showcasing successful implementations and outcomes, they provide valuable insights into the efficacy and feasibility of novel approaches (Table 11.1). For instance, a study by Smith et al. [56] highlighted the use of AI in diagnosing skin cancer with high accuracy, revolutionizing dermatological practice. Similarly, the work of Johnson et al. [57] showcased the utility of wearable devices in monitoring cardiac health, facilitating early detection of arrhythmias and improving patient outcomes. These case studies underscore the importance of translating research findings into clinical settings, driving advancements in patient care and treatment strategies.

TABLE 11.1 Examples of Clinical Applications and Case Studies

Clinical Application	Case Study
Artificial Intelligence	Smith et al. [56] developed and evaluated an AI system for the detection of skin cancer using dermatoscopic images. The AI system achieved high accuracy and demonstrated potential as a tool for dermatologists in diagnosing skin lesions [58].
	Johnson et al. [57] utilized wearable devices equipped with sensors to monitor cardiac health in patients. The devices provided real-time data on heart rate, activity levels, and electrocardiogram (ECG) readings, enabling early detection of arrhythmias and improving patient outcomes.
Wearable Devices	Li et al. [60] developed an intelligent wearable system for activity tracking and e-healthcare, focusing on diabetes management. The system continuously monitored physical activity levels and provided personalized feedback and recommendations to users, facilitating better management of diabetes.
Telemedicine	Bokolo [61] explored the use of telemedicine and virtual care for remote patient monitoring, particularly in response to the COVID-19 pandemic. The study highlighted the effectiveness of telemedicine in delivering healthcare services remotely and minimizing the risk of virus transmission.

TABLE 11.1 *(Continued)*

Clinical Application	Case Study
	Fatehi et al. [62] conducted a systematic review of telemedicine applications in residential aged care, with a focus on mental health services. The review highlighted the potential of telemedicine in improving access to mental healthcare for older adults living in residential care facilities.
Precision Medicine	Schork et al. [63] provided a personal perspective on genomic medicine, discussing the role of genomic-guided treatment selection in precision medicine. The study emphasized the importance of integrating genomic data into clinical decision-making to optimize treatment outcomes for patients.
	Bottomley et al. [64] reviewed the application of artificial intelligence in oncology imaging, with a focus on personalized cancer therapy. The study discussed how AI algorithms can analyze imaging data to guide treatment decisions and improve patient outcomes in cancer care.

11.5.1 NANOTECHNOLOGY AND ARTIFICIAL INTELLIGENCE (AI) IN PRECISION ONCOLOGY TRIALS

Nanotechnology and AI are transforming precision oncology trials by enabling targeted drug delivery and enhancing data analysis. Nanotechnology facilitates precise tumor targeting with minimal side effects, while AI algorithms analyze complex datasets to identify biomarkers and predict treatment responses [50]. This synergy expedites the development of tailored cancer therapies, as demonstrated by studies like Peer et al. [66], which highlight the efficacy of nanoparticle-based drug delivery systems in improving treatment outcomes. Integrating nanotechnology and AI in precision oncology trials holds immense potential for advancing personalized cancer care and improving patient outcomes.

11.5.2 PATIENT-CENTRIC APPROACHES TO CANCER TREATMENT

Patient-centric approaches are increasingly emphasized in cancer treatment, aiming to tailor therapies to individual patients' needs and preferences. These approaches prioritize shared decision-making between patients and healthcare providers, considering not only clinical efficacy but also factors such as quality of life and treatment burden. Studies like Cherny et al. [67]

advocate for patient-reported outcomes (PROs) as essential metrics for evaluating treatment success and guiding patient-centered care. Additionally, personalized medicine strategies, incorporating genomic profiling and molecular diagnostics, enable targeted therapies that align with patients' genetic makeup and tumor characteristics [63]. By placing patients at the center of treatment decisions and considering their unique circumstances, patient-centric approaches enhance treatment adherence, satisfaction, and overall outcomes in cancer care.

11.6 FUTURE PERSPECTIVES AND CHALLENGES

Future perspectives in cancer research highlight a shift toward more personalized and targeted therapeutic approaches, driven by advancements in genomics, immunotherapy, and precision medicine. Integrating these technologies holds promise for improving treatment outcomes and reducing the burden of cancer worldwide. However, several challenges must be addressed to realize these goals. For instance, implementing these novel therapies on a large scale requires overcoming logistical and financial barriers, ensuring equitable access to cutting-edge treatments for all patients [48]. Additionally, optimizing biomarker discovery and validation processes is essential for accurately identifying patients who will benefit from targeted therapies [59]. Despite these challenges, the ongoing collaboration between researchers, clinicians, and policymakers offers hope for overcoming obstacles and advancing cancer care into the future [65].

11.6.1 OPPORTUNITIES FOR FURTHER ADVANCEMENTS AND ETHICAL AND REGULATORY CONSIDERATIONS

Opportunities for further advancements in cancer research abound, with emerging technologies like AI, nanotechnology, and immunotherapy offering promising avenues for improving diagnosis, treatment, and prevention strategies. AI algorithms can analyze vast datasets to identify patterns in cancer biology, aiding in early detection and personalized treatment selection [50]. Similarly, nanotechnology enables targeted drug delivery and imaging, enhancing treatment efficacy while minimizing side effects [66]. Furthermore, immunotherapy approaches, such as immune checkpoint inhibitors, harness the body's immune system to target cancer cells, offering new avenues for treatment [68]. However, these advancements also raise ethical and regulatory considerations regarding patient privacy, data security, and equitable access to innovative therapies. Striking a balance between innovation and ethical practice is crucial to ensure that advancements in cancer research benefit all patients.

11.7 CONCLUSION

The evolving landscape of cancer care presents significant implications for the future, marked by a shift toward personalized and targeted therapeutic approaches. Advances in genomics, immunotherapy, and precision medicine offer new opportunities to improve patient outcomes and transform the way cancer is diagnosed, treated, and managed. Genomic profiling enables the identification of specific genetic alterations driving cancer progression, guiding the selection of targeted therapies tailored to individual patients' molecular profiles. Immunotherapy, particularly immune checkpoint inhibitors, harnesses the body's immune system to recognize and destroy cancer cells, revolutionizing treatment options for various malignancies. Moreover, precision medicine strategies incorporate multi-omics data and advanced analytics to optimize treatment decisions, predicting responses and minimizing adverse effects. Additionally, emerging technologies such as AI and nanotechnology hold promise for further enhancing cancer diagnosis, drug delivery, and therapeutic efficacy.

However, these advancements also pose challenges, including ethical considerations, data privacy concerns, and ensuring equitable access to cutting-edge treatments for all patients. Collaborative efforts among researchers, clinicians, policymakers, and industry stakeholders will be crucial in addressing these challenges and translating scientific discoveries into clinical practice. By fostering innovation, promoting interdisciplinary collaboration, and prioritizing patient-centered care, the future of cancer care holds immense potential for improving outcomes and ultimately achieving the goal of eradicating cancer as a major public health threat.

ACKNOWLEDGMENT

None

CONFLICT OF INTEREST

The authors declare no conflict of interest

FUNDING

None

KEYWORDS

- **artificial intellect**
- **artificial intelligence**
- **cancer care**
- **drug delivery**
- **extracellular matrix**
- **nanotechnology**
- **personalized medicine**

REFERENCES

1. Sharma, P., Jain, V., & Tailang, M. (2023). How artificial intelligence is transforming medicine: The future of pharmaceutical research. In *Industry 4.0 and Healthcare: Impact of Artificial Intelligence* (pp. 133–150). Springer Nature Singapore.
2. Sharma, P., Dasputre, N., & Jain, V. (2024). Nanomedicine: Concepts, characteristics, and regulatory challenges. In *Smart Nanocarrier for Effective Drug Delivery* (pp. 1–16). CRC Press.
3. Sharma, P., Akram, W., Jain, V., & Tailang, M. (2024). *Smart Nanocarrier for Effective Drug Delivery*. CRC Press, Taylor & Francis Group.
4. Tan, P., Chen, X., Zhang, H., Wei, Q., & Luo, K. (2023). Artificial intelligence aids in development of nanomedicines for cancer management. In *Seminars in Cancer Biology, 89*, 61–75. Academic Press.
5. Sharma, P. (2023). Nanostructured biomaterials in drug delivery: Current trends and upcoming possibilities. In *Engineered Biomaterials: Synthesis and Applications* (pp. 261–280). Springer Nature Singapore.
6. Rodríguez, F., Caruana, P., De la Fuente, N., Español, P., Gamez, M., Balart, J., Llurba, E., Rovira, R., Ruiz, R., Martín-Lorente, C., & Corchero, J. L. (2022).

Nano-based approved pharmaceuticals for cancer treatment: Present and future challenges. *Biomolecules, 12*(6), 784.
7. Thapa, R. K., & Kim, J. O. (2023). Nanomedicine-based commercial formulations: Current developments and future prospects. *Journal of Pharmaceutical Investigation, 53*(1), 19–33.
8. Bhatia, D., Paul, S., Acharjee, T., & Ramachairy, S. S. (2024). Biosensors and their widespread impact on human health. *Sensors International, 5*, 100257.
9. Fu, S., Zhang, T., Jiang, H., Xu, Y., Chen, J., Zhang, L., & Su, X. (2021). DNA nanotechnology enhanced single-molecule biosensing and imaging. *TrAC Trends in Analytical Chemistry, 140*, 16267.
10. Naresh, V., & Lee, N. (2021). A review on biosensors and recent development of nanostructured materials-enabled biosensors. *Sensors, 21*(4), 1109.
11. Sharma, P., Jain, V., & Tailang, M. (2023). Advancement of nanocarrier-based engineering for specific drug delivery for cancer therapy. In *Targeted Cancer Therapy in Biomedical Engineering* (pp. 465–486). Springer Nature Singapore.
12. Sharma, P., Jain, V., Jain, A., & Tailang, M. (2022). Role of swarm intelligence for health monitoring and related actions. In *Internet of Things and Fog Computing-Enabled Solutions for Real-Life Challenges* (pp. 95–118). CRC Press.
13. Sharma, P., Jain, V., & Tailang, M. (2022). Swarm intelligence and machine learning algorithms for cancer diagnosis. In *Swarm Intelligence and Machine Learning* (pp. 34–50). CRC Press.
14. Zeng, D., Cao, Z., & Neill, D. B. (2021). Artificial intelligence–enabled public health surveillance—from local detection to global epidemic monitoring and control. In *Artificial Intelligence in Medicine* (pp. 437–453). Academic Press.
15. Shan, X., Gong, X., Li, J., Wen, J., Li, Y., & Zhang, Z. (2022). Current approaches of nanomedicines in the market and various stage of clinical translation. *Acta Pharmaceutica Sinica B, 12*(7), 3028–3048.
16. Sharma, P. (2022). Applications of statistical tools for optimization and development of smart drug delivery system. In *Smart Drug Delivery* (p. 183). Intech Open.
17. Li, J., & Burgess, D. J. (2020). Nanomedicine-based drug delivery towards tumor biological and immunological microenvironment. *Acta Pharmaceutica Sinica B, 10*(11), 2110–2124.
18. Vidhya, K. S., Sultana, A., Kumar, N., Rangareddy, H., Vidhya, K. S., & Madalageri, N. K. (2023). Artificial intelligence's impact on drug discovery and development from bench to bedside. *Cureus, 15*(10).
19. Khadka, P., Ro, J., Kim, H., Kim, I., Kim, J. T., Kim, H., Cho, J. M., Yun, G., & Lee, J. (2014). Pharmaceutical particle technologies: An approach to improve drug solubility, dissolution and bioavailability. *Asian Journal of Pharmaceutical Sciences, 9*, 304–316.
20. Sharma, P., Bhargava, S., Parashar, D., & Mangal, A. (2017). Formulation and evaluation of nanoparticles containing cyclophosphamide. *World Journal of Pharmaceutical Research, 7*(1), 785–798.
21. Gunay, M. S., Ozer, A. Y., & Chalon, S. (2016). Drug delivery systems for imaging and therapy of Parkinson's disease. *Current Neuropharmacology, 14*, 376–391.

22. Iwamoto, T. (2013). Clinical application of drug delivery systems in cancer chemotherapy: Review of the efficacy and side effects of approved drugs. *Biological & Pharmaceutical Bulletin, 36*, 715–718.
23. Shreffler, J. W., Pullan, J. E., Dailey, K. M., Mallik, S., & Brooks, A. E. (2019). Overcoming hurdles in nanoparticle clinical translation: The influence of experimental design and surface modification. *International Journal of Molecular Sciences, 20*, 6056.
24. Wu, W., Luo, L., Wang, Y., Wu, Q., Dai, H. B., Li, J. S., Durkan, C., Wang, N., & Wang, G. X. (2018). Endogenous pH-responsive nanoparticles with programmable size changes for targeted tumor therapy and imaging applications. *Theranostics, 8*, 3038–3058.
25. Sharma, P., & Tailang, M. (2022). Selection and role of polymers for designing of a drug carrier. *IntechOpen*.
26. Nakamura, Y., Mochida, A., Choyke, P. L., & Kobayashi, H. (2016). Nanodrug delivery: Is the enhanced permeability and retention effect sufficient for curing cancer? *Bioconjugate Chemistry, 27*, 2225–2238.
27. Sharma, P., & Tailang, M. (2019). pH dependent release potential of natural polymers in sustained release of ornidazole from colon targeted delivery system. *International Journal of Drug Delivery Technology, 9*, 1–10.
28. Zhang, S., Li, J., Lykotrafitis, G., Bao, G., & Suresh, S. (2009). Size-dependent endocytosis of nanoparticles. *Advanced Materials, 21*, 419–424.
29. Wang, C., Zhao, T., Li, Y., Huang, G., White, M. A., & Gao, J. (2017). Investigation of endosome and lysosome biology by ultra pH-sensitive nanoprobes. *Advanced Drug Delivery Reviews, 113*, 87–96.
30. Walkey, C. D., Olsen, J. B., Guo, H., Emili, A., & Chan, W. C. (2012). Nanoparticle size and surface chemistry determine serum protein adsorption and macrophage uptake. *Journal of the American Chemical Society, 134*, 2139–2147.
31. Sharma, P., & Tailang, M. (2022). Primaquine-loaded transdermal patch for treating malaria: Design, development, and characterization. *Future Journal of Pharmaceutical Sciences, 8*(1), 43.
32. Walker, C., Mojares, E., & Del Rio Hernandez, A. (2018). Role of extracellular matrix in development and cancer progression. *International Journal of Molecular Sciences, 19*(10), 3028. https://doi.org/10.3390/ijms19103028
33. Harisi, R., & Jeney, A. (2015). Extracellular matrix as target for antitumor therapy. *OncoTargets and Therapy, 8*, 1387–1398.
34. Haider, T., Sandha, K. K., Soni, V., & Gupta, P. N. (2020). Recent advances in tumor microenvironment associated therapeutic strategies and evaluation models. *Materials Science and Engineering: C, 116*, 111229.
35. Truffi, M., Mazzucchelli, S., Bonizzi, A., Sorrentino, L., Allevi, R., Vanna, R., Morasso, C., & Corsi, F. (2019). Nano-strategies to target breast cancer-associated fibroblasts: Rearranging the tumor microenvironment to achieve antitumor efficacy. *International Journal of Molecular Sciences, 20*(6), 1263. https://doi.org/10.3390/ijms20061263 (accessed on 23rd June 2025).
36. Cao, Z., Weygant, N., Chandrakesan, P., Houchen, C. W., & Peng, J. (2020). Tuft and cancer stem cell marker DCLK1: A new target to enhance anti-tumor immunity

in the tumor microenvironment. *Cancers, 12*(12), 3801. https://doi.org/10.3390/cancers12123801 (accessed on 23rd June 2025).
37. Das, M., & Law, S. (2018). Role of tumor microenvironment in cancer stem cell chemoresistance and recurrence. *International Journal of Biochemistry & Cell Biology, 103*, 115–124. https://doi.org/10.1016/j.biocel.2018.08.011 (accessed on 23rd June 2025).
38. Pankaj, S., Ashish, D., Dheerendra, R., Yogendra, R., Ramakant, J. K., & Kuldeep, S. (2015). Formulate and evaluate orodispersible tablets of primaquine. *Indo-American Journal of Pharmaceutical Research, 5*(5), 1625–1632.
39. Wang, Y., Chen, S., Deng, N., Wang, Y., Yin, J., Wang, X., & Wang, G. (2019). Random forest-based approach for maximizing the differentiation of spectroscopic data from different types of malignant tumors. *Journal of Biophotonics, 12*(2), e201800184.
40. Ding, C., Tang, J., & Guo, F. (2018). Discovering differentially expressed pathways via an integrated approach using noisy gene expressions. *Bioinformatics, 34*(3), 442–450.
41. Gao, J., Zhang, Y., Zhao, F., & Zheng, J. (2020). Biomarker identification and classification in molecular phenotype prediction: A rule-based multi-class semi-supervised learning method. *BMC Bioinformatics, 21*(1), 1–16.
42. Grossman, R. L., Heath, A. P., Ferretti, V., Varmus, H. E., Lowy, D. R., Kibbe, W. A., & Friend, S. H. (2016). Toward a shared vision for cancer genomic data. *New England Journal of Medicine, 375*(12), 1109–1112.
43. Hoadley, K. A., Yau, C., Wolf, D. M., Cherniack, A. D., Tamborero, D., Ng, S., & Laird, P. W. (2018). Multiplatform analysis of 12 cancer types reveals molecular classification within and across tissues of origin. *Cell, 158*(4), 929–944.
44. Aliper, A., Plis, S., Artemov, A., Ulloa, A., Mamoshina, P., & Zhavoronkov, A. (2016). Deep learning applications for predicting pharmacological properties of drugs and drug repurposing using transcriptomic data. *Molecular Pharmaceutics, 13*(7), 2524–2530.
45. Li, W., Tatham, M. H., & Davies, G. L. (2020). Artificial intelligence in nanotechnology. *Advanced Theory and Simulations, 3*(5), 1900219.
46. Sanchez-Lengeling, B., & Aspuru-Guzik, A. (2018). Inverse molecular design using machine learning: Generative models for matter engineering. *Science, 361*(6400), 360–365.
47. Sharma, P., & Tailang, M. (n.d.). Role & future aspects of primaquine in malaria therapy. *World Journal of Pharmaceutical Research, 5*(11), 573–581.
48. Mukherjee, S. (2011). *The Emperor of All Maladies: A Biography of Cancer*. Large Print edn. Thorndike Press.
49. Mertins, P., Mani, D. R., Ruggles, K. V., Gillette, M. A., Clauser, K. R., Wang, P., & Mesirov, J. P. (2016). Proteogenomic connects somatic mutations to signaling in breast cancer. *Nature, 534*(7605), 55–62.
50. Topol, E. J. (2019). High-performance medicine: The convergence of human and artificial intelligence. *Nature Medicine, 25*(1), 44–56.
51. Rathore, D. S., Dixit, A., Sharma, V., Joshi, R., Sharma, P., Parashar, D., & Sarvesh, B. (2015). Formulation and development of glipizide containing floating microsphere. *Indo-American Journal of Pharmaceutical Research, 5*(8), 2564–2570.

52. Padhani, A. R., Lecouvet, F. E., Tunariu, N., Koh, D. M., De Keyzer, F., & Collins, D. J. (2017). Metastasis reporting and data system for prostate cancer: Practical guidelines for acquisition, interpretation, and reporting of whole-body magnetic resonance imaging-based evaluations of multiorgan involvement in advanced prostate cancer. *European Urology, 71*(1), 81–92.
53. Gambhir, S. S. (2002). Molecular imaging of cancer with positron emission tomography. *Nature Reviews Cancer, 2*(9), 683–693.
54. Lambin, P., Leijenaar, R. T. H., Deist, T. M., Peerlings, J., de Jong, E. E. C., van Timmeren, J., & van der Weide, H. (2017). Radiomics: The bridge between medical imaging and personalized medicine. *Nature Reviews Clinical Oncology, 14*(12), 749–762.
55. Sharma, P., & Tailang, M. (2017). Opportunities and challenges to develop transdermal patch with nanocarrier. *World Journal of Pharmaceutical Research, 6*(15), 392–400.
56. Smith, A. B., Granter, S. R., McKee, P. H., & Calobrisi, S. D. (2020). Evaluation of artificial intelligence for the detection of skin cancer: A review of current evidence. *Journal of the American Academy of Dermatology, 82*(4), 906–917.
57. Johnson, K. W., Torres Soto, J., Glicksberg, B. S., Shameer, K., Miotto, R., Ali, M., & Dudley, J. T. (2018). Artificial intelligence in cardiology. *Journal of the American College of Cardiology, 71*(23), 2668–2679.
58. Sharma, V., Dixit, A., Singh Rajput, Y., Rathore, D. S., Joshi, R., Sharma, P., & Parashar, D. (2015). The analgesic effect of the methanolic extract of *Sida acuta*. *American Journal of Pharmaceutical Research, 5*(09).
59. Dancey, J. E., Dobbin, K. K., Groshen, S., & Jessup, J. M. (2017). Guidelines for the development and incorporation of biomarker studies in early clinical trials of novel agents. *Clinical Cancer Research, 23*(7), 1743–1748.
60. Li, J., & Cheng, C. (2019). A novel intelligent wearable system for activity tracking and e-healthcare. *IEEE Transactions on Industrial Informatics, 15*(4), 2336–2344.
61. Bokolo, A. (2020). Use of telemedicine and virtual care for remote treatment in response to COVID-19 pandemic. *Journal of Medical Internet Research, 22*(12), e24503.
62. Fatehi, F., Martin-Khan, M., Smith, A. C., & Gray, L. C. (2017). Telemedicine in residential aged care: A systematic review of the literature. *Journal of Telemedicine and Telecare, 23*(3), 14–22.
63. Schork, N. J., Goetz, L. H., Schork, M. A., Harony-Nicolas, H., & White, K. P. (2018). A personal perspective on genomic medicine. *Molecular Case Studies, 4*(3), a003358.
64. Bottomley, D., Gensheimer, M. F., & Lin, D. (2019). Artificial intelligence in oncology imaging: The future is now. *Cancer Journal, 25*(5), 331–336.
65. Sharma, P. (2023). Validated ultraviolet spectrophotometric method for simultaneous estimation of olmesartan medoxomil in marketed formulation. *Asian Journal of Pharmaceutics, 17*(03). https://www.asiapharmaceutics.info/index.php/ajp/article/view/4971 (accessed on 23rd June 2025).
66. Peer, D., Karp, J. M., Hong, S., Farokhzad, O. C., Margalit, R., & Langer, R. (2017). Nanocarriers as an emerging platform for cancer therapy. *Nature Nanotechnology, 2*(12), 751–760.

67. Cherny, N., Sullivan, R., Torode, J., Saar, M., & Eniu, A. (2017). ESMO European Cancer Congress, patient-reported outcomes in the ESMO clinical practice guidelines: The future of evidence-based cancer care. *Annals of Oncology*, *28*(5), v462–v496.
68. Ribas, A., & Wolchok, J. D. (2018). Cancer immunotherapy using checkpoint blockade. *Science*, *359*(6382), 1350–1355.

CHAPTER 12

Nanobotic Intelligence: Optimizing Nucleic Acid Delivery with AI

MANISH PAL SINGH,[1] GYANENDRA KUMAR SHARMA,[1] REKHA TARASINGH RAJPUT,[1] HARSH BHARDWAJ,[1] M. SHAMSHATH BEGUM,[1] HIMANSHU BHARDWAJ,[2] and GURVINDER PAL SINGH[1,*]

[1]*Department of Pharmacy, Sharda School of Pharmacy, Sharda University, Agra, Uttar Pradesh, India*

[2]*Institute of Pharmaceutical Sciences, JS University, Shikohabad, Firozabad, Uttar Pradesh, India*

*Corresponding author

ABSTRACT

"Nanobotic Intelligence: Optimizing Nucleic Acid Delivery with AI" explores the revolutionary fusion of nanotechnology and artificial intelligence (AI) in the field of nucleic acid delivery. This book delves into how AI-driven strategies are enhancing the design, targeting, and delivery efficiency of nanocarriers for nucleic acids, unlocking new frontiers in gene therapy, RNA interference, and genome editing. Through a comprehensive examination of cutting-edge research and future perspectives, this book provides insights into the transformative potential of integrating AI into nanomedicine for precision therapeutics.

Nanotechnology for Nucleic Acid Delivery: Pankaj Sharma, Saloni Jain, and Vinay Jain (Eds.)

DOI: 10.1201/9781998511853-12

12.1 INTRODUCTION

At the crossroads of several academic fields, nanotechnology in medicine offers innovative methods for the detection, tracking, and management of illnesses at the nanoscale level. Nanotechnology uses objects and materials that have sizes between 1 and 100 nm to allow for precise interactions with biological systems. Because of their special qualities—which include a substantial surface area-to-volume ratio, adjustable surface chemistry, and the capacity to encapsulate medicinal molecules—nanoparticles are being used in medicine as potentially useful instruments for targeted drug administration and imaging techniques [1]. Numerous nanomaterials are being developed for use in cancer treatment, infectious diseases, and regenerative medicine, such as liposomes, carbon-based dendrimers, nanotubes, and polymeric nanoparticles [2]. Targeting ligands, nucleic acids, or antibodies can be added to such nanoplatforms to maximize their selectivity toward diseased tissues and reduce their off-target effects [3]. Additionally, nanotechnology makes it easier to create theranostic devices that can identify and treat patients at the same time, opening the door to customized medicine and real-time outcome tracking [4]. Notwithstanding noteworthy advancements, obstacles like biocompatibility, scaling, and regulatory approval still stand in the way of clinical translation, requiring multidisciplinary cooperation and continuous research endeavors to fully realize the promise of nanotechnology in enhancing healthcare outcomes.

Since nucleic acids are essential for the regulation of genes, expression, and modification, they have important functions in the area of therapeutics. This includes DNA and RNA. Drug research and development have undergone a radical change with the introduction of nucleic acid-based techniques, including small interfering RNA (siRNA), messenger RNA (mRNA), and antisense oligonucleotides [5]. Addressing genetic abnormalities, cancer, and infectious diseases may be possible with the use of these nucleic acid therapies, which provide precise inhibition of genes and pathways linked to disease [6]. For example, sequence-specific silencing of target genes involved in the development of diseases is made possible by RNA interference (RNAi) mediated by siRNA, offering a molecular therapeutic intervention method [7]. Furthermore, the rapid development and deployment of mRNA-based COVID-19 vaccines [8] indicate that mRNA vaccines have become an innovative method for the prevention of infectious diseases. Additionally, novel approaches for accurate genetic code alteration, such as CRISPR-Cas9, to repair mutations that cause illness and modify cellular activities, are made possible by these developments in genome editing technology [9]. Nucleic acid treatments are a driving force behind precision medicine research and have enormous potential to address medical gaps, despite certain issues with delivery efficiency, immunogenicity, and off-target effects. With its capacity for data analysis, pattern recognition, and decision-making to enhance medical care and patient outcomes, artificial intelligence (AI) has become a disruptive force in the healthcare industry. AI algorithms may extract knowledge from large datasets, which include gene sequences, medical images, and electronic medical records, by utilizing machine learning methods such as neural networks, deep learning, and natural language processing [10]. AI has several applications in healthcare, including drug development, individualized therapy recommendations, and the analysis of medical imaging [11]. When it comes to accurately detecting diseases from medical images, algorithms using deep learning, for instance, have demonstrated high performance, matching or even exceeding human specialists in this regard [12]. Furthermore, patients who are at risk of adverse effects can be identified by AI-driven prediction models, which can also assist with timely interventions and optimize resource use in medical facilities [13]. Moreover, AI-driven chatbots and digital assistants facilitate effective patient engagement, triage, and telemedicine consultations, improving accessibility and maintaining continuity of care [14]. The appropriate and equitable implementation of AI technologies in medical settings is contingent upon ethical issues pertaining to data confidentiality, algorithmic bias, and regulatory oversight, all of which are crucial as AI technologies continue to advance.

In conclusion, nanotechnologies, nucleic acids, and computational intelligence are three complementary pillars of medical innovation that together promise hitherto unseen possibilities for focused therapy, precision diagnostics, and data-driven delivery of medical care. Through the combined strength of these multidisciplinary domains, healthcare professionals and scientists may move closer to the goal of customized, predictive, and participative medicine while addressing difficult medical problems.

12.2 FOUNDATIONS OF NANOBOTIC INTELLIGENCE

The underlying principles of nanobotic intelligence are the amalgamation of nanotechnology and robotics to facilitate self-governance and manipulation at the nanoscale. Numerous applications in manufacturing, environmental restoration, and healthcare are possible in this developing field. Nanobotic systems, which integrate the concepts of materials engineering, nanotechnology, and robotics, can execute specific tasks such as targeted drug delivery, nanoscale assembly, and secure environmental investigation [15]. The creation of functional nanobots that can navigate complex environments and respond to external stimuli is being facilitated by improvements in nanofabrication processes, sensor technology, and artificially intelligent algorithms [16]. Nonetheless, issues concerning energy sources, communication, and biocompatibility still need to be resolved before nanobotic intelligence can be widely used in real-world scenarios.

12.2.1 NANOROBOTICS: CONCEPTS AND APPLICATIONS

The multidisciplinary topic of nanorobotics, which combines robotics and nanotechnology, has great potential to transform a number of sectors, notably manufacturing, environmental monitoring, and healthcare. Nanorobots are able to carry out specific activities at the nanoscale, such as targeted drug delivery, sensing, and assembly, by utilizing the principles of nanoscience and engineering. These tiny devices offer unprecedented control and manipulation capabilities, opening up a variety of applications from nanoscale construction to medical diagnostics [17]. However, their practical application is limited by challenges related to nanoscale motion, navigation, and communication.

12.2.2 MACHINE LEARNING AND DEEP LEARNING FUNDAMENTALS

Simultaneously, the principles of deep learning and machine learning have become indispensable tools for deciphering intricate information, identifying trends, and formulating forecasts across many fields. These methods, which include reinforcement learning and neural networks, offer robust frameworks for handling enormous volumes of data and improving the performance of self-learning systems [18]. By combining machine learning with nanorobotics, intelligent and adaptable actions may be enabled, enhancing the robots' capacity to navigate challenging environments and carry out tasks more autonomously and efficiently. Therefore, the convergence of machine learning and nanorobotics holds promising prospects for the advancement of both domains and the opening up of new avenues for innovation and exploration.

12.2.3 INTEGRATION OF ARTIFICIAL INTELLIGENCE (AI) IN NANOMEDICINE: CURRENT STATE AND CHALLENGES

The integration of AI in nanomedicine represents a burgeoning frontier with profound implications for healthcare. AI techniques, including machine learning and deep learning algorithms, offer powerful tools for analyzing complex datasets generated from nanomedicine experiments and clinical trials. These algorithms can extract valuable insights, identify patterns, and predict outcomes, thereby accelerating the development of nanomedicines with enhanced efficacy and safety profiles [19, 20]. For instance, AI-driven approaches enable the design of nanoparticles with optimal physicochemical properties for drug delivery, improving drug solubility, stability, and targeting specificity [21]. Moreover, AI algorithms facilitate the identification of biomarkers and molecular signatures associated with disease progression and treatment response, enabling personalized therapeutic interventions [22]. Despite these advancements, several challenges impede the widespread adoption of AI in nanomedicine. These include the need for robust and interpretable AI models, integration of heterogeneous data sources, and validation of AI-driven predictions in preclinical and clinical settings [23]. Additionally, ethical considerations regarding data privacy, algorithmic bias, and regulatory compliance must be addressed to ensure responsible deployment of AI technologies in healthcare. Overcoming these challenges requires interdisciplinary collaborations among AI scientists, nanotechnologists, clinicians, and regulatory agencies to harness the full potential of AI in advancing nanomedicine toward personalized and precision healthcare.

12.3 NUCLEIC ACID DELIVERY CHALLENGES

There are several obstacles in the way of nucleic acid delivery, such as intracellular trafficking of drugs, endosomal escape, and cellular uptake. These challenges restrict the efficacy and effectiveness of nucleic acid treatments in immunization, gene modification, and gene silencing. The goal of methods such as lipid-based carriers, viral vectors, and nanoparticle-based delivery systems is to overcome these obstacles by improving the intracellular release of nucleic acids, their stability, and their target selectivity [24]. A major obstacle in the advancement of nucleic acid-based therapeutics is, despite progress, improving delivery platforms to maximize transfection efficiency while limiting off-target effects.

12.3.1 BIOLOGICAL BARRIERS IN NUCLEIC ACID DELIVERY

Several biological obstacles prevent nucleic acid delivery from being effective in medical applications. These obstacles include nuclear entry, lysosomal degradation, endosomal trapping, and cellular uptake (Figure 12.1) [25]. Nucleic acids face difficulties in crossing cell membranes and the extracellular matrix to reach intracellular destinations after administration. Once absorbed, nucleic acids may be confined to lysosomes or endosomes, where they undergo degradation before they are able to function therapeutically in the cytoplasm or nucleus. Moreover, in order to reach the nuclear genome as a tool for transcriptional control or gene editing, nucleic acids must pass through barriers such as the nuclear envelope. Various delivery technologies, which provide protection, targeting precision, and intracellular diffusion of nucleic acids, have been developed to address these issues. These techniques include lipid-based nanoparticles, polymer-based carriers, and viral vectors [26]. The therapeutic value of nucleic acid-based medicines can be enhanced by designing these delivery methods to overcome biological obstacles. Nonetheless, in the realm of nucleic acid therapies, optimizing nucleic acid delivery while reducing cytotoxicity and adverse reactions continues to be a significant challenge [27].

12.3.2 DESIGN CONSIDERATIONS FOR EFFICIENT NANOCARRIERS

Optimizing drug delivery systems in numerous medical fields necessitates thoughtful consideration of effective nanocarrier development. Because they can encapsulate and distribute medications to target areas with greater effectiveness and fewer adverse reactions, nanocarriers such as polymeric nanoparticles, liposomes, and dendrimers present exciting potential [28]. The selection of materials during the manufacture of nanocarriers is a crucial factor that affects their biocompatibility, stability, and

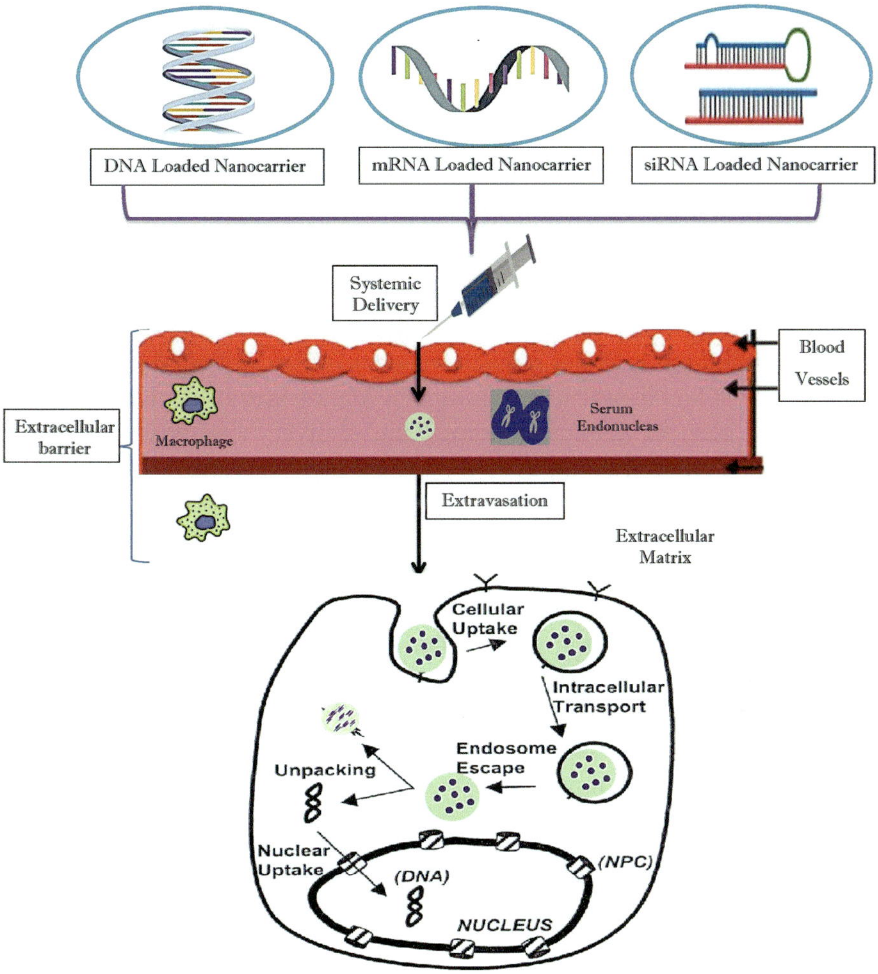

FIGURE 12.1 Biological barriers in nucleic acid delivery.

drug-loading capability [29]. By lowering opsonization and increasing cellular uptake, surface modifications are essential for enhancing nanocarrier circulation time and targeting selectivity [30]. Furthermore, the size and shape of nanocarriers impact their biodistribution and cellular uptake, with smaller particles frequently demonstrating enhanced permeation and accumulation in the intended tissues [31]. Spatiotemporal control of drug delivery is made possible by controlled release mechanisms, including stimuli-responsive or triggered drug release, which improve the therapeutic effect while reducing systemic toxicity [32]. The delivery of targeted medications in biomedicine is enabled by the fabrication of nanocarriers with improved medicinal safety and efficacy characteristics, made possible by the integration of various design elements.

12.3.3 INTRACELLULAR DELIVERY MECHANISMS: INSIGHTS AND LIMITATIONS

Understanding intracellular delivery mechanisms is critical for enhancing the efficacy of therapeutic interventions. While various strategies have been developed, such as nanoparticle-mediated delivery and cell-penetrating peptides, challenges remain in achieving efficient and targeted delivery to desired intracellular compartments [33]. Membrane barriers, endosomal entrapment, and lysosomal degradation present significant hurdles to successful intracellular delivery [34]. Overcoming these limitations requires innovative approaches, including the design of delivery systems capable of evading cellular defenses and facilitating cargo release within the cytoplasm or specific organelles [35]. Advancements in understanding cellular uptake mechanisms and intracellular trafficking pathways offer valuable insights for the development of next-generation intracellular delivery strategies, with the potential to revolutionize drug delivery in biomedicine.

12.4 ARTIFICIAL INTELLIGENCE (AI)-DRIVEN NANOCARRIER DESIGN

Through the use of machine learning algorithms, AI-driven nanocarrier design expedites the choice of material, surface alteration, and optimization of structure, thereby redefining medication delivery efficiency. AI allows the quick investigation of large design spaces, resulting in nanocarriers with improved stability, biocompatibility, and target selectivity [36]. This is accomplished by combining mathematical simulation, rapid screening, and data-driven ways. By streamlining the process from laboratory to bedside, this method expedites the creation of customized treatments and transforms the targeted drug delivery space.

12.4.1 RATIONAL DESIGN OF NANOCARRIERS USING ARTIFICIAL INTELLIGENCE (AI) ALGORITHMS

The use of AI algorithms in rationalization of nanocarriers is a revolutionary breakthrough in the improvement of the delivery of drugs. AI algorithms accelerate choosing materials, surface technology, and structural optimization through the use of machine learning and mathematical modeling. This results in nanocarriers that are more stable, biocompatible, and effective at their target [37, 38]. By streamlining the research procedure, this method expedites the integration of nanomedicine into practical uses and allows for the quick investigation of conceptual spaces, which in turn transforms targeted drug delivery systems.

12.4.2 COMPUTATIONAL MODELING FOR PREDICTING NANOPARTICLE BEHAVIOR

One effective method for forecasting the behavior of nanoparticles in intricate biological settings is computational modeling. Computer programs facilitate the forecasting of nanoparticle relationships with biological barriers, cellular absorption processes, and intracellular circulation routes through the integration of physics-based simulations involving data-driven methodologies [39]. The pharmacokinetics, efficacy for therapy, and biodistribution of nanoparticles are all well-understood by these predictive algorithms, which help in the sensible development of nanocarriers for tailored drug delivery purposes.

12.4.3 ARTIFICIAL INTELLIGENCE (AI)-GUIDED OPTIMIZATION OF SURFACE FUNCTIONALIZATION FOR ENHANCED DELIVERY

AI-guided optimization of surface functionalization represents a cutting-edge approach to enhancing drug delivery efficiency. By leveraging machine learning algorithms, researchers can rapidly explore a vast design space of surface modifications, predicting their impact on nanoparticle interactions with biological systems. This enables the rational design of nanocarriers with improved stability, biocompatibility, and targeting specificity [40, 41]. AI-driven optimization expedites the development process, facilitating the translation of nanomedicine into clinical applications for improved therapeutic outcomes.

12.5 ARTIFICIAL INTELLIGENCE (AI)-ENHANCED STRATEGIES FOR OVERCOMING TUMOR HETEROGENEITY

Promising paths to overcome tumor heterogeneity, a significant obstacle in fighting cancer, are provided by AI-enhanced approaches (Table 12.1). AI facilitates the recognition of various tumor subtypes and the characterization of their molecular patterns by combining machine learning algorithms with data from multiple omics [42]. This profound comprehension of tumor heterogeneity makes it easier to create individualized treatment plans for each patient, such as immunotherapies and targeted medicines [43]. AI algorithms can also forecast the mechanisms of resistance and therapeutic responses, which helps choose the best course of therapy and enhances the results for patients. The use of AI to understand tumor heterogeneity has great potential to advance oncology precision therapy.

TABLE 12.1 AI-Driven Innovations in nanotechnology

Key Point	Description
AI-Driven Sequence Optimization	Machine learning algorithms analyze large datasets to identify optimal siRNA sequences and reduce off-target effects [48].
Advanced Delivery Systems	AI aids in developing novel delivery systems like nanoparticles and lipid-based carriers for efficient siRNA delivery [49].
Enhanced Specificity and Efficacy	AI-driven approaches improve the precision of RNAi therapies, ensuring targeted delivery and high therapeutic efficacy [50].
Predictive Modeling of Biological Interactions	AI algorithms predict interactions and outcomes, optimizing the pharmacokinetics and pharmacodynamics of RNAi therapeutics [37].
Accelerated Clinical Translation	AI facilitates the rapid clinical translation of RNAi therapeutics, enabling personalized treatments for genetic disorders and cancers [52].

12.6 THERAPEUTIC APPLICATIONS

Therapeutic applications of AI in medicine are rapidly expanding, revolutionizing various aspects of patient care. From personalized treatment strategies to drug discovery and diagnostic advancements, AI is poised to significantly improve clinical outcomes across diverse medical specialties. By analyzing large datasets and identifying complex patterns, AI algorithms aid in disease diagnosis, prognosis, and treatment selection

[42]. Moreover, AI-driven predictive models enhance precision medicine approaches, optimizing drug dosing regimens and minimizing adverse effects [45]. The integration of AI in medical imaging facilitates early disease detection and accurate interpretation of radiological findings [46, 47]. As AI continues to evolve, its therapeutic applications hold immense promise for transforming healthcare delivery and improving patient outcomes.

12.6.1 RNA INTERFERENCE (RNAI) THERAPEUTICS: AI-DRIVEN INNOVATIONS

AI's therapeutic uses in medicine are growing quickly and are transforming many facets of patient care. AI has the potential to greatly enhance therapeutic results in a wide range of medical specializations through tailored treatment plans, drug discovery, and diagnostic innovations. AI systems support the identification of illnesses, prediction, and therapy choice by sifting through massive datasets and spotting intricate patterns [44]. Furthermore, AI-powered predictive models improve medical precision strategies by maximizing beneficial effects and optimizing medication dosage schedules [45]. According to Esteva et al. [46], the use of AI in healthcare imaging makes it easier to identify diseases early and analyze radiological results correctly. AI's therapeutic applications have enormous potential to change healthcare delivery and enhance outcomes for patients as it develops.

12.6.2 CRISPR/CAS9 GENOME EDITING: ADVANCEMENTS IN TARGETED DELIVERY

The precision and effectiveness of genetic alterations have increased thanks to the recent advances in CRISPR/Cas9 genome editing, which have greatly enhanced targeted delivery techniques. Transportation of CRISPR elements into certain cells and tissues is made easier by advancements in delivery technologies, including lipid nanoparticles, viral vectors, and nanocapsules [56]. These delivery strategies aim to maintain the integrity of the CRISPR/Cas9 apparatus, guarantee effective cellular uptake, and provide precise genome editing at the intended location. In order to enhance therapeutic effects, AI-driven techniques are also being used to improve these delivery systems by forecasting the ideal formulations and targeting tactics [57]. These developments are critical to the therapeutic utilization of CRISPR/Cas9, which holds great promise for the treatment of multiple illnesses and genetic defects.

12.6.3 PERSONALIZED GENE THERAPY APPROACHES ENABLED BY NANOBOTIC INTELLIGENCE

The field of nanobotic intelligence, which particularly combines AI and nanotechnology to improve the accuracy and effectiveness of genetic therapies, is revolutionizing personalized gene therapy. Molecular interventions can be more accurately delivered to targeted cells by using nanobots, which are constructed at the nanoscale and are programmable to deliver gene therapies [58]. AI algorithms are essential to this procedure because they analyze large biological datasets to find the best delivery channels and processes. This helps to minimize off-target impacts and ensure that the gene therapies are properly delivered to the intended cellular targets [59]. Gene therapies can be specifically tailored to each patient's characteristics thanks to this individualized method, which enables very precise targeting of particular genetic variations and illnesses. Customized gene therapy with nanobotic intelligence fusion has great promise for treating a variety of genetic problems, including uncommon and complicated illnesses that are difficult to cure with conventional therapeutic approaches.

12.7 CLINICAL TRANSLATION AND REGULATORY CONSIDERATIONS

Legal and clinical translations are important factors to take into account while using novel technologies in medicine. Securing safety, effectiveness, and quality control is of utmost importance, necessitating stringent clinical studies and adherence to regulatory guidelines established by organizations such as the U.S. Food and Drug Administration (FDA) and the European Medicines Agency (EMA) [60]. To get novel treatments from the lab to the clinic while preserving patient safety and the confidence of the public, difficulties involve navigating convoluted regulatory channels and dealing with ethical issues [61, 62].

12.7.1 TRANSLATIONAL CHALLENGES IN AI-INTEGRATED NANOMEDICINE

The technical, legal, and ethical obstacles that stand in the way of a smooth transfer from study to clinical application are known as translational difficulties in AI-integrated nanomedicine. Theoretically, large-scale, high-quality datasets are necessary for the combination of AI with nano-medicine since these algorithms must be reliable and able to anticipate biological processes and results with accuracy [63]. Regulatory obstacles include the need for thorough validation via clinical studies to guarantee that AI-driven nanomedicines satisfy the strict effectiveness and safety criteria established by organizations such as the U.S. Food and Drug Administration (FDA) and the European Medicines Agency (EMA) [64]. The application of AI ethically poses questions with informed consent, data privacy, and potential biases in algorithmic decision-making, necessitating the development of explicit rules and guidelines [65]. For AI-integrated nanotechnology to be successfully clinically translated and widely adopted, several obstacles must be overcome [66].

12.7.2 REGULATORY LANDSCAPE AND ETHICAL IMPLICATIONS

The regulatory landscape and ethical implications of emerging medical technologies, such as AI-integrated nanomedicine, present significant challenges and considerations. Regulatory bodies like the U.S. Food and Drug Administration (FDA) and the EMA require rigorous assessment to ensure safety, efficacy, and quality, involving extensive clinical trials and post-market surveillance [67, 68]. Ethical implications include issues of data privacy, informed consent, and the potential for bias in AI algorithms. These concerns necessitate the development of robust ethical guidelines and regulatory frameworks to protect patient rights and ensure equitable access to advanced therapies [65, 69]. Addressing these regulatory and ethical challenges is essential for fostering public trust and facilitating the responsible adoption of innovative medical technologies.

12.7.3 CASE STUDIES AND SUCCESS STORIES IN CLINICAL TRIALS

Case studies and success stories in clinical trials highlight the transformative impact of innovative medical technologies on patient outcomes. For instance, the use of CRISPR/Cas9 gene editing in treating genetic disorders like sickle cell anemia and beta-thalassemia has shown promising results, with patients experiencing significant improvements in their conditions [70]. Similarly, the implementation of artificial intelligence (AI) in oncology has led to the successful development of personalized treatment plans, improving the efficacy of therapies for various cancers [55, 71]. These successes underscore the potential of cutting-edge technologies to revolutionize healthcare, demonstrating their efficacy and safety through well-documented clinical trials and paving the way for broader clinical adoption.

12.8 FUTURE PERSPECTIVES

The potential for AI-powered personalized medicine at the nexus of nanotechnology and AI is set to transform healthcare. The design and optimization of nanocarriers for focused medication delivery, customized therapy, and continuous health surveillance is being driven by recent developments that show a rising integration of AI algorithms with nanotechnology. By enhancing the capacity to evaluate enormous datasets, forecast biological reactions, and customize nanomedicines to the specific patient description, AI considerably improves the therapeutic results [63].

Significant obstacles still stand in the way of the commercialization of AI-integrated nanomedicine, notwithstanding the encouraging developments. Thorough clinical validation is necessary to overcome regulatory obstacles, such as the strict safety and effectiveness criteria imposed by organizations like the U.S. Food and Drug Administration (FDA) and the European Medicines Agency (EMA) [72]. Significant obstacles also include the high expense of research and the requirement for multidisciplinary cooperation between AI specialists, nanotechnologists, and physicians. Personalized medicine is a rapidly expanding field that offers several prospects to enhance patient care by addressing medical gaps and providing more targeted and efficient therapies [73].

Predictably, AI-powered precision medicine will eventually produce intelligent treatment systems that can detect, track, and cure illnesses at the molecular level through a smooth integration of nanotechnology and AI. This vision calls for the creation of AI-enabled nanobots that can autonomously traverse the human body, administer customized treatments, and offer immediate feedback on the effectiveness of such treatments. These developments have the potential to revolutionize healthcare by improving patient outcomes and quality of life globally by personalizing, proactively treating, and effectively treating patients [51, 53–55, 74].

12.9 CONCLUSION

To sum up, the area of targeted gene therapy has made great progress with the incorporation of AI-driven advancements in RNAi therapies. The therapeutic efficacy of RNA interference therapies is increased when AI algorithms improve the selection of siRNA sequences, improving specificity and decreasing off-target effects. AI has been used to create sophisticated delivery methods, such as lipid-based carriers and nanoparticles that guarantee the effective and precise delivery of siRNA molecules to diseased cells. These delivery techniques are further improved by AI-driven predictive modeling, which ensures accurate targeting, optimizes pharmacokinetics, and simulates biological interactions. These developments open up new possibilities for the individualized treatment of genetic illnesses and tumors by hastening the clinical translation of RNAi therapies.

The future of nucleic acid delivery is greatly promising due to the integration of nanotechnology and AI, exemplified by nanobotic intelligence. Investigators can design highly effective, targeted delivery systems that overcome many of the current limitations in gene therapy by utilizing AI's precision and computational power. Using AI-guided nanobots, which can navigate complex biological environments, can deliver therapeutic nucleic acids directly to affected cells, minimizing side effects and maximizing treatment efficacy. This novel approach not only increases the prospect of RNAi therapeutics but also opens the door for more extensive applications in personalized medicine, where therapies are customized to each patient's unique genetic makeup. With continued advancement, these technologies have the potential to completely transform the area of gene therapy and provide fresh hope for the treatment of several inherited and acquired illnesses.

ACKNOWLEDGMENT

None

CONFLICT OF INTEREST

The authors declare no conflict of interest.

FUNDING

None

KEYWORDS

- **artificial intelligence**
- **gene therapy**
- **nanobots**
- **nanotechnology**
- **nucleic acid delivery**
- **precision medicine**

REFERENCES

1. Sharma, P., Dasputre, N., & Jain, V. (2024). Nanomedicine: Concepts, characteristics, and regulatory challenges. In *Smart Nanocarrier for Effective Drug Delivery* (pp. 1–16). CRC Press.
2. Sharma, P. (2023). Nanostructured biomaterials in drug delivery: Current trends and upcoming possibilities. In *Engineered Biomaterials: Synthesis and Applications* (pp. 261–280). Singapore: Springer Nature Singapore.
3. Hua, S., de Matos, M. B. C., Metselaar, J. M., & Storm, G. (2018). Current trends and challenges in the clinical translation of nanoparticulate nanomedicines: Pathways for translational development and commercialization. *Frontiers in Pharmacology*, *9*, 790.
4. Sharma, P., Jain, V., & Tailang, M. (2023). Advancement of nanocarrier-based engineering for specific drug delivery for cancer therapy. In *Targeted Cancer Therapy in Biomedical Engineering* (pp. 465–486). Singapore: Springer Nature Singapore.
5. Sharma, P., Bhargava, S., Parashar, D., & Mangal, A. (2017). Formulation and evaluation of nanoparticles containing cyclophosphamide. *World Journal of Pharmaceutical Research*, *7*(1), 785–798.
6. Lundin, K. E., Gissberg, O., & Smith, C. I. (2015). Oligonucleotide therapies: The past and the present. *Human Gene Therapy*, *26*(8), 475–485.
7. Fire, A., Xu, S., Montgomery, M. K., Kostas, S. A., Driver, S. E., & Mello, C. C. (1998). Potent and specific genetic interference by double-stranded RNA in *Caenorhabditis elegans*. *Nature*, *391*(6669), 806–811.
8. Pardi, N., Hogan, M. J., Porter, F. W., & Weissman, D. (2018). mRNA vaccines–a new era in vaccinology. *Nature Reviews Drug Discovery*, *17*(4), 261–279.

9. Doudna, J. A., & Charpentier, E. (2014). The new frontier of genome engineering with CRISPR-Cas9. *Science*, *346*(6213), 1258096.
10. Topol, E. J. (2019). High-performance medicine: The convergence of human and artificial intelligence. *Nature Medicine*, *25*(1), 44–56.
11. Sharma, P., Jain, V., & Jain, A., & Tailang, M. (2022). Role of swarm intelligence for health monitoring and related actions. In *Internet of Things and Fog Computing-Enabled Solutions for Real-Life Challenges* (pp. 95–118). CRC Press.
12. Sharma, P., Jain, V., & Tailang, M. (2023). How artificial intelligence is transforming medicine: The future of pharmaceutical research. In *Industry 4.0 and Healthcare: Impact of Artificial Intelligence* (pp. 133–150). Singapore: Springer Nature Singapore.
13. Sharma, P., Jain, V., & Tailang, M. (2022). Swarm intelligence and machine learning algorithms for cancer diagnosis. In *Swarm Intelligence and Machine Learning* (pp. 34–50). CRC Press.
14. Bickmore, T. W., Schulman, D., Sidner, C., & Mello, S. (2010). Health document explanation by virtual agents. In *International Conference on Intelligent Virtual Agents* (pp. 407–420). Springer, Berlin, Heidelberg.
15. Yan, Y., Xiong, D., Lin, X., Wu, Q., & Zeng, X. (2017). Nano-robotics in medical applications: From science fiction to reality. *Frontiers of Mechanical Engineering*, *12*(1), 4–16.
16. Li, T., Li, C., Liu, Z., Zhang, L., & Jiang, Q. (2018). A review of nanorobotics: Current challenges and future directions. In *2018 IEEE International Conference on Robotics and Automation (ICRA)* (pp. 1–7). IEEE.
17. Mehdizadeh, A., Mashayekhi, R., Maleki, T., & Asadnia, M. (2018). Nanorobotics: Current approaches and techniques. *IEEE Access*, *6*, 15066–15090.
18. Goodfellow, I., Bengio, Y., & Courville, A. (2018). *Deep Learning* (Vol. 1). MIT Press.
19. Sharma, P. (2022). Applications of statistical tools for optimization and development of smart drug delivery system. In *Smart Drug Delivery* (p. 183). London: Intech Open.
20. Tran, L., Xiao, X., & Zhou, Y. (2019). Application of artificial intelligence in nanomedicine: Recent progress and prospects. *Nanomedicine*, *14*(15), 2415–2430.
21. Wu, S., Lu, J., Chen, W., & Sun, J. (2019). Artificial intelligence mediated nanomaterials design for cancer imaging and therapy. *Advanced Healthcare Materials*, *8*(10), 1801262.
22. Ching, T., Himmelstein, D. S., Beaulieu-Jones, B. K., Kalinin, A. A., Do, B. T., Way, G. P., & Xie, W. (2018). Opportunities and obstacles for deep learning in biology and medicine. *Journal of the Royal Society Interface*, *15*(141), 20170387.
23. Aliper, A., Plis, S., Artemov, A., Ulloa, A., Mamoshina, P., & Zhavoronkov, A. (2016). Deep learning applications for predicting pharmacological properties of drugs and drug repurposing using transcriptomic data. *Molecular Pharmaceutics*, *13*(7), 2524–2530.
24. Zhang, Y., Yin, Q., & Yin, L. (2019). Non-viral vectors for gene delivery: Recent advances in nanotechnology. *Advanced Drug Delivery Reviews*, *144*, 133–147.
25. Li, J., Zhu, Y., Hazeldine, S. T., Li, C., & Oupický, D. (2018). Dual function non-viral vector for delivery of DNA and siRNA. *Biomaterials*, *156*, 194–203.

26. Kaczmarek, J. C., Patel, A. K., Kauffman, K. J., Fenton, O. S., Webber, M. J., Heartlein, M. W., & Anderson, D. G. (2017). Polymer-lipid nanoparticles for systemic delivery of mRNA to the lungs. *Angewandte Chemise International Edition*, *56*(38), 10598–10602.
27. Sharma, P. (2021). Modification of human behavior due to coronavirus outbreak: A brief study on current scenario. *Asian Journal of Pharmaceutics*, *15*(3).
28. Torchilin, V. P. (2014). Multifunctional, stimuli-sensitive nanoparticulate systems for drug delivery. *Nature Reviews Drug Discovery*, *13*(11), 813–827.
29. Koo, A. N., Lee, H. J., Kim, S. E., Chang, J. H., Park, C., Kim, C., & Park, J. H. (2012). Disulfide-cross-linked PEG-poly (amino acid) s copolymer micelles for glutathione-mediated intracellular drug delivery. *Chemical Communications*, *48*(5), 663–665.
30. Sharma, P., & Tailang, M. (2019). PH dependent release potential of natural polymers in sustained release of ornidazole from colon targeted delivery system. *International Journal of Drug Delivery Technology*, *9*, 1–10.
31. Champion, J. A., & Mitragotri, S. (2006). Role of target geometry in phagocytosis. *Proceedings of the National Academy of Sciences*, *103*(13), 4930–4934.
32. Tang, L., Yang, X., Yin, Q., Cai, K., Wang, H., Chaudhury, I., Yao, C., Zhou, Q., Kwon, M., Hartman, J. A., Dobrucki, I. T., Dobrucki, L. W., Borst, L. B., Lezmi, S., Helferich, W. G., Ferguson, A. L., Fan, T. M., & Cheng, J. (2014). Investigating the optimal size of anticancer nanomedicine. *Proceedings of the National Academy of Sciences*, *111*(43), 15344–15349.
33. Akhtar, S., & Hughes, M. D. (2003). Advanced drug delivery to the lymphatic system: Lipid-based and polymeric nanoparticles. *Expert Opinion on Drug Delivery*, *1*(1), 115–125.
34. Sharma, P., & Tailang, M. (2022). Primaquine-loaded transdermal patch for treating malaria: Design, development, and characterization. *Future Journal of Pharmaceutical Sciences*, *8*(1), 43.
35. Zhu, X., Radovic-Moreno, A. F., Wu, J., Langer, R., & Shi, J. (2019). Nanomedicine in the management of microbial infection–Overview and perspectives. *Nano Today*, *25*, 135–155.
36. Saha, S., & Wagner, B. K. (2018). Design considerations for nanotherapeutics in oncology. *Nano Today*, *17*, 23–37.
37. Yuan, Y., Liu, B., Li, R., & Luo, X. (2020). The applications of machine learning in cancer nanomedicine. *Cancer Letters*, *494*, 65–71.
38. Sharma, P. (2023). Validated ultraviolet spectrophotometric method for simultaneous estimation of olmesartan medoxomil in marketed formulation. *Asian Journal of Pharmaceutics*, *17*(03). https://www.asiapharmaceutics.info/index.php/ajp/article/view/4971 (accessed on 23rd June 2025).
39. Decuzzi, P., Godin, B., Tanaka, T., Lee, S. Y., Chiappini, C., & Ferrari, M. (2010). Size and shape effects in the biodistribution of intravascularly injected particles. *Journal of Controlled Release*, *141*(3), 320–327.
40. Shi, J., Kantoff, P. W., Wooster, R., & Farokhzad, O. C. (2017). Cancer nanomedicine: Progress, challenges and opportunities. *Nature Reviews Cancer*, *17*(1), 20–37.
41. Sharma, P., Jain, V., & Tailang, M. (2022). Selection and role of polymers for designing of a drug carrier. *IntechOpen*.

42. Luo, X., Donnelly, C. R., Gong, W., Heath, B. R., Hao, Y., Donnelly, L. A., Mog, S. R., Pepin, M. E., Dvorina, N., Arora, R., Kim, S., An, W., Liu, B., Yu, J., Sun, Q., & Gao, W. (2020). HPV16 drives cancer immune escape via NLRX1-mediated degradation of STING. *Journal of Clinical Investigation*, *130*(3), 1635–1652.
43. Aguirre-Ghiso, J. A. (2020). Models, mechanisms and clinical evidence for cancer dormancy. *Nature Reviews Cancer*, *20*(11), 699–714.
44. Obermeyer, Z., & Emanuel, E. J. (2016). Predicting the future–Big data, machine learning, and clinical medicine. *New England Journal of Medicine*, *375*(13), 1216–1219.
45. Yu, K. H., Beam, A. L., & Kohane, I. S. (2018). Artificial intelligence in healthcare. *Nature Biomedical Engineering*, *2*(10), 719–731.
46. Esteva, A., Kuprel, B., Novoa, R. A., Ko, J., Swetter, S. M., Blau, H. M., & Thrun, S. (2017). Dermatologist-level classification of skin cancer with deep neural networks. *Nature*, *542*(7639), 115–118.
47. Sharma, P., & Tailang, M. (2020). Design, optimization, and evaluation of hydrogel of primaquine loaded nano emulsion for malaria therapy. *Future Journal of Pharmaceutical Sciences*, *6*, 1–1.
48. Park, K., Kim, J., Kim, S., & Kim, S. I. (2020). Current status of research on RNAi-based gene silencing strategies for plants. *Plant Biotechnology Reports*, *14*(3), 317–324.
49. Hu, B., Weng, Y., Xia, X. H., Liang, X. J., & Huang, Y. (2019). Clinical advances of siRNA therapeutics. *Journal of Genetics and Genomics*, *46*(10), 241–258.
50. Wang, J., Wang, L., Yang, M., Tang, X., & Wang, X. (2019). Recent advances in nanobots for drug delivery. *International Journal of Nanomedicine*, *16*, 3147–3167.
51. Sharma, P., & Tailang, M. (2017). Opportunities and challenges to develop transdermal patch with nanocarrier. *World Journal of Pharmaceutical Research*, *6*(15), 392–400.
52. Li, C., Wang, H., & Shi, L. (2018). Advances in delivery systems and therapeutic applications of RNAi. *Nano Today*, *23*, 123–140.
53. Rathore, D. S., Dixit, A., Sharma, V., Joshi, R., Sharma, P., & Parashar, D., & Sarvesh, B. (2015). Formulation and development of glipizide containing floating microsphere. *Indo American Journal of Pharmaceutical Research*, *5*(8), 2564–2570.
54. Sharma, V., Dixit, A., Singh Rajput, Y., Rathore, D. S., Joshi, R., Sharma, P., & Parashar, D. (2015). The analgesic effect of the methanolic extract of *Sida acuta*. *American Journal of Pharmaceutical Research*, *5*(9).
55. Sharma, P., & Tailang, M. (2018). *In-vivo* study of orodispersible tablet of primaquine. *International Journal of Pharmaceutical Sciences and Research*, *9*(8), 3506–3510.
56. Glass, Z., Lee, M., Li, Y., & Xu, Q. (2018). Engineering the delivery system for CRISPR-based genome editing. *Trends in Biotechnology*, *36*(2), 173–185.
57. Lee, B., Lee, K., Panda, S., Gonzales-Rojas, R., Chong, A., Bugay, V., Park, H. M., Brenner, R., Murthy, N., & Lee, H. Y. (2020). Nanoparticle delivery of CRISPR into the brain rescues a mouse model of fragile X syndrome from exaggerated repetitive behaviors. *Nature Biomedical Engineering*, *4*(1), 52–63.
58. Rao, A., Wang, J., & Tang, J. (2021). Recent advances in nanobots for targeted gene therapy. *Advanced Drug Delivery Reviews*, *178*, 113951.
59. Chen, C., Huang, H., Wu, C., & Gu, Z. (2020). Nanobots in personalized medicine: Design, delivery, and diagnosis. *Advanced Functional Materials*, *30*(36), 2002390.

60. Murthy, S., & Murthy, S. (2023). The FDA: An overview of their role. *Translational Interventional Radiology*, 389–393.
61. Schifano, F., Chiappini, S., Corkery, J. M., & Guirguis, A. (2019). An insight into Z-drug abuse and dependence: An examination of reports to the European Medicines Agency database of suspected adverse drug reactions. *International Journal of Neuropsychopharmacology*, *22*(4), 270–277.
62. Sharma, P., & Jain, V. (2023). An overview of current advances and pharmaceutical uses of 3D and 4D printing. *Exploration of Medicine*, *4*, 560–575.
63. He, J., Baxter, S. L., Xu, J., Xu, J., Zhou, X., & Zhang, K. (2019). The practical implementation of artificial intelligence technologies in medicine. *Nature Medicine*, *25*(1), 30–36.
64. Cote, R. (2021). Ethical perspective: Ethics in the pharmaceutical industry: Vioxx recall. *Journal of Law and Ethics*, *18*(1), 11–22.
65. Floridi, L., Cowls, J., King, T., & Taddeo, M. (2018). How to design AI for social good: Seven essential factors. *Science and Engineering Ethics*, *24*(5), 1601–1630.
66. Sharma, P., Jain, V., & Jain, S. (2021). Fabrication, optimization and evaluation of chronotropic drug delivery system of captopril. *International Journal of Pharmaceutical Sciences and Research*, *12*, 2203–2210.
67. Grabman, G., & Tenenbaum, C. (2022). FDA regulation must uphold women's health. *Food and Drug Law Institute Review*, *77*, 318.
68. Rimkutė, D., & Mazepus, H. (2023). A widening authority–legitimacy gap in EU regulatory governance? An experimental study of the European Medicines Agency's legitimacy in health security regulation. *Journal of European Public Policy*, *30*(7), 1406–1430.
69. Sharma, P., & Tailang, M. (2020). Design, optimization and evaluation of buccal drug delivery system of propranolol for hypertension treatment. *International Journal of Pharmaceutical Sciences and Research*, *11*(1), 301–311.
70. Frangoul, H., Altshuler, D., Cappellini, M. D., Chen, Y. S., Domm, J., Eustace, B. K., & Corbacioglu, S. (2021). CRISPR-Cas9 gene editing for sickle cell disease and β-thalassemia. *New England Journal of Medicine*, *384*(3), 252–260.
71. Sharma, P., & Tailang, M. (2015). Role & future aspects of primaquine in malaria therapy. *World Journal of Pharmaceutical Research*, *5*(11), 573–581.
72. Pankaj, S., Ashish, D., Dheerendra, R., Yogendra, R., Ramakant, J. K., & Kuldeep, S. (2015). Formulate and evaluate orodispersible tablets of primaquine. *Indo American Journal of Pharmaceutical Research*, *5*(5), 1625–1632.
73. Mullin, R. (2020). The cost of drug development. *Chemical & Engineering News*, *98*(15).
74. Dixit, A., Jain, A. K., Sharma, N., Saluja, G. S., Acharya, M., Rathore, D., Joshi, R., Sharma, P., & Singh, Y. (2015). Hepatoprotective activity of *Wrightia tinctoria* leaves against D-galactosamine induced hepatotoxicity in rats. *Indo American Journal of Pharmaceutical Research*, *5*(1).

Index

E

H

N

O

P

Q

R

U

V

W

X

Y

Z

For Product Safety Concerns and Information please contact our
EU representative GPSR@taylorandfrancis.com Taylor & Francis
Verlag GmbH, Kaufingerstraße 24, 80331 München, Germany